17TH EDITION

The Comprehensive NCLEX-PN® Review

Contributors

Lawrette Axley, PhD, RN, CNE

Bridgette Bryan, MS, RN

Nicole Camp, MSN, RN

Alison DeLong, MS, RN

Jo Ellen Greischar-Billiard, MS, RN

Dianne Harris, MSN, RN, CNE

Rochelle Hughes, MSN, RN

Teresa LaFave, NP, MS, RN

Archae Laubmeier, MS, RN

Kathryn Meglitsch, MSN, RN

Japonica Morris, MSN, RN

Shari Payne, MSN, RN

Lynn Schneider, FNP, MSN, RN

Faye Sigman, PhD, MSN, RN

Editorial and Publishing

Derek Prater

Spring Lenox

Mandy Tallmadge

Kelly Von Lunen

Intellectual Property Notice

ATI Nursing is a division of Assessment Technologies Institute®, LLC

Copyright © 2014 Assessment Technologies Institute, LLC. All rights reserved.

The reproduction of this work in any electronic, mechanical or other means, now known or hereafter invented, is forbidden without the written permission of Assessment Technologies Institute, LLC. All of the content in this publication, including, for example, the cover, all of the page headers, images, illustrations, graphics, and text, are subject to trademark, service mark, trade dress, copyright, and/or other intellectual property rights or licenses held by Assessment Technologies Institute, LLC, one of its affiliates, or by third parties who have licensed their materials to Assessment Technologies Institute, LLC.

Important Notice to the Reader

Assessment Technologies Institute, LLC, is the publisher of this publication. The content of this publication is for informational and educational purposes only and may be modified or updated by the publisher at any time. This publication is not providing medical advice and is not intended to be a substitute for professional medical advice, diagnosis, or treatment. The publisher has designed this publication to provide accurate information regarding the subject matter covered; however, the publisher is not responsible for errors, omissions, or for any outcomes related to the use of the contents of this book and makes no guarantee and assumes no responsibility or liability for the use of the products and procedures described or the correctness, sufficiency, or completeness of stated information, opinions, or recommendations. The publisher does not recommend or endorse any specific tests, providers, products, procedures, processes, opinions, or other information that may be mentioned in this publication. Treatments and side effects described in this book may not be applicable to all people; likewise, some people may require a dose or experience a side effect that is not described herein. Drugs and medical devices are discussed that may have limited availability controlled by the Food and Drug Administration (FDA) for use only in a research study or clinical trial. Research, clinical practice, and government regulations often change the accepted standard in this field. When consideration is being given to use of any drug in the clinical setting, the health care provider or reader is responsible for determining FDA status of the drug, reading the package insert, and reviewing prescribing information for the most up-to-date recommendations on dose, precautions, and contraindications and determining the appropriate usage for the product. Any references in this book to procedures to be employed when rendering emergency care to the sick and injured are provided solely as a general guide. Other or additional safety measures may be required under particular circumstances. This book is not intended as a statement of the standards of care required in any particular situation, because circumstances and a patient's physical condition can vary widely from one emergency to another. Nor is it intended that this book shall in any way advise personnel concerning legal authority to perform the activities or procedures discussed. Such specific determination should be made only with the aid of legal counsel. Some images in this book feature models. These models do not necessarily endorse, represent, or participate in the activities represented in the images. THE PUBLISHER MAKES NO REPRESENTATIONS OR WARRANTIES OF ANY KIND, WHETHER EXPRESS OR IMPLIED, WITH RESPECT TO THE CONTENT HEREIN. THIS PUBLICATION IS PROVIDED AS-IS, AND THE PUBLISHER AND ITS AFFILIATES SHALL NOT BE LIABLE FOR ANY ACTUAL, INCIDENTAL, SPECIAL, CONSEQUENTIAL, PUNITIVE, OR EXEMPLARY DAMAGES RESULTING, IN WHOLE OR IN PART, FROM THE READER'S USE OF, OR RELIANCE UPON, SUCH CONTENT.

User's Guide and Organization

Congratulations, graduate! You have successfully completed your program of nursing studies and are now eligible to take the licensing exam created by the National Council of State Boards of Nursing (NCSBN®).

Understanding the organizational format of this review book will help guide you through a focused review in preparation for NCLEX®. The book is intended to accompany a live review presentation and then used as an outline for continued review prior to taking NCLEX. Each unit focuses on a specific area of nursing care. Unit 1 offers practical information about the exam, including how to prepare, along with test-taking strategies. The next eight units review essential content for the exam:

1. **Coordinated Care**
1. **Community Health Nursing**
2. **Pharmacology in Nursing**
3. **Fundamentals for Nursing**
4. **Adult Medical-Surgical Nursing**
5. **Mental Health Nursing**
6. **Maternal and Newborn Nursing**
7. **Nursing Care of Children**

Tables and graphics are provided throughout to simplify more challenging content.

The content provided in this book is organized by specific areas of nursing and focuses on descriptions, contributing factors, manifestations, and collaborative care, which includes nursing interventions, diagnostics, medications, therapeutic measures, client education, and referral. The information is presented in a manner that promotes analysis and application of knowledge and reinforces priority of care when managing client care.

It is important for new graduates to stay connected to content and practice questions until the NCLEX is taken. Implementing a focused review will create success on the NCLEX.

Feedback is always welcome. Therefore, please send suggestions for improvement, any noted errors, and personal testimonials of effectiveness to: *LRAdmin@atitesting.com*.

Table of Contents

UNIT FIVE   FUNDAMENTALS FOR NURSING   65

UNIT SIX   ADULT MEDICAL-SURGICAL NURSING   77

Review of Test-Taking Strategies for the NCLEX-PN® Exam

Information About NCLEX®

A. **General Information**

1. The purpose of the NCLEX-PN® is to determine that a candidate is prepared to safely practice entry-level nursing.

2. The exam is designed to test essential nursing knowledge and a candidate's ability to apply that knowledge to clinical situations.

3. The new test plan will bring the exam in line with current nursing behaviors (the nursing process and decision making).

4. The exam is pass/fail, and no other score is given.

B. **Computerized Adaptive Testing (CAT)**

1. CAT is a system that selects test items for you based on your ability to answer previous items.

2. When a question is answered, CAT determines the next question based on its estimate that you will have a 50% chance of answering the question correctly.

3. Passing or failing is determined when you reach a point in the test when minimal competency has been demonstrated.

C. **Exam Schedule**

1. The exam is given all year long.

2. Candidates must wait a minimum of 45 or 90 days between each examination as determined by the board of nursing.

D. **Number of Questions and Time Allowed**

1. There is not a minimum amount of time for the exam, and the maximum time allowed is 5 hr. The average time for a candidate is 2.3 hr.

2. A candidate must answer a minimum of 85 test questions with a maximum of 205 test questions. The average candidate takes around 117 questions. There is no time limit per question.

3. The computer will automatically stop as soon as one of the following occurs.

   a. The candidate's measure of competency is determined to be above or below the passing standard.

   b. The candidate has answered all 205 test questions.

   c. The maximum amount of time has expired.

4. It is not possible to skip questions or return to previous questions.

5. The exam includes 25 unmarked experimental questions that do not affect the final score.

6. Breaks are optional and count as part of the total 5 hr. Remember, a fresh mind is more alert!

7. About 2% of NCLEX® candidates run out of time on their exams. So be aware of the time, but be sure to give every question your best effort. Do not randomly answer questions to finish quickly, as this can hinder your chance of passing.

The NCLEX-PN® Test Plan

A. **The NCLEX-PN test plan is revised every 3 years.** The current test plan, available at www.ncsbn.org, identifies the major categories and nursing activities that guide the exam's content and questions.

B. **NCLEX® questions are distributed and weighted according to client need categories in the 2014 test plan.**

C. **The NCLEX-PN® Registration Process**

1. Apply for licensure with one board of nursing (BON).

2. Register and pay fees with Pearson VUE via the Internet (www.pearsonvue.edu), phone, or mail.

3. Receive acknowledgement of receipt of registration from Pearson VUE.

4. The BON makes you eligible in the Pearson VUE system.

5. Receive authorization to test (ATT) email from Pearson VUE. Candidates must test within the validity dates. There are no extensions.

6. Schedule an exam appointment by accessing your online account or calling 1-866-496-2539. (International scheduling can only be done via telephone).

7. Arrive for exam appointment and present your acceptable identification (ID). The only acceptable forms of ID for test centers in the U.S., American Samoa, Guam, Northern Mariana Islands, and U.S. Virgin Islands are:

   a. U.S. driver's license (Department of Motor Vehicle-issued; if expired, a renewal slip that includes a photograph and a signature must be presented as well).

   b. U.S. state identification (Department of Motor Vehicle-issued).

   c. U.S. military identification.

   d. Passport. (The only acceptable form of ID for international test centers is a passport.)

8. Receive results from the BON approximately 4 weeks after the exam.

9. If you are not successful on NCLEX, contact ATI for continued assistance and support.

It is recommended that you visit the Pearson Vue website to take the online NCLEX® tutorial at www.pearsonvue.edu.

You may learn more about the NCLEX® at www.ncsbn.org.

NCLEX-PN® Item Types

A. **Multiple Choice**

1. Most common type of question on the exam.

2. Has four options, only one of which is correct.

3. The correct answer is the **best** answer.

4. The other three options are distractors.

5. Distractors are options made to look like correct answers. They are intended to distract you from selecting the correct answer.

B. **Fill-in-the-Blank**

1. Fill-in-the-blank items are primarily calculation problems. The question may ask for an answer in a specific unit amount or a rounded decimal.

2. To answer these questions, a number should be typed into the answer box on the screen.

3. When answering the question, solve for the correct unit value.

4. Write out the calculations on material provided.

5. Bring up the drop-down calculator and double-check your work.

C. **Drag-and-Drop/Ordered Response**

1. Drag-and-drop/ordered response items list steps that must be placed in a correct sequence as indicated by the prompt.

2. To answer these questions, drag options in the left-hand column into the appropriate order of performance in the right-hand column.

3. There is only one correct sequence.

D. **Multiple Response: Select All That Apply**

1. Multiple response items have five or six options with a minimum of two correct (key) options.

2. To answer these questions, click on all the answers that apply.

3. Credit will only be given for completely correct answers. No partial credit is given.

4. Consider each response as a true-false question.

E. **Hot Spot**

1. Hot spot items use a "point-and-click" method that presents the candidate with a problem and a figure. The test taker selects the correct location on the figure.

2. An "x" will appear on the area selected. Click on the area that constitutes the landmark to correctly answer the item.

3. Read the question carefully, then analyze the image.

4. The exam will allow the test taker to reclick on the image as many times as necessary.

5. It is very important to remember that the screen is not a mirror image. If the question asks for an answer on the right or left side of the body, make sure to click on the appropriate side.

F. **Exhibit Items**

1. Standard multiple-choice questions may also include chart exhibits that must be analyzed and understood to answer the question. The chart/exhibit question cannot be answered without obtaining further information; this is where the chart comes in to play. On-screen tabs, similar to the tabs either in a client's chart or computerized medical record, will allow the test taker to select various client documents. For example, one tab may say "Medication Administration Record," another may be labeled "Vital Signs," and another may say "Laboratory Results." These documents will contain information that the test taker must analyze to correctly answer the question.

2. First, read the question carefully. Then, analyze the charts or exhibit. Use the mouse to click on each tab to open the document. When the tab is clicked, a separate window will open to display the data contained in the selected section of the client's chart. Analysis of the data in each of these documents provides the information necessary to answer the question.

G. **Graphic Option**

1. The item and/or answer options are presented as graphics instead of text.

2. The answers to these items are preceded by circles. Be sure to click on the circle to select the answer.

H. **Audio Format Items**

1. Audio items may test knowledge of audible breath and heart sounds, change-of-shift client reports, or unit-transfer reports.

2. When an audio item is presented on NCLEX®, the candidate is prompted to apply headphones. The volume of the audio may be adjusted and replayed as often as needed.

Assess and Remediate

A. **New nursing graduates should review content and questions daily until they take the exam.** Adequate review depends on scores obtained on practice assessments, and NCLEX® preparation after a live review may take from 2 to 8 weeks.

B. **For content review, use this NCLEX-PN® review book that outlines content.** Use other nursing reference materials for more detailed information.

C. **Your practice assessment score reports will identify and help direct review of content.**

D. **Begin with areas that are most difficult or least familiar.**

E. **When studying body systems and the associated diseases:**

1. Define the disease in terms of the pathophysiological process that is occurring.

2. Identify a client's early and late manifestations.

3. Identify the most important or life-threatening complications.

4. Review the prescribed medical plan including ordered diagnostic and laboratory tests, expected lab value alterations, medications, and ordered treatments.

5. Identify and prioritize the nursing interventions associated with early and late manifestations.

6. Identify client teaching that the nurse should provide to the client/family to prevent or adapt to the disease process and/or clinical condition.

SECTION 5

Test-Taking Strategies

NOTE: Although the majority of NCLEX-PN® items are written at the application and analysis level, there are some knowledge and comprehension items on the test. Make certain that you have a broad knowledge in all Client Need categories so that you can demonstrate a minimal level of competency when asked to apply your knowledge to the care of the clients in the scenario presented on the exam.

A nurse is preparing to administer medications to a client who has asthma. Which of the following should the nurse recognize as an adverse effect of bronchodilator therapy?

1. **Limited routes of administration**
2. **Hyperkalemia**
3. **Increased myocardial oxygen use**
4. **Hypoglycemia**

NOTE: Knowledge-based questions test recall and recognition.

An older adult client reports recurring calf pain after walking one to two blocks that disappears with rest. The client has weak pedal pulses, and the skin on the lower legs is shiny and cool to touch. Which of the following nursing interventions is appropriate?

1. **Position the legs dependently.**
2. **Elevate the legs above the heart.**
3. **Immobilize the legs to prevent further injury.**
4. **Assess dorsiflexion and extension of the feet.**

NOTE: Application and analysis questions require use of nursing knowledge to solve client problems.

A. **The amount of information in the stem and distractors can be overwhelming.** A useful approach is to break the analysis of the question into a series of steps. Remember to focus on the fact that there is always something you know in the question and answer options. This helps you stay in control of the exam.

B. **Use the STOP approach.**

1. **Story:** Identify the Issue and Client in the Question

   a. The issue in a question is the problem that is presented. Examples of the issue:

   1) Medication: digoxin (Lanoxin)

   2) Nursing problem: a client who is at risk for infection or in pain

   3) Behavior: restlessness, agitation

   4) Disorder: diabetes mellitus, ulcerative colitis

   5) Procedure: glucose tolerance test, cardiac catheterization

   6) The client in the question usually has a health problem.

   7) The client may be a relative, significant other, or another member of the health care team with whom the nurse is interacting.

   8) The correct answer to the question must relate to the client in the question.

2. **Think:** About the Type of Stem and Key Words

   a. Identify the type of stem in the question.

   1) True-response stem requires an answer that is a true statement.

      a) Example: A nurse is preparing to administer a bolus feeding to a client through a nasogastric (NG) tube and observes the exit mark on the tube has moved since the last feeding. Which of the following actions should the nurse take?

   2) False-response stem requires an answer that is a false statement.

      a) Example: A nurse demonstrates safe body mechanics when repositioning a client by avoiding which of the following actions?

   3) Answering questions that focus on priorities.

      a) The majority of NCLEX® questions will be priority-setting questions, which ask the test taker to identify what comes first, is most important, or gets the highest priority.

      b) The NCLEX® will use distractors, which ask, "What will the nurse do **first**?" For example:

      (1) What is the nurse's initial response?

      (2) A nurse should give immediate consideration to which of the following?

      (3) Which of the following nursing actions should receive the highest priority?

      (4) Which of the following actions should the nurse take first? Example: A nurse is preparing an automated external defibrillator (AED) for a client receiving CPR after a cardiac arrest. Which of the following actions should the nurse perform first?

b. Key words focus attention on important details.

   1) During the **early** period, which of the following nursing **procedures** is **best**?

   2) The nurse should **expect** to find which of the following characteristics in an **adult** who has **diabetes mellitus**?

   3) Which of the following nursing **actions** is **essential**?

   4) Which of the following nursing **actions** should the nurse take **first**?

3. **Options:** Consider Potential Responses/Answers

  a. Develop answers in your mind before looking at the options provided.

  b. Review each answer option one at a time.

4. **Pick:** The Correct Answer

  a. Identify the option that best matches your answer or best answers the question.

  b. Make your selection and do not change it.

C. **Use Priority-Setting Guidelines to answer questions.**

1. **Maslow's Hierarchy of Needs** indicates that physiological needs come first, followed by safety and security; love and belonging; self-esteem; and self-actualization.

2. **"ABCs"**—airway, breathing, circulation needs will frequently take priority. Never perform ABC checks blindly without considering whether ABC issues are acute vs. chronic or stable vs. unstable. For example, a client who is quadriplegic and receiving ventilation has chronic airway/breathing problems. However, if there is not an acute consideration such as pneumonia, the client should be considered chronic and stable. This client would not be the nurse's first priority.

3. **Sources of safety and risk reduction** issues need to be identified.

4. **The nursing process** indicates that data collection is a priority.

5. Consider options that are **least restrictive or least invasive**.

6. Determine the survival potential of the client. Is the issue emergent, urgent, nonurgent, or expectant. It is not unusual to want to care for the client who, in your mind, is the sickest. However, this may be an inappropriate choice in triage situation. Clients who are so sick that they cannot be saved should not be treated first.

7. **Acute** client problems are priority over **chronic** problems.

8. Determine if the client is **stable** or **unstable**.

D. **Default Test Taking Strategies help you make decisions.**

1. Use time to your advantage

  a. **Early vs. late signs and symptoms:** Early clinical manifestations are generalized and nonspecific, whereas late signs are specific and serious. Eliminate incorrect answer choices using this strategy.

   1) Example: A client who is exhibiting early signs of hemorrhage. **The nurse should anticipate which of the following findings?**

     1. Blood pressure 80/60 mm Hg

     2. Heart rate 120/min

     3. Weak thready pulse

     4. Cold, clammy skin

  b. **Pre, post, intra:** You may be asked about complications associated with certain procedures. What should you do if you know little or nothing about the procedure? Pay attention to whether the question is asking about "preprocedural," or "postprocedural" concerns. Eliminate the options that do not correspond to what is being asked.

   1) Example: A nurse is caring for a client who is scheduled for a positron emission tomography (PET). **The nurse should recognize which of the following medications is contraindicated?**

     1. Glucophage (Metformin)

     2. Phenytoin (Dilantin)

     3. Levofloxacin (Levaquin)

     4. Duragesic (Fentanyl)

  c. **Time elapsed:** The priority nursing action will change based on the time interval stipulated. The closer the client is to the origination of risk, the higher the risk for complications. The time issue may be stated in terms of hours or days. In other instances, the physical location of the client will tell you how long it has been since the origination of risk. Pay attention. Is the client in the PACU, postsurgical unit, or somewhere else? The time issue buried in those words should help you eliminate incorrect answers that don't match what is being asked.

   1) Example: During a visit to the medical clinic a nurse collects data from a client who had a knee arthroplasty 1 week ago. **Which of the following client statements should concern the nurse most?**

     1. "I am so glad to be off those blood thinners."

     2. "I will keep a pillow under my knee when I am in bed."

     3. "I am planning to use a wheelchair to help me get around."

     4. "I plan to take Motrin instead of the prescribed Lortab for pain control."

d. Remember: the **most complete answer** = least room for error.

   1) You'll encounter questions on NCLEX® that will ask you to choose the instruction or documentation that is most accurate. What should you do if you don't remember much about the subject matter? Choosing an answer that is most complete will typically result in the least room for error and subsequent delivery of safe and effective care.

   2) To help you determine which answer is the most complete, evaluate answer options based on how much objectivity (fact) vs. subjectivity (opinion) there is in the answer choices. A specific value, like a blood pressure, is factual, whereas a client's report of past incidences of "high" blood pressure is subjective. Responses that are subjective are generally not correct.

      a) Example: A client has not voided 8 hr following the removal of an indwelling bladder catheter. Which of the following should be the nurse's initial action?

         1. Increase fluids.

         2. Perform bladder scan.

         3. Place indwelling catheter.

         4. Provide assistance to bathroom.

e. Read the question and options closely for words asking about **direction** or **magnitude**. For instance, stop and concentrate on the terms intra vs. inter; hyper vs. hypo; increase vs. decrease; lesser vs. greater; and gain vs. lose. It is common to misread these terms by simply skimming over them too quickly.

   1) Example: A nurse irrigates a postoperative client's NG tube twice with 30 mL normal saline solution. At the end of the shift, the NG collection device contains 475 mL. Record the amount of NG drainage.

f. When in doubt, always choose a nursing action that could **prevent harm to the client**. Even if you don't know whether it is related to the stem, it is still a life-saving maneuver that, in all likelihood, is correct.

   1) Example: A nurse is caring for a client who has a chest tube. The nurse notes that the chest tube has become disconnected from the chest drainage system. Which of the following actions should the nurse take?

      1. Reposition the client to a high-Fowler's position.

      2. Increase the suction to the chest drainage system.

      3. Place the client on low flow oxygen via nasal cannula.

      4. Immerse the end of the chest tube in a bottle of sterile water.

g. Seldom will a correct answer have the nurse physically leave the client. Choose an answer that **keeps the nurse with a client**.

   1) Example: When an older adult client dies from complications of a cerebral vascular accident (CVA), the client's partner is present at the bedside. Which of the following nursing actions should the nurse take?

      1. Escort the partner to the hallway outside the room.

      2. Ask the chaplain to come be with the partner.

      3. Stay with the partner at the bedside.

      4. Give the partner time alone.

h. In some instances, rule out an option if you know it is associated with something else. For example, you may not know about the laboratory values for warfarin therapy, but you do know the laboratory values for heparin and aspirin. Those values can be eliminated because you are **using what you know**.

   1) Example: A client who has just been diagnosed with rheumatoid arthritis is required to receive 3 months of methotrexate therapy. The nurse recognizes that which of the following are associated with the therapy? (Select all that apply.)

      1. WBC count 1,200 mm^3

      2. Weight gain 2.27 kg (5 lb)

      3. Oral temperature of 37.2° C (99° F)

      4. Urine specific gravity 1.003

      5. Platelets 5,000 mm^3

i. **Safe and effective delegation** of tasks and client care assignments are extremely important when setting priorities for client care.

   1) RNs perform all initial client teaching. The licensed practical nurse (LPN) may reinforce teaching performed by the RN.

   2) RNs should perform all admission assessments and vital signs so that an accurate baseline is established.

   3) Client care assignments are made by the RN, not by support staff.

      a) Example: A nurse is organizing care for a group of clients. Which of the following should the nurse assign to the assistive personnel (AP)?

         1. Record a client's vital signs during the transfusion of blood.

         2. Assist a client who is requesting a bedpan 1 day postpartum following hysterectomy.

         3. Offer a pamphlet regarding advanced directives to a newly admitted client.

         4. Ask a client if pain was relieved after administration of acetaminophen (Tylenol).

j. You may want to answer questions based on the way you saw procedures done while you were in a clinical setting at school, during summer employment, or working as an intern. NCLEX® items must be answered to be consistent with nationwide practice standards, not necessarily with what may have been done within your particular institution or geographic area.

The Day of the Exam

A. **Plan for everything.**

B. **Assemble everything needed for the exam the night before.**

C. **Identification:** When candidates arrive at the test center, they will be required to present one form of acceptable identification. The first and last names on the ID must exactly match the first and last names on the application sent to the board of nursing. Visit the NCSBN website (www.ncsbn.org) for acceptable forms of ID.

D. **Plan to arrive at the test site early.**

E. **Verify the route to the exam site, and take a test drive several days prior.**

F. **Pay close attention to your physiological needs.**

   1. Dress in layers to accommodate your comfort in the testing center.

   2. Get a good night's sleep the night before the exam.

   3. Eat a nourishing meal that includes protein and long-acting carbohydrates.

   4. Avoid stimulants and depressants.

   5. Meet elimination needs prior to beginning the exam.

G. **During the exam:**

   1. Listen to and carefully read the instructions.

   2. Don't let yourself become distracted. Focus on answering one question at a time.

   3. Think positive.

H. **Manage your anxiety level.**

   1. Mild levels of anxiety increase effectiveness.

   2. Avoid cramming the night before the exam.

   3. Do something enjoyable and relaxing the night before the exam.

   4. Learn and practice measures to manage your anxiety level during the exam, as needed.

      a. Take a few deep breaths.

      b. Tense and relax muscles.

      c. Visualize a peaceful scene.

      d. Visualize your success.

UNIT TWO

Coordinated Care

Coordinated Care

ꞏ Concepts of Management

A. **Leadership**: A way of behaving that influences others to respond, not because they have to, but because they want to. Leaders help others to identify and focus on goals and the achievement of them. Leadership is a personal interaction that focuses on the personal development of the members of the group.

1. Essential components of leadership

   a. Knowledge

   b. Self-awareness

   c. Communication

   d. Energy

   e. Goals

   f. Action

2. **Nursing Interventions**: All nurses will need leadership skills to manage other nurses, assistive personnel, and clients. It is essential to the nursing role to identify and implement effective leadership practices.

B. **Management**: A problem-oriented process with a focus on the activities needed to achieve a goal; supplying the structure, resources, and direction for the activities of the group. Management involves personal interaction, but the focus is on the group's process. The most effective managers are also effective leaders.

1. Phases of the management process

   a. Planning

   b. Organizing

   c. Staffing

   d. Directing

   e. Controlling

2. Management styles

   a. Autocratic

   b. Laissez-faire

   c. Democratic

3. **Nursing Interventions**: Nurses should learn management skills and identify their own personal leadership styles. Nurses should know the differences between being an autocratic and democratic leader. The most effective management style in a health care environment is the democratic leader who uses an interdisciplinary approach to encourage open communication and collaboration, which will promote individual autonomy and accountability.

DETERMINE THE LEADERSHIP STYLE
(AUTOCRATIC, DEMOCRATIC, OR LAISSEZ-FAIRE) USED IN EACH SCENARIO

Scenario 1: A nurse manager does not participate, but delegates the staff scheduling to the nurses on the unit.	☐ AUTOCRATIC ☐ LAISSEZ-FAIRE ☐ DEMOCRATIC
Scenario 2: A nurse manager allows the staff nurses to participate in trial use of new IV pumps and contribute input when choosing a new product.	☐ AUTOCRATIC ☐ LAISSEZ-FAIRE ☐ DEMOCRATIC
Scenario 3: A nurse manager makes a decision for the staff to wear blue scrubs without consulting the staff nurses.	☐ AUTOCRATIC ☐ LAISSEZ-FAIRE ☐ DEMOCRATIC
Scenario 4: A nurse manager allows the staff to choose which holiday they would prefer to take off before completing the work schedule.	☐ AUTOCRATIC ☐ LAISSEZ-FAIRE ☐ DEMOCRATIC
Scenario 5: A nurse manager instructs the staff nurses to "work out the problem between yourselves" when a conflict arises between two nurses.	☐ AUTOCRATIC ☐ LAISSEZ-FAIRE ☐ DEMOCRATIC
Scenario 6: A nurse manager changes the policy regarding sterile dressing changes and directs the staff to follow the new procedure.	☐ AUTOCRATIC ☐ LAISSEZ-FAIRE ☐ DEMOCRATIC

Answer key: 1. Laissez-faire; 2. Democratic; 3. Autocratic; 4. Democratic; 5. Laissez-faire; 6. Autocratic

Reference: Marquis, B. L. & Huston, C. J. (2012). *Leadership Roles and Management Functions in Nursing.* 7th edition. Philadelphia, PA: Lippincott Williams & Wilkins. (p. 38).

C. **Communication**: Involves sending, receiving, and interpreting written, face-to-face, and nonverbal information between at least two people

1. Functional components of communication

   a. Referent

   b. Sender

   c. Message

   d. Channel

   e. Receiver

   f. Environment

   g. Feedback

   h. Interpersonal variables

2. **Therapeutic communication**: The purposeful use of communication to build and maintain helping relationships with clients, families, and significant others. Therapeutic communication is client-centered, purposeful, planned, and goal-directed.

3. Effective communication skills and techniques
   a. Active listening
   b. Open-ended questions
   c. Clarifying techniques
   d. Offering general leads, broad opening statements
   e. Showing acceptance and recognition
   f. Focusing
   g. Asking questions
   h. Giving information
   i. Presenting reality
   j. Summarizing
   k. Offering self
   l. Touch

4. **Nursing Interventions**: Effective communication requires commitment, effort, focus, and cooperation, especially when dealing with complex clinical issues and people who have diverse backgrounds and perspectives. It is essential to understand and use effective communication skills to successfully manage others.

D. **Conflict**: Arises when there are two opposing views, feelings, expectations, or other divergent issues. It can occur within an individual, between individuals, or between groups and organizations. Conflict can be managed.
   1. Sources of conflict
      a. Lack of resources and/or economics
      b. Differences in values, feelings, beliefs, backgrounds, goals, economic values, and professional values
      c. Struggles for power or influence
      d. Sexual harassment
   2. Types of conflict management strategies (optimal goal is creating a win-win solution for all involved)
      a. Avoiding
      b. Cooperating/accommodating
      c. Compromising
      d. Competing
      e. Collaborating
      f. Smoothing

   3. **Nursing Interventions**: A nurse manager's role is to identify the source of conflict, understand the issues that have developed, and work toward conflict resolution while maintaining positive regard for each individual. It is essential to address the person with whom there is conflict before going to superiors (use the chain of command). The most important conflict strategy involves collaboration that results in a win-win solution for everyone.
   4. **SBAR**: A communication model used in conflict resolution that incorporates the **s**ituation, **b**ackground, **a**ssessment, and **r**ecommendation to improve communication between clinicians

ll Power vs. Influence

Power: ability, strength, and capacity to do something
Influence: control over people and their actions

A. **Types of Power**
   1. **Reward**: the ability to control resources
   2. **Coercive**: the ability to inflict aversive outcomes or punishment
   3. **Legitimate**: based on one's position
   4. **Referent**: based on attractive characteristics
   5. **Expert**: based on expertise or knowledge

B. **Influence Tactics**
   1. **Ingratiation**: the ability to manipulate others through flattery and style
   2. **Conformity pressure**: the pressure to conform to the group; this pressure increases as group size increases to greater than six, or as familiarity with the topic decreases
   3. **Foot-in-the-door**: a small request followed by a larger request
   4. **Door-in-the-face**: a large request that is intended to be denied, followed by a smaller request that is intended to be granted
   5. **Guilt**: the practice of inducing guilt before making a request; granting the request reduces the feeling of guilt

C. **Nursing Interventions**: The power of influence is aimed at accomplishing well-defined goals, preferably as a cohesive team.

lll Team Building

Activities or efforts intended to unify people into a team to more effectively accomplish the overall objectives and mission of the organization

A. **Components of Team Building**
   1. **Clear expectations**: Expectations should be clearly defined and communicated to members of the team.
   2. **Context**: Members should understand why they are participating on the team.
   3. **Commitment**: Members should feel valued, excited, and challenged, and should be committed to the success of the team.
   4. **Competence**: Team should feel like it has the resources, strategies, and support it needs to meet its goals.
   5. **Collaboration**: Rules of conduct should be followed for conflict resolution and cooperative decision-making.
   6. **Communication**: There should be a clear, honest, and respectful dialogue between team members.
   7. **Creativity**: New and innovative ideas should be encouraged and welcomed.
   8. **Consequences**: Contributions and success should be recognized and rewarded.

B. **Nursing Interventions**
   1. Foster a culture that values collaboration and cooperation.
   2. Communicate that teamwork is expected.
   3. Publicly celebrate team success.
   4. Bring a sense of play and fun to the team.

IV Continuity of Care

Focuses on the experience of the client as the client moves through the health care system; guiding the client through this experience requires coordination, integration, collaboration, and facilitation of all the events along the continuum.

A. **Nursing's Role in Continuity of Care**

   1. Facilitate the continuity of care provided.

   2. Act as a liaison and be a client advocate.

   3. Complete admission, transfer, discharge, and post-discharge.

   4. Initiate, revise, and evaluate the plan of care.

   5. Report the client's status.

   6. Coordinate discharge planning.

   7. Facilitate referrals and use of community resources.

V Quality

A. **Total Quality Improvement Model (Continuous Quality Improvement)**: A philosophy that doing the right thing, the right way, the first time, with problem-prevention planning (not reactive problem-solving) leads to quality outcomes.

B. **Performance Improvement (Quality Improvement, Quality Control)**: The process used to identify and resolve performance deficiencies focusing on assessment of outcomes to improve delivery of quality care. All employees are involved in this process.

   1. Steps in the performance improvement process

      a. A standard is developed and approved by facility committee.

      b. Standards are made available to employees by way of policies and procedures.

      c. Quality issues are identified by staff, management, or risk management department.

      d. An interdisciplinary team is developed to review the issue.

      e. The current state of structure and process related to the issue is analyzed.

      f. Data collection methods are determined.

      g. Quantitative methods

      h. Audits

      i. Data is collected, analyzed, and compared with the established benchmark.

      j. If the benchmark is not met, possible influencing factors are determined. A root cause analysis may be done.

         1) Investigates the consequence and possible causes

         2) Analyzes the possible causes and relationships that may exist

         3) Determines additional influences at each level of relationship

         4) Determines the root cause or causes

      k. Potential solutions or corrective actions are analyzed and one is selected for implementation.

      l. Educational or corrective action is implemented.

      m. The issue is re-evaluated at a pre-established time to determine the efficacy of the solution or corrective action.

VI Variance/Incident/Occurrence Reports

A variance or incident is an event that occurs outside the usual expected normal events or activities of the client's stay, unit functioning, or organizational processes.

 A. **Nursing Interventions**: Incident or variance reports are not intended to point blame, just document the facts. Their purpose is to identify situations or system issues that contributed to the occurrence and to engage strategies to prevent reoccurrence or to correct the situation. Generally, the report is confidential communication and cannot be subpoenaed. However, if it is inadvertently disclosed, it can be subpoenaed. The report should not be placed in the chart.

B. **Reportable Incidents**

   1. Client injury

   2. Unanticipated client death

   3. Malfunction of equipment

   4. Unanticipated adverse reactions

   5. Inability to meet client needs—system problem, order problem, lack of qualified staff, or client/family refusal of care

   6. Unethical, illegal, or incompetent practice

   7. Client/family complaint about care

   8. Toxic spills, fires, and/or other environmental emergencies

   9. Violent behavior by the client/family

   10. Loss of property

VII Resource Management

A. **Health Care Reimbursement Methods**

   1. Retrospective vs. prospective payment

   2. Health maintenance organizations

B. **Budgeting**

   1. Types of budgets

      a. **Personnel budget**: Worked time and benefit time

      b. **Operating budget**: Electricity, maintenance, and supplies

      c. **Capital budget**: Buildings or major equipment

   2. The budget process

      a. **Planning**: Assess what the needs are.

      b. **Preparation**: Develop a plan (time frame).

      c. **Modification and approval**: Implement (ongoing monitoring and analysis).

      d. **Monitoring**: Evaluate (revise and modify as needed).

 C. **Nursing Interventions**: A nurse manager must be aware of economic issues in health care. Budgetary terms are fundamental to understanding the financial management of facilities. The more information available to the nurse, the better the decisions and input into long-range planning for the facility.

VIII Case Management

Case management is a collaborative process of assessment, planning, facilitation, and advocacy for options and services to meet an individual's health needs through communication and available resources to promote quality, cost-effective outcomes.

A. **Nursing Interventions:** A nurse's role in case management is to coordinate services that respond to the hierarchy of the client's individual needs. This system provides care that minimizes fragmentation and maximizes holistic individualized client care.

IX Consultation and Referral

A. **Consultation:** A professional provides expert advice in a particular area and determines what treatment or services the client requires.

1. Examples of consultation: an orthopedic surgeon for a client with a hip fracture; a psychiatrist for a client whose risk for suicide must be assessed

2. **Nursing Interventions:** Notify the primary care provider of the client's needs, provide the consultant with pertinent information, include consultant's information into the plan of care, and facilitate coordination with other health care providers in order to protect the client from conflicting and potentially dangerous prescriptions.

B. **Referral:** A formal request for a special service by another care provider so that the client can access the care identified by the primary care provider or consultant. The intervention becomes that specialist's responsibility, but the nurse continues to be responsible for monitoring the client's response and progress.

1. Examples of referrals: inpatient—physical therapy, wound care nurse; outside of the facility—hospice

C. **Nursing Interventions:** The processes of consultation and referral are integral for effective use of services along the continuum, and they establish collaboration with the interdisciplinary team. The nurse should support the client/family with appropriate consultation and referral to contacts in the community.

SECTION 2

Delegation and Prioritization

I Delegation/Assignment/ Supervision/Accountability

A. **Delegating:** Transferring the authority to perform a selected nursing task in a selected situation to another team member while maintaining accountability.

B. **Assigning:** Transferring the authority, accountability, and responsibility to another member of the health care team (e.g., when a PN directs another PN to administer medication the second PN is already authorized to perform the assignment in the PN scope of practice).

C. **Supervising:** Monitoring the progress toward completion of delegated tasks; the amount of supervision required depends on the direction of the delegation, the abilities of the person being delegated to, and the location of the ultimate responsibility for outcomes.

D. **Accountability:** Moral responsibility for consequences of actions

E. **Five Rights of Delegation**
1. Right person
2. Right task
3. Right circumstances
4. Right direction and communication
5. Right supervision and evaluation

F. **Nursing Interventions:** It is essential for a nurse to understand legal responsibilities when managing and delegating nursing care to a wide variety of health care workers. The nurse must delegate activities thoughtfully, taking into account individual job descriptions, knowledge base, and skills demonstrated. Remember, the professional nurse is accountable for determining the extent and complexity of client needs and for assigning work that is consistent with the individual's position, description, and duties.

G. **The RN Cannot Delegate**
1. Nursing process
2. Client education
3. Tasks that require nursing judgment (including care of unstable clients)

DELEGATION WORKSHEET

Which tasks are most appropriately delegated to a licensed practical nurse (LPN) or assistive personnel (AP)?

1. Shave a client.	☐ LPN	☐ AP
2. Transfer a client from the bed to a chair.	☐ LPN	☐ AP
3. Perform tracheostomy care.	☐ LPN	☐ AP
4. Perform oral suctioning.	☐ LPN	☐ AP
5. Assist a client who has visual impairment with meals.	☐ LPN	☐ AP
6. Reposition a client.	☐ LPN	☐ AP
7. Insert an indwelling urinary catheter.	☐ LPN	☐ AP
8. Feed a client via NG tube.	☐ LPN	☐ AP
9. Monitor IV infusion.	☐ LPN	☐ AP
10. Collect a clean-catch urine specimen.	☐ LPN	☐ AP
11. Obtain vital signs during a blood transfusion.	☐ LPN	☐ AP
12. Record intake and output.	☐ LPN	☐ AP
13. Contribute to client plan of care.	☐ LPN	☐ AP
14. Monitor response to medication.	☐ LPN	☐ AP
15. Remove antiembolism stockings.	☐ LPN	☐ AP

Answer Key: 1. AP; 2. AP; 3. LPN; 4. LPN; 5. AP; 6. AP; 7. LPN; 8. LPN; 9. LPN; 10. LPN; 11. LPN; 12. AP; 13. LPN; 14. LPN 15. AP

Reference: Marquis, B. L. & Huston, C. J. (2012). Leadership Roles and Management Functions in Nursing. 7th edition. Philadelphia, PA: Lippincott Williams & Wilkins. (p. 453–456).

II Roles and Responsibilities for Levels of Staff

A. **Assistive Personnel (AP)/Unlicensed Assistive Personnel (UAP)**
   1. Training is often on the job.
   2. An AP may complete a certification program—certified nursing assistant.
   3. An AP functions under the direction of the licensed practical nurse (LPN) or RN.
   4. Skills
      a. Performs basic hygiene care and grooming.
      b. Reports to the LPN or RN.
      c. Provides assistance with ADLs such as nutrition, elimination, and mobility.
      d. Performs basic skills such as taking vital signs, including pulse oximetry, and calculating I&O.
      e. Emphasis is on maintaining a safe environment and recognizing situations to report to immediate superior.

B. **Licensed Practical Nurse (LPN)/ Licensed Vocational Nurse (LVN)**
   1. Education is approximately 12 to 18 months in an accredited program.
   2. LPNs must complete and pass the NCLEX-PN® exam for licensure.
   3. Supervised by the RN or provider.
   4. Scope of practice is determined by nurse practice acts, which vary by state (requirements to maintain an active license are determined by each state).
      a. Meets the health needs of clients
      b. Cares for clients whose condition is considered to be stable and/or chronic with an expected outcome
      c. Performs reinforcement teaching
      d. Contributes to care plan
      e. Administers IVPB medications
      f. Monitors IV fluids

C. **Registered Nurse (RN)**
   1. May be diploma, associate degree, baccalaureate degree, or higher.
   2. Education ranges from 2 or more years.
   3. RNs must complete and pass the NCLEX-RN® exam for licensure.
   4. Functions under the direction of the health care provider.
   5. Advanced clinical skills in caring for the acute client with complex care needs; outcome uncertain.
   6. Scope of practice is determined by nurse practice acts, which vary by state (requirements to maintain an active license are determined by each state).

D. **Advanced Practice Nurse**
   1. May be nondegree, master's degree, or higher.
   2. Education ranges from 18 months to more than 4 years (in addition to basic RN program).
   3. Must complete and pass a certification exam (in addition to the NCLEX-RN® exam) applicable to the specialty and practice (adult nurse practitioner, diabetic educator).
   4. Functions vary according to the state practice act, which may be either autonomous or under the direct or indirect supervision of a provider.
   5. Skills vary according to the state practice act, and may include the ability to prescribe, diagnose, and treat.

E. **Health Care Provider**
   1. May be a provider, provider's assistant, or nurse practitioner.
   2. In general, only an attending provider has admitting privileges to a facility, although another care provider in the practice may direct the care given to the client.

III Prioritization Principles

A. **Nurses must continuously set and reset priorities in order to safely care for multiple clients.**
   1. Assessment and data collection is completed
   2. Interventions are provided.
   3. Steps in a client procedure are completed.
   4. Components of client care are completed.

B. **Establishing priorities in nursing practice requires that decisions be made based on evidence obtained:**
   1. During shift reports and other communications with members of the health care team.
   2. Through careful review of documents.
   3. By continuously and accurately collecting client data.

PRIORITIZATION PRINCIPLES IN CLIENT CARE

PRINCIPLE	EXAMPLES
Prioritize systemic before local ("life before limb").	Prioritizing interventions for a client in shock over interventions for a client with a localized limb injury
Prioritize acute (less opportunity for physical adaptation) before chronic (greater opportunity for physical adaptation).	Prioritizing the care of a client with a new injury/illness (e.g., mental confusion, chest pain) or an acute exacerbation of a previous illness over the care of client with a long-term chronic illness
Prioritize actual problems before potential future problems.	Prioritizing administration of medication to a client experiencing acute pain over ambulation of a client at risk for thrombophlebitis
Prioritize according to Maslow's Hierarchy of Needs.	Prioritizing the care of the client needs according to Maslow's Hierarchy (e.g., physiological needs such as nutrition is a higher priority than self esteem)
Recognize and respond to trends vs. transient findings.	Recognizing a gradual deterioration in a client's level of consciousness and/or Glasgow Coma Scale score
Recognize signs of emergencies and complications vs. "expected client findings."	Recognizing signs of increasing intracranial pressure in a client newly diagnosed with a stroke vs. the clinical findings expected following a stroke
Apply clinical knowledge to procedural standards to determine the priority action.	Recognizing that the timing of administration of antidiabetic and antimicrobial medications is more important than administration of some other medications

PRIORITIZATION WORKSHEET

Review each of the following client assignments. Place each group of clients in the correct priority. Select a principle of prioritization used for your decision from the list below.

- ABCs
- Maslow's Hierarchy of Needs
- Chronic/acute
- Expected/unexpected
- Least restrictive/least invasive

Group A

☐ 1. A client receiving morphine sulfate via a PCA pump who has respirations of 8/min

☐ 2. A client who had a thyroidectomy 2 hr ago with respiratory stridor upon inspiration

☐ 3. A client who had a left below-the-knee amputation and has difficulty with body image

☐ 4. A client who received an albuterol inhalation treatment 15 min ago and has a heart rate of 180/min

Group B

☐ 1. A client who is having difficulty looking at a newly placed colostomy

☐ 2. A client who has an oral temperature of 103.6 °F and had a colon resection 2 days ago

☐ 3. A client who is 1 day postpartum and does not want to hold her newborn

☐ 4. A client who needs to assistance to ambulate the length of the hallway following a hip replacement

Group C

☐ 1. A client who has chronic kidney disease and a creatinine level of 2.3 mg/dL

☐ 2. A client who is 2 hr postoperative right knee replacement with capillary refill less than 3 seconds

☐ 3. A client who has a swollen, reddened, and painful IV site after receiving gentamicin sulfate

☐ 4. A client who develops a rash after receiving IV contrast for a CT scan

Answer Key

Group A (ABCs): The client who has respiratory stridor upon inspiration after a thyroidectomy indicates swelling of tissues and a compromised airway, which places this client at highest priority (A). The client receiving morphine sulfate via PCA pump has decreased respirations of 8/min, thus ineffective breathing (B). The client who has a heart rate of 180/min has a circulation problem (C). The client having difficulty with body image does not have any issues with airway, breathing, or circulation, thus placing him at lowest priority.

Group B (Maslow): The client who has a temperature of 103.6 °F 2 days postoperative is the highest priority. Physiological needs are the highest and include food, oxygen, water, sleep, sex, and constant body temperature. Safety is the next highest priority. The client who had a hip replacement is at high risk for emboli , so it is imperative that the client walk to prevent complications. Love and belonging is the next priority according to Maslow, which includes the need for intimate relationships and experiencing love and affection. The client is in the "taking-in" phase, and bonding with her newborn falls under this category. The client having difficulties accepting a new colostomy falls under self-esteem, which is a lesser priority than the other clients.

Group C (Expected/unexpected): The client who has a rash takes highest priority because her condition indicates a systemic allergic reaction, which could cause respiratory and circulatory collapse. The inflamed intravenous site with antibiotics is considered a local reaction, and therefore is second in priority. The client who has CKD has an elevated creatinine, which is consistent and expected with the condition. The creatinine is abnormal, placing the client at higher priority than the client who has a normal capillary refill following knee replacement.

References: Varcarolis, E. M., Carson, V. B., & Shoemaker, N. C. (2010). *Foundations of psychiatric mental health nursing: A clinical approach* (6th ed.). St. Louis, MO: Saunders. (p. 38–40). Marquis, B. L. & Huston, C. J. (2012). *Leadership Roles and Management Functions in Nursing.* 7th edition. Philadelphia, PA: Lippincott Williams & Wilkins. (p. 186–187).

Ethical Issues

I Ethical Practice

A. **Basic Ethical Principles**

1. **Autonomy:** The right to make one's own decisions
2. **Beneficence:** The obligation to do good for others
3. **Confidentiality:** The obligation to observe the privacy of another and maintain strict confidence
4. **Fidelity:** The obligation to be faithful to an agreement and responsibilities, to keep promises
5. **Justice:** The obligation to be fair to all people (when allocating limited resources)
6. **Nonmaleficence:** The obligation not to harm others (Hippocrates states, "First, do no harm.")
7. **Paternalism:** Assuming the right to make decisions for another
8. **Veracity:** The obligation to tell the truth

B. **Ethical Dilemmas:** Ethical dilemmas are problems for which more than one choice can be made, and the choice is influenced by the values and beliefs of the decision makers. Ethical dilemmas are very common in health care, and nurses must be prepared to apply ethical theory and decision making.

C. **The American Nurses Association's (ANA)** *Code of Ethics for Nurses*: Sets guidelines to use when providing client care, outlines the nurse's responsibility to the client and the profession of nursing, and assists the nurse in making ethical decisions.

D. **Ethical Decision-Making:** A process in which the nurse, client, client's family, and health care team make decisions, taking into consideration personal and philosophical viewpoints, the ANA Code of Ethics for Nurses, and ethical principles. Frequently this requires that a balance be struck between science and morality.

E. **Advocacy:** A process by which the nurse assists the client to grow and develop toward self-actualization. Advocacy is a critical leadership role and emphasizes the values of caring, autonomy, respect, and empowerment.

II Organ Donation

A. **Organ and tissue donation is regulated by state and federal laws.** Facilities will have specific policies and procedures to follow during the process.

B. **Determination of death**

C. **Nursing role**

D. **Family needs**

1. **Nursing Interventions:** Nurses have an ethical responsibility to participate in the donation process by presenting the option of organ donation to all suitable clients and families. Families in this situation may be receptive to organ donation because they want something positive to come from their loss. The nurse should be comfortable when discussing this and be able to provide appropriate information about it.

III Advance Directive

A document in which a client who is competent is able to express wishes regarding future acceptable health care (including the desire for extraordinary lifesaving measures: resuscitation, intubation, and artificial hydration and nutrition) and/or designate another person to make decisions when the client becomes physically or mentally unable to do so.

A. **Planning guides for seriously ill clients**

1. **Living will:** Legal document that instructs health care providers and family members about what, if any, life-sustaining treatment an individual wants if at some time the individual is unable to make decisions.

2. **Durable power of attorney for health care:** Legal document that designates another person to make health care decisions for the client when the client becomes unable to make decisions independently.

3. **Nursing Interventions:** It is important for a nurse to identify clients who do not have advance directives, inform them of their rights, and ensure that clients who have advance directives have copies placed in their medical records.

Legal Issues

I Informed Consent

Obtained after a client receives complete disclosure of all pertinent information regarding the surgery or procedure to be performed. Obtained only if the client understands the potential benefits and risks associated with the surgery or procedure.

A. **Elements of Informed Consent**

1. Individual giving consent must fully understand the procedure that will be performed, the risks involved, expected/desired outcomes, expected complications/side effects, and alternate treatments or therapies available.

2. Consent is given by a competent adult, legal guardian, or designated power of attorney (DPOA), emancipated or married minor, parent of a minor, or a court order.

B. **Nurse's Role:** Witness the client's signature, provide clarification to information already given by the provider (do not give new information), and advocate for the client by protecting the client's rights

II Client Rights

A. **Patient Bill of Rights:** Right to humane care and treatment

B. **Americans with Disabilities Act (ADA):** Eliminates discrimination against Americans who have physical or mental disabilities

C. **Confidentiality:** The right to privacy with respect to one's personal medical information

1. **Legislation:** Health Insurance Portability and Accountability Act (HIPAA) of 1996

   a. A uniform, federal act provides privacy protection for health consumers.

   b. State laws that may provide additional protections to consumers are not affected by HIPAA.

   c. Guarantees that clients are able to access their medical records.

   d. Provides clients with control over how their personal health information is used and disclosed.

   e. Outlines limited circumstances in which personal health information can be disclosed without first obtaining consent of the client or the client's family:

      1) Suspicion of child or elder abuse

      2) When otherwise required by law (such as suspicion of criminal activity due to gunshot wounds)

      3) Incidences of state agencies or health department requirements; reportable communicable disease

III Legal Responsibilities

A. **Sources of Law:** The Constitution, statutes, administrative agencies, and court decisions

B. **Types of Laws and Courts**

1. Criminal law

   a. Felony—major

   b. Misdemeanor—minor

2. Civil laws

   a. Tort law

      1) **Unintentional torts:** negligence, malpractice

      2) **Quasi-intentional torts:** breach of confidentiality, defamation of character

      3) **Intentional torts:** assault, battery, false imprisonment

3. State laws: Nursing practice is regulated by state law. Each state's board of nursing has rules, regulations, and standards that vary by state.

   a. Federal regulations: HIPAA, ADA, etc.

C. **Nurse Practice Act**

1. Varies from state to state

D. **Good Samaritan Law**

1. Health care providers are protected from potential liability if volunteering away from their place of employment, as long as the nurses' actions are not grossly negligent.

E. **Mandatory Reporter of Abuse of Clients of All Ages and Communicable Diseases**

F. **Impaired Coworker**

1. A nurse who suspects a coworker of using drugs or alcohol while working has the duty to report to the appropriate supervisory personnel according to institutional policy.

G. **Malpractice**

1. The failure of a person with professional training to act in a reasonable and prudent manner

H. **Negligence**

1. The omission to do something that a reasonable person would do, or doing something that a reasonable person would not do

2. Standard of professional practice developed by professional organizations

 I. **Nursing Interventions:** Nurses who are able to recognize the rights and responsibilities in legal matters are better able to protect themselves against liability or loss of licensure.

! Point to Remember

One of the most vital and basic functions of a professional nurse is the duty to intervene when the safety or well-being of a client or another person is obviously at risk.

Information Systems and Technology

I Impact of Technology on the Nursing Profession

A. Allows candidates to test for nursing licensure (NCLEX®) with rapid results

B. Permits verification of licensure online for nurses and other health care professionals

C. Improves communication within and between departments through the use of e-mail, intranet, and the Internet

D. Eases the retrieval of medical histories to optimize decision making

E. Automates medication delivery systems to help prevent error

F. Automates distribution of client-care supplies

G. Facilitates client-centered care with portable and wireless terminals, workstations, and laptops

H. Improves and facilitates client education through the use of multimedia software, including graphics, photographs, videos, and 3D visuals

I. Supports continuing education with distance learning

    1. Videoconferencing via satellite

    2. Online degrees and certification programs

    3. Computer-mediated instruction

J. Increases client monitoring capabilities

K. Decreases deviation from standards of practice

L. Allows electronic documentation

II Future Impact of Technology

A. Federally mandated electronic transferable medical records

B. Virtual and augmented reality allowing for simulated client teaching activities

III Data Security

A. Passwords are necessary to prevent improper access to computers and medication systems.

B. Only individuals who have a professional relationship with a client may access the client's personal health information, per HIPAA regulations.

C. Computer terminals must be logged off and locked when not in immediate use.

D. Monitor screens must be shielded or situated so that unauthorized individuals cannot see the information.

! Point to Remember

A nurse should not share computer passwords with another person, including coworkers and family members.

UNIT THREE

Community Health Nursing

The Nurse's Role in Community Nursing

I Community Nurse Assessment

A comprehensive assessment clarifying the client problem by evaluating

A. Biological factors.

B. Social factors.

C. Cultural factors.

D. Physical factors.

E. Environmental factors.

F. Social systems.

G. Financial constraints. (The client's eligibility for service and situational constraints must also be considered.)

II Community Nurse Referrals

Assist in linking the community resource with the client to provide holistic care; must have thorough knowledge of resource individuals and organizations.

A. Use computerized records, databases, and telecommunication technologies for physical, audio, and visual data

B. Responsible for coordination, providing continuity of care, and evaluating the outcome

C. Examples of community nursing referrals

1. Psychological services

2. Support groups

3. Medical equipment providers

4. Meal delivery services

5. Transportation services

6. Life care planner

D. Examples of community health nurse practice

1. Home health nurse

2. Hospice nurse

3. Occupational health nurse

4. Parish nurse

5. School nurse

6. Case managers

Disaster Planning

I Disaster

A serious disruption of the functioning of a community that causes widespread human, material, economic, or environmental losses that exceeds the ability of the affected community or society to cope with using its own resources

A. **Internal disasters** are events in the health care facility that threaten to disrupt the care environment.

1. Structural (fire, loss of power)

2. Personnel-related (strike, high absenteeism)

B. **External disasters** may be man-made or natural.

1. Man-made disasters

a. Transportation-related incidents (e.g., car, train, plane, and subway crashes)

b. Terrorist attacks, including bombs (e.g., suicide bombs and dirty bombs), and bioterrorism

c. Industrial accidents

d. Chemical spills or toxic gas leaks

e. Structural fires

2. Natural disasters

a. Extreme weather conditions, including blizzards, ice storms, hurricanes, tornadoes, and floods

b. Ecological disasters, including earthquakes, landslides, tsunamis, volcanoes, and forest fires

c. Microbial disasters, such as epidemics and pandemics

d. A combined internal/external disaster situation can arise when an external disaster, such as a severe weather condition, both causes mass casualties and prevents health care providers from getting to the facility, perhaps due to traffic or road conditions.

II Disaster Planning

A. **Interagency cooperation within the community is essential in a disaster and requires:**

1. Community-wide planning for emergencies and/or hazards that can affect the local area.

2. Coordination between community emergency system and health care facilities.

3. Developing a local emergency communications plan and/or network.

4. Identification of potential emergency public shelters.

B. **Role of the nurse**

1. In the health care facility

a. The Joint Commission mandates specific standards for hospital preparedness.

b. Disaster plans.

c. Disaster drills (at least two annually; one involving community-wide resources and actual or simulated clients).

2. In the community

  a. Education provided to families about disaster planning

    1) A family disaster plan should include:

      a) What to do in an evacuation.

      b) Plans for family pets.

      c) Where to meet in case of an emergency.

    2) A family disaster kit should include:

      a) A flashlight with extra batteries.

      b) A battery-powered radio.

      c) Nonperishable food that requires no cooking (along with a nonelectric can opener).

      d) One gallon of water per person.

      e) Basic first-aid supplies.

      f) Matches in a waterproof container.

      g) Household liquid bleach for disinfection.

      h) Emergency blanket and/or sleeping bag and pillow.

      i) Rain gear.

3. **Nursing Interventions**

  a. Collect data about risks in the community.

III Disaster Management

A. **Emergency management system**

  1. Provides public access to immediate health care (911)

  2. Dispatch communication center

  3. Trained first responders: emergency medical technicians

  4. Transportation to medical resources: ground (ambulance) and/or air (helicopter)

B. **Declaration of a disaster**

  1. **Disaster area:** Local officials request that the governor of the state take appropriate action under state law and the state's emergency plan and declare a disaster area.

  2. **Federal disaster area:** The governor of the affected state requests declaration of a disaster area by the president to qualify the affected area for federal disaster relief.

  3. **Internal disaster:** The nursing or administrative supervisor may declare an internal disaster in case of a facility-related issue.

C. **Disaster relief organizations**

  1. Federal Emergency Management Agency (FEMA)

    a. FEMA is part of the U.S. Department of Homeland Security.

      1) Manages federal response and recovery efforts

  2. American Red Cross

    a. Not a government agency, but authorized by the government to provide disaster relief

    b. The American Red Cross provides:

      1) Shelter and food to address basic human needs.

      2) Health and mental services.

      3) Food to emergency and relief workers.

      4) Blood and blood products to disaster victims.

    c. The American Red Cross also handles inquiries from concerned family members outside the disaster area.

  3. Hazardous material response team (Hazmat)

    a. Hazardous materials may be radioactive, flammable, explosive, toxic, corrosive, or biohazardous, or may have other characteristics that make them hazardous in specific circumstances.

    b. Hazmat team members are specially trained to respond to these situations and wear protective equipment.

    c. In a toxic exposure disaster, Hazmat will coordinate the decontamination effort.

IV Role of the Nurse

A. **Triage:** Process of prioritizing which clients should receive care first

  1. **Non-mass-casualty situation:** The nurse prioritizes client care so that clients who have conditions of the highest acuity are evaluated and treated first. Emergency services are presented with a large number of casualties. However, they are still functional and able to provide care to victims on all three levels.

    a. **Nonurgent:** minor injuries that do not require immediate treatment; slightly injured

    b. **Urgent:** major injuries that require immediate treatment

    c. **Emergent:** immediate threat to life; critically injured

  2. **Mass casualty disaster triage:** The field and/or emergency services are presented with a number of casualties and/or ground conditions and are unable to treat everyone. The staff must provide the greatest good for the greatest number. Consists of four levels:

    a. **Emergent or Class I (red tag):** immediate threat to life; do not delay treatment

    b. **Urgent or Class II (yellow tag):** major injuries that require treatment; can delay treatment 1 to 2 hr

    c. **Nonurgent or Class III (green tag):** minor injuries that do not require immediate treatment, can delay treatment 2 to 4 hr

    d. **Expectant or Class IV (black tag):** expected and allowed to die; prepare for morgue

MASS CASUALTY DISASTER TRIAGE

Select the appropriate triage category after a mass casualty disaster triage (red, yellow, green, black).

1. Client who is choking	☐ RED ☐ GREEN ☐ YELLOW ☐ BLACK
2. "Walking wounded"	☐ RED ☐ GREEN ☐ YELLOW ☐ BLACK
3. Requires immediate attention	☐ RED ☐ GREEN ☐ YELLOW ☐ BLACK
4. Sprained ankle	☐ RED ☐ GREEN ☐ YELLOW ☐ BLACK
5. Shock	☐ RED ☐ GREEN ☐ YELLOW ☐ BLACK
6. Expected and allowed to die	☐ RED ☐ GREEN ☐ YELLOW ☐ BLACK
7. Contusions	☐ RED ☐ GREEN ☐ YELLOW ☐ BLACK
8. Profound hemorrhage	☐ RED ☐ GREEN ☐ YELLOW ☐ BLACK
9. Need treatment within 30 min to 2 hr	☐ RED ☐ GREEN ☐ YELLOW ☐ BLACK
10. Cardiac arrest	☐ RED ☐ GREEN ☐ YELLOW ☐ BLACK
11. Femur protruding through skin	☐ RED ☐ GREEN ☐ YELLOW ☐ BLACK
12. Treatment can be delayed more than 2 hr	☐ RED ☐ GREEN ☐ YELLOW ☐ BLACK

Answer Key: 1. Red, 2. Green, 3. Red, 4. Green, 5. Red, 6. Black, 7. Green, 8. Black, 9. Yellow, 10. Black, 11. Yellow, 12. Green

Reference: Ignatavicius, D. & Workman, M. (2013). Medical-surgical nursing. (7th ed.). St. Louis, MO: Saunders. (p. 158).

B. Health care facility disaster plan

1. A nursing or administrative supervisor may implement the disaster plan due to extreme weather conditions or an anticipation of mass casualties.

2. Plans to implement

   a. Establishment of an incident command center

   b. Premature discharge of clients who are stable from the facility

   c. Transfer of clients who are stable from the intensive care unit

   d. Postponement of scheduled admissions and elective operations

   e. Mobilization of personnel (call in off-duty individuals)

   f. Protection of personnel and visitors

   g. Evacuation plan

3. Role of the charge nurse during a disaster

   a. Preparation of a discharge list that features clients who can safely and quickly be discharged

   b. Personnel sent to the command center, if required

   c. Off-duty personnel called in, if requested

   d. Disaster victims prepared for admittance

v Psychosocial Aftermath of a Disaster

A. Crisis intervention

1. Mental health response team employs advanced crisis intervention techniques to help victims, survivors, and their families better handle the powerful emotional reactions associated with crises and disasters.

2. Goals

   a. Reduce the intensity of an individual's emotional reaction

   b. Assist individuals in recovering from the crisis

   c. Help to prevent serious long-term problems from developing

B. Posttraumatic stress disorder (PTSD): A mental health condition that can develop following any traumatic or catastrophic life experience

1. PTSD symptoms can develop in survivors of a disaster weeks, months, or even years following the catastrophic event.

C. Critical incident stress debriefing

1. Health care providers who respond to a highly stressful event that is extremely traumatic or overwhelming can experience significant stress reactions.

2. The critical incident stress debriefing process is designed to prevent the development of posttraumatic stress among first responders and health care professionals.

   a. Defusing: discussion of feelings shortly after the disaster/critical incident (such as at the end of a shift)

   b. Formal debriefing: discussion some hours or days after the disaster/critical incident, in a large group setting, with mental health teams of peer support personnel serving as the leaders

Culturally Competent Care

ı Nursing Process for Culturally Competent Care

A. Data Collection

1. What is the client's ethnic affiliation?

2. What is its importance in the client's daily life?

3. How well does the client speak, write, read, and understand English?

4. What dietary preferences or prohibitions does the client follow?

5. Are there rituals or customs that the client wishes to keep related to transitions such as birth and death?

6. Does the client want or need to have family involved in care?

7. Is the client using herbal or other traditional remedies?

 B. Nursing Interventions

1. Remain sensitive to the client's spiritual beliefs, even if they are in opposition to your personal beliefs.

2. Provide a trained, bilingual interpreter if necessary.

3. Provide a diet that is consistent with the client's customs.

4. Allow family to be involved in the client's care, if desired.

5. Be respectful of the client's cultural preferences for personal space.

6. Be aware of the meaning of eye contact in the client's culture.

7. Check the client's herbal and/or alternative methods to make sure they are not interacting with the medications that the facility is providing.

II African American

African Americans comprise a very diverse population that varies considerably by geographic region and age.

A. **Spiritual beliefs**

1. Church and religious life are typically very important.

2. Primary religious/spiritual affiliation: Most are Christian (primarily Baptist or from other Protestant sects) or Muslim.

3. Illness may have both natural and supernatural causes.

4. Mental illness may be viewed as a lack of spiritual balance.

5. Some chronic or congenital illnesses may be considered God's will.

B. **Practices associated with life transitions**

1. Death
   a. The deceased are highly respected.
   b. Cremation is avoided.
   c. Organ donation is unusual except in the case of an immediate family member.

C. **Cultural variations**

1. **Eye contact**: Viewed as a sign of respect and trust.

2. **Time orientation**: Primarily focused on the present with a flexible time frame.

3. **Personal space**: Affection is shown by touching, hugging, and being close.

4. **Family**: Nuclear, extended, frequently matriarchal (women head the household); grandparents often involved in the care and raising of children.

5. **Sick role**: Attention from family and relatives is expected.

D. **Healing practices**

1. Home and folk remedies are often used first. It is usually the role of the mother or wife to obtain the remedy from a knowledgeable person.

2. Prayer and visits from a minister may be important.

3. There may be some mistrust of the medical establishment.

E. **Health risks**

1. Hypertension

2. Coronary artery disease

3. Sickle-cell anemia

4. Diabetes mellitus

5. Prostate, breast, colorectal cancer

6. Renal disease

III Asian American

Asian Americans comprise a very diverse population including ethnic groups of Pacific Islanders, Southeast Asians, Chinese, Japanese, Koreans, and others, each of which have their own customs and practices.

A. **Spiritual beliefs**

1. Primary religious or spiritual affiliations: Buddhism, Christianity, and Hindu

B. **View of illness**

1. Chinese traditionally believe that illnesses are caused by imbalances in the yin and yang.

2. External influences block the circulation of vital energy (chi).

C. **Practices associated with life transitions**

1. Birth
   a. May want female family members at bedside during labor.
   b. Breastfeeding is the norm.
   c. Genetic defects may be blamed on something the mother did during pregnancy.
   d. New mother may be expected to eat a special diet and remain at home to recuperate for several weeks.
   e. Circumcision is a decision that depends on religious and ethnic practice.

2. Death
   a. Organ donation is uncommon.
   b. An autopsy is discouraged.

D. **Dietary preferences**

1. Depending on the individual ethnic group, food may be considered important in maintaining a healthy balance, and the client may believe that certain foods are "hot" or "cold."

2. Chinese traditionally believe that food is critical to maintaining the balance of yin (cold) and yang (hot) in the body.

E. **Cultural variation**

1. **Language**: Many different dialects exist for most major Asian languages, and English competence varies considerably. Use a trained, bilingual interpreter if the client has limited English skills.

2. **Eye contact**: Avoided with authority figures as a sign of respect.

3. **Time orientation**: Present oriented; punctuality is not a traditional value, except in Japanese culture where promptness is important.

4. **Personal space**: Client may be very modest, and public display of affection (physical touching) is not typical; the head may be considered sacred, so touching someone on the head may be disrespectful.

5. **Family**: Patriarchal, extended families are common; wife may become a part of husband's family; filial piety (duty and obedience to one's parents and ancestors) is expected.

6. **Sick role**: People who are sick usually assume a passive role; the client may not ask questions, as this is seen as disrespectful; however, she may nod politely at everything that is said; the client may be stoic in regard to pain.

F. **Healing practices**

1. May want to use traditional and herbal remedies in addition to medical care.

2. Older adult immigrants might have a strong belief in traditional folk medicine, while second-generation Asian Americans are often more oriented toward Western medicine.

3. Chinese traditionally believe that health is achieved by restoring balance between yin and yang.

4. Other specific health practices may depend on religion or ethnicity.

G. **Health risks**

1. Hypertension

2. Stomach, cervical, liver cancer

3. Osteoporosis

4. Thalassemia anemia

5. Tuberculosis

IV Hispanic

Also known as Latino; comprised of a very diverse population including individuals of Mexican, Cuban, Central American, South American, Spanish, and Puerto Rican heritage.

A. **Spiritual beliefs**

1. Traditionally very religious.

2. Primary religious/spiritual affiliation is Catholic/Christian.

3. Traditional belief is that health is controlled by fate, environment, and the will of God.

B. **Practices associated with life transitions**

1. Birth

   a. May want female family members present for labor.

   b. Most breastfeed.

   c. New mother may be expected to eat a special diet and remain at home to recuperate for several weeks.

   d. Circumcision is not the traditional practice.

2. Death

   a. Extended family may want to tend to the sick and dying.

   b. The body is respected, and organ donation is discouraged.

   c. An autopsy is discouraged.

   d. Women who are pregnant may be excluded from attending a funeral.

C. **Dietary preferences**

1. Traditional diet contains fresh ingredients; processed foods may be distrusted.

D. **Cultural variation**

1. **Language:** Majority are bilingual Spanish/English, although English competence varies significantly; use a trained, bilingual interpreter if the client's English skills are limited; considered respectful to address individuals formally until a rapport has been established.

2. **Eye contact:** Direct eye contact is avoided with authority figures.

3. **Time orientation:** Primarily oriented in the present with a flexible time frame.

4. **Personal space:** Handshaking is considered polite, but other touching by a stranger is generally considered inappropriate; embracing is common among family and friends.

5. **Family:** Family is believed to come first, and members are expected to have a strong sense of family loyalty; most live in nuclear families with extended families and godparents.

6. **Sick role:** Clients will often assume a passive role and may be stoic with regard to pain.

E. **Healing practices**

1. Soup and herbal teas may be thought to speed healing process.

2. Siesta is a traditional period of rest after the midday meal thought to be important for maintaining health.

3. The client may seek medical care for severe symptoms while using traditional folk healing measures for chronic illnesses.

F. **Health risks**

1. Diabetes mellitus

2. Childhood obesity

3. Hypertension

4. Vitamin B_{12} deficiency anemia

V Native American

There are more than 500 Native American tribal groups, each with its own culture, beliefs, and practices.

A. **Spiritual beliefs**

1. Belief in the Creator; sacred myths and legends provide spiritual guidance.

2. Primary religious/spiritual affiliation: Specific tribes follow rituals referred to in a general way by the tribal name; for example, the Navajo Indians follow "The Navajo Way."

3. Illness results from not living in harmony, or being out of balance with nature.

B. **Practices associated with life transitions**

1. Birth

   a. May desire female family members to be present at birth

   b. No circumcision

2. Death

   a. Organ donation is usually not desired.

   b. An autopsy is usually not desired.

   c. Some tribes avoid contact with a person who is dying (a hospital is preferable to home).

C. **Dietary preference**

1. May vary with tribal affiliation, although most are assimilated to a U.S.-style diet.

D. **Cultural variation**

1. **Language:** Most speak English.

2. **Eye contact:** Respect is communicated by avoiding eye contact.

3. **Time orientation:** Primarily oriented in the present with a flexible time frame; rushing a client is considered rude and disrespectful.

4. **Personal space:** Keep a respectful distance.

5. **Family:** Some tribes are matrilineal, meaning they trace ancestral descent through the mother's line instead of the father's line; the mother may be the head of the family or clan.

6. **Sick role:** Usually quiet and stoic.

E. **Healing practices**

1. A person who is ill may seek both modern medical attention and the services of a traditional medicine man/woman.

2. Home and herbal remedies may be used.

3. A medicine bag is a leather pouch that is worn around the neck, and the contents of it are considered sacred; it is improper to ask about the contents of the bag, and every effort should be made not to remove it.

4. Health practices are intertwined with religious and cultural beliefs.

F. **Health risks**

1. Alcohol use disorder
2. Gallbladder disease
3. Diabetes mellitus
4. Coronary artery disease
5. Tuberculosis
6. Maternal-infant mortality
7. Obesity
8. Hypertension

RELIGIOUS PRACTICES

	BIRTH PRACTICES	DEATH PRACTICES	DIETARY RESTRICTIONS	HEALTH PRACTICES
Buddhism	Believe in reincarnation. Contraception to prevent conception is acceptable.	Ensure a calm, peaceful environment. Chanting is common. Monk delivers last rites. Organ donation is encouraged. Cremation is common.	Vegetarian diet practiced by many. Avoidance of alcohol.	A quiet peaceful environment allows client to rest and practice meditation and prayer.
Catholicism	Contraception, abortion, and sterilization are prohibited. Baptism is required.	Priest administers last rites. Organ donation is acceptable. Suicide may prevent burial in Catholic cemetery.	Some may abstain from eating meat on Ash Wednesday and on Fridays during Lent.	Most want to see a priest when hospitalized. May request communion or confession to aid in healing. May wear cross or medal or display religious statues.
Christian Science	Abortion is prohibited. A client may choose to give birth at home.	Unlikely to seek medical help to prolong life. Organ donation is discouraged.	Must abstain from alcohol.	Medications and blood products are avoided. Healing ministers practice spiritual healing and do not use medical or psychological techniques.
Hinduism	Contraception is acceptable. Abortion may be prohibited. Males are not circumcised. Child is not named till the 10th day of life.	Believe in reincarnation. Allowing a natural death is traditional. Client may want to lie on floor while dying. A thread is placed around the neck/wrist. Organ donation is acceptable. Prefer cremation.	Vegetarian diet is encouraged. Most abstain from beef and pork. Right hand is used for eating and left hand for toileting and hygiene. Several days a year are set aside for fasting.	Personal hygiene is very important. Future lives are influenced by how one faces illness, disability, and death.

RELIGIOUS PRACTICES (CONTINUED)

	BIRTH PRACTICES	DEATH PRACTICES	DIETARY RESTRICTIONS	HEALTH PRACTICES
Islam	Contraception is acceptable. Abortion is permitted in certain circumstances. A prayer is said into the infant's ear at birth. Circumcision is customary.	Client may want to confess sins prior to death. A dying client may wish to be placed facing Mecca (usually east). Organ donation is acceptable. An autopsy is permitted. Rituals include traditional bathing with burial within 24 hr. Cremation is prohibited.	Food must be halal (lawful). Pork, alcohol, and some shellfish are prohibited. Ramadan is a period of fasting during the ninth lunar month.	A client may wish to pray five times a day, facing Mecca, and may have a prayer rug. Privacy during prayer is important. Women are very modest and wear clothes that cover their entire body.
Judaism	Abortion is permitted. Ritual circumcision of males is called a bris, performed on the 8th day of life.	An autopsy is discouraged. Organ donation is permitted. Someone stays with the body at all times. Ritual bathing and burial within 24 hr. Cremation is prohibited.	Food is required to be kosher. Milk and meat cannot be served at the same meal. Pork and shellfish prohibited. Fasting required on Yom Kippur. Lactose intolerance is common among Jews of European origin.	Saving a life overrides nearly all religious obligations. Prayers of well-being of the sick may be said. Anything that can be done to ease the client's suffering is encouraged.
The Church of Jesus Christ of Latter-day Saints	Contraception and abortion are forbidden. Infants are not baptized.	Organ donation is permitted. An autopsy is permitted. Life continues beyond death.	Alcohol, coffee, and tea are prohibited. Fasting is required once a month.	May want to use herbal remedies in addition to medical care. When blessing the sick, a person is anointed with oil by two elders.
Seventh-Day Adventist	Abortion is acceptable in some circumstances. Opposed to infant baptism.	An autopsy is acceptable. Organ donation is acceptable.	Vegetarian diet is encouraged. Alcohol, coffee, and tea are prohibited.	Healing accomplished through medical intervention and divine healing. Prayer and anointing with oil may be performed.

UNIT FOUR

Pharmacology in Nursing

Calculations and Conversions

Basic medication dose conversion and calculation skills are essential to providing safe nursing care. Standard conversions are used to solve dosage calculation problems. Nurses are responsible for the administration of the correct amount of medication based on the type of medication being administered.

A. **Standard Conversion Factors**

1. 1 mg = 1,000 mcg
2. 1 g = 1,000 mg
3. 1 kg = 1,000 g
4. 1 kg = 2.2 lb
5. 60 mg = 1 gr
6. 30 mL = 1 oz
7. 1 L = 1,000 mL
8. 5 mL = 1 tsp
9. 15 mL = 1 tbsp
10. 1 tbsp = 3 tsp

B. **Temperature Conversions**

1. $37.0°C = 98.6°F$
2. $°C = (°F - 32) \times (5/9)$
3. $°F = (°C \times 9/5) + 32$

C. **Calculations for IV Administration**

1. Number of hours = total volume/mL/hr
2. gtt per min = total volume × gtt/mL in administration set/ total number of minutes

D. **Calculations for Dosage**

1. Dosage on hand (H)/mL = Dosage desired (D)/mL

PRACTICE TEST QUESTIONS

1. A client has the following food for lunch: 6 oz ice chips, 1 cup tea, 2 cups coffee, and 240 mL milk. The client eats the ice chips, and drinks all of the tea, coffee, and half of the milk. The total intake for lunch is how many milliliters?

2. A client has a prescription for 0.25 mg lanoxin (Digoxin). The dose on hand is 0.5 mg tablets of lanoxin. How many tablets will the client receive?

3. A client's IV infusion rate is 75 mL/hr. How many hours will it take for a 500 mL bag of IV fluid to infuse?

4. The IV rate is 100 mL/hr and the administration set is 15 drops/mL. How many drops per minute will deliver the required fluids?

5. A client has a prescription for heparin sodium 8,000 units IV. The vial contains 10,000 units/mL. How many milliliters of heparin will the nurse administer?

6. A nurse is preparing 300,000 units of procaine penicillin (Wycillin). The vial contains 1,500,000 units/2 mL. How many milliliters will the nurse administer?

7. A client weighs 170 lb and has a prescription for 0.5 mL of medication per kilogram of body weight. How many milliliters of medication will the client receive? (Round the answer to the nearest whole number.)

8. A client is receiving dextrose 5% in water at 50 mL/hr in one IV and D$_5$W 75 mL/hr in another IV. The client also receives IV piggyback medication every 8 hr prepared in 100 mL of fluid. What is the total amount of IV fluid the client will receive in 8 hr?

9. The IV administration set delivers 15 drops/mL. The rate of flow in drops/min for 1,000 mL dextrose 5% in water to infuse over 10 hr is _____.

10. When measuring a client's output, the nurse records 300 mL of urine at 0800, 450 mL of liquid stool at 1130, 225 mL of urine at 1300, and 35 mL of emesis at 1430. What is the client's total output for this shift?

11. A client receiving an IV infusion has a prescription for 1,000 mL in 12 hr. Using a microdrip system that delivers 60 microdrops/mL, the nurse should regulate the infusion for how many drops per minute?

    A. 45

    B. 68

    C. 83

    D. 96

12. A client's temperature is 37.8°C. What is this temperature in degrees Fahrenheit?

13. A nurse has available meperidine (Demerol) 50 mg/mL. The order is to administer meperidine 35 mg. How many milliliters should the nurse administer?

14. A nurse is preparing an IV antibiotic in 100 mL dextrose 5% in water to infuse over 30 min. The infusion set is calibrated for 10 gtt/mL. What drip rate should the nurse use?

Answer Key: 1. 930; 2. 0.5; 3. 6.7; 4. 25; 5. 0.8; 6. 0.4; 7. 39; 8. 1,100; 9. 25; 10. 1,010; 11. C; 12. 100; 13. 0.7; 14. 33

Medication Therapies

I Medication Actions, Interactions, and Reactions

A. **Medication Properties (pharmacokinetics):** The absorption, distribution, metabolism, and excretion of a medication; describes the onset of action, peak level, duration of action, and bioavailability

B. **Medication Interaction:** When a medication is given with another medication and alters the effect of either or both medications

C. **Adverse Reactions:** Negative effects experienced by a client as the result of a specific medication; can be hazardous, tolerated, or subside with continued use

II Pharmacotherapy Across the Life Span

A. **Medications and Pregnancy:** A majority of medications cross the placental barrier, thereby increasing the risk of teratogenicity. All medications should be given with extreme caution to ensure safety to the developing fetus.

B. **Medications and Breastfeeding:** Most medications taken by a mother who is breastfeeding appear in breast milk. Medication levels tend to be the highest in the newborn immediately after the medication is administered to the mother. Mothers who are breastfeeding are advised to breastfeed before taking the medication.

C. **Medication in Children:** Pharmacokinetics are influenced by a child's age, size, and maturity of the targeted organ. To reduce the risk of toxicity, these factors must be considered: safe calculation of the child's dosage (mg/kg/day), medication that is age-appropriate, monitoring of IV medications to prevent fluid overload (smaller solution containers should be used to avoid infusing too much fluid), and the administration of inhalants using a metered-space device.

D. **Intramuscular Injections for Children**

1. A eutectic mix of lidocaine and prilocaine (EMLA) or liposomal lidocaine cream (LMX) may be applied topically if time permits and is congruent with facility practice guidelines.

2. Vastus lateralis (anterolateral thigh) is the site for IM injections in children who are less than 2 years of age.

3. Needle length must be sufficient to penetrate the subcutaneous tissue and deposit the medication in the body of the muscle.

4. Maximum dose is not to exceed 0.5 mL for small infants or 1 mL for small children.

E. **Medication in Older Adults:** Age-related changes affect therapeutic effects of medications in older adult clients. Older adult clients experience twice as many adverse effects as younger adults due to aging body systems. Confusion, lethargy, falls, and weakness may be mistaken for senility, rather than adverse reactions. If the adverse reaction is not identified, unnecessary medication may be prescribed to treat complications caused by the medication. As the client continues to receive medications, the risk for toxicity increases, especially in cases of polypharmacy.

III Safe Medication Administration

A. **The PN is prepared to administer medications using the enteral, parenteral, and transcutaneous routes.**

1. The PN is prepared to calculate and monitor IV flow rate.

2. The PN is prepared to administer IV secondary medications.

B. **The PN must validate the client's:**

1. allergies and adverse effects.

2. current medication regimen for potential interactions.

3. physiologic status compared to baseline assessment data.

C. **The PN follows the six rights of medication administration** (right client, right drug, right dose, right route, right time, right documentation) to protect the safety of the client and follow the scope of practice to maintain professional licensure.

IV Laboratory Profiles in Pharmacology

Laboratory testing may be indicated for specific medications. The nurse is accountable for collaborating with the health care provider in ensuring client safety when laboratory testing is ordered.

A. **Therapeutic Drug Monitoring**

1. Measures blood drug levels to determine effective medication dosages and prevent medication toxicity. The test may also be used to identify noncompliance with medication regimens.

2. Blood testing is preferred because it provides information about current therapeutic levels, whereas urine levels reflect the presence of a drug over several days.

B. **Peak levels** reflect the highest concentration.

AVERAGE TIMES FOR DRAWING PEAK LEVELS

ROUTE OF ADMINISTRATION	TIME SPECIMEN IS DRAWN AFTER ADMINISTRATION
Oral intake	1 to 2 hr
Intramuscular	1 hr
Intravenous	30 min

C. **Trough levels** reflect the lowest concentration or residual level and are usually obtained within 15 min prior to administration of the next scheduled dose. The scheduled dose of medication should not be administered until the trough level is confirmed.

> **NOTE:** The timing for drawing a peak and trough level varies based on the half-life (time required for the body to decrease the medication blood level by 50%) for the medication.

D. **Culture and Sensitivity:** Cultures are obtained to detect the presence of pathogens within the specimen collected. If a culture produces organisms, testing is performed in the laboratory to identify the appropriate antibiotic therapy (sensitivity). Begin antibiotic therapy after obtaining lab sample.

> **NOTE:** When ordered, cultures should be obtained prior to initiating antibiotic therapy (definitive therapy). When cultures cannot be drawn prior, the provider will prescribe a broad-spectrum antibiotic (empirical therapy). Monitoring culture results is imperative to ensure proper antimicrobial treatment.

v Intravenous Therapy

Administration of fluids via an intravenous catheter (peripheral or central vein access) for the purpose of providing medication, fluid, electrolyte, or nutrient replacement

A. **Guidelines for Safe IV Administration**

1. Review medication guidelines for precautions related to IV administration for compatibility, rate of administration, necessity of infusion pump, and serious adverse reactions.

2. Never administer medications through tubing being used for blood administration.

3. Implement standard precautions and follow policies related to IV site changes.

4. Fluids should be infused within 24 hr (discard unused portion) to prevent infection.

5. Maintain patency of IV access.

B. **Prevent complications associated with IV infusion.**

COMPLICATIONS ASSOCIATED WITH IV INFUSION

COMPLICATION	NURSING INTERVENTIONS
Infiltration	**Prevention:** use smallest catheter for prescribed therapy, stabilize port-access, monitor blood return **Treatment:** stop infusion, remove peripheral catheters, apply cold compress, elevate extremity, insert new catheter in opposite extremity
Extravasation	**Prevention:** know vesicant potential before giving medication **Treatment:** stop infusion, discontinue administration set, aspirate drug if possible, apply cold compress, document condition of site (may photograph)
Phlebitis/ thrombophlebitis	**Prevention:** rotate sites every 72 to 96 hr, secure catheter, use aseptic technique; for PICCs, avoid excessive activity with the extremity **Treatment:** stop infusion, remove peripheral IV catheters, apply heat compress, insert new catheter in opposite extremity
Hematoma	**Prevention:** avoid veins not easily seen or palpated; obtain hemostasis after insertion **Treatment:** remove IV device and apply light pressure if bleeding; monitor for signs of phlebitis and treat
Venous spasm	**Prevention:** allow time for vein diameter to return after tourniquet removed; infuse fluids at room temperature **Treatment:** temporarily slow infusion rate; apply warm compress

vi Total Parenteral Nutrition (TPN)

Hypertonic solution containing dextrose, proteins, electrolytes, minerals, trace elements, and insulin prescribed according to the client's needs and administered via central venous device (PICC line, subclavian, or internal jugular vein)

A. **Care and Maintenance of TPN**

1. Infusion pump must be used.

2. Monitor weight daily.

3. Monitor and record I&O, noting fluid balance.

4. Monitor serum glucose levels every 4 to 6 hr.

5. Monitor for signs of infection.

6. Change dressing every 48 to 72 hr per facility protocol.

7. IV tubing and fluid should be changed every 24 hr.

8. If TPN solution is temporarily unavailable, dextrose 10% in water should be administered to prevent hypoglycemia.

B. **Complications Associated with Central Venous Catheters**

COMPLICATIONS OF CENTRAL VENOUS CATHETERS

COMPLICATION	NURSING INTERVENTIONS
Pneumothorax (during insertion)	**Prevention:** use ultrasound to locate veins, avoid subclavian insertion when possible **Treatment:** administer oxygen, assist provider with chest tube insertion
Air embolism	**Prevention:** have client lie flat when changing administration set or needleless connectors, ask client to perform Valsalva maneuver if possible **Treatment:** place client in left lateral Trendelenburg, administer oxygen
Lumen occlusion	**Prevention:** flush promptly with NS between, before, and after each medication **Treatment:** use 10 mL syringe with a pulsing motion
Bloodstream infection	**Prevention:** maintain sterile technique **Treatment:** change entire infusion system, notify provider, obtain cultures, and administer antibiotics

VII Antidote/Reversal Agents

A. **Acetaminophen:** acetylcysteine (Mucomyst)
B. **Benzodiazepine:** flumazenil (Romazicon)
C. **Curare:** edrophonium (Tensilon)
D. **Cyanide poisoning:** methylene blue
E. **Digitalis:** digoxin immune FAB (Digibind)
F. **Ethylene poisoning:** fomepizole (Antizol)
G. **Heparin and enoxaparin (Lovenox):** protamine sulfate
H. **Iron:** deferoxamine (Desferal)
I. **Lead:** succimer (Chemet)
J. **Magnesium sulfate:** calcium gluconate 10% (Kalcinate)
K. **Narcotics:** naloxone (Narcan) Warfarin: phytonadione (vitamin K)
L. **Gentamicin:** greater than 12 mcg/mL
M. **Lidocaine:** greater than 5 mcg/mL
N. **Lithium:** greater than 2.0 mEq/L
O. **Magnesium sulfate:** greater than 9 mg/dL
P. **Methotrexate:** greater than 10 mcmol over 24 hr
Q. **Phenobarbital:** greater than 40 mcg/mL
R. **Phenytoin:** greater than 30 mcg/mL
S. **Quinidine:** greater than 10 mcg/mL
T. **Salicylate:** greater than 300 mcg/mL
U. **Theophylline:** greater than 20 mcg/mL
V. **Tobramycin:** greater than 12 mcg/mL

VIII Common Drug Class Suffixes

COMMON DRUG CLASS SUFFIXES

SUFFIX	MEDICATION CATEGORY
-dipine	Ca$^+$ channel blocker
-afil	Erectile dysfunction
-caine	Anesthetic
-pril	ACE inhibitor
-pam, -lam	Benzodiazepine
-statin	Antilipidemic
-asone, -solone	Corticosteroid
-olol	Beta blocker
-cillin	Penicillin
-ide	Oral hypoglycemic
-prazole	Proton pump inhibitor
-vir	Antiviral
-ase	Thrombolytic
-azine	Antiemetic
-phylline	Bronchodilator
-arin	Anticoagulant
-tidine	Antiulcer
-zine	Antihistamine
-cycline	Antibiotic
-mycin	Aminoglycoside
-floxacin	Antibiotic
-tyline	Tricyclic antidepressant
-pram, -ine	SSRI

MEDICATION CATEGORIES

This worksheet will build on your overall knowledge of medications. Learning medications by categories will help you group medications and reduce the number you have to memorize. This list is not all-inclusive, but is a great place to start. NCLEX® will expect you to know entry level pharmacology. Column one lists generic medication categories or classifications. In column two, write the commonly used "ending" for the medication classification. In column three, write an example of a medication that would be included in the classification.

MEDICATION CATEGORY	"ENDING"	MEDICATION
ACE inhibitors		
Antivirals		
Antifungals		
Antilipidemics		
Angiotensin II receptor blockers (ARBs)		
Beta blockers		
Calcium channel blockers		
Erectile dysfunction medications		
Histamine$_2$ receptor blockers		
Proton pump inhibitors		

Answer Key for Endings: 1. –pril; 2. –vir; 3. –azole; 4. –statin; 5. –sartan; 6. –olol; 7. –dipine; 8. –afil; 9. –dine; 10. –prazole
Medications: Answers for medications may vary.

Reference: Lehne, R. A. (2013). *Pharmacology for nursing care.* (8th ed). St. Louis, MO: Saunders. (p. 504, 1150, 1137, 608, 508, 171, 517, 838, 987, 999).

PHARMACOLOGICAL THERAPIES: EXPECTED ACTIONS/OUTCOMES

Choose the medication a PN should administer to achieve the expected client action/outcome. Each medication should be used once.

____ 1. Reduction of edema and pulmonary congestion	A. Carbamazepine (Tegretol)
____ 2. Relief of chest pain	B. Meningococcal vaccine (MCV4)
____ 3. Relief of an acute asthma attack	C. Metronidazole (Flagyl)
____ 4. Long-term control of asthma in combination with a glucocorticoid	D. Furosemide (Lasix)
____ 5. Decrease in the risk of infection in a client undergoing chemotherapy	E. Albuterol (Proventil, Ventolin)
____ 6. Improvement in cognition, behavior, and function	F. Methotrexate (Rheumatrex)
____ 7. Control of seizure activity in a client who has epilepsy	G. Morphine sulfate
____ 8. Reduction of joint pain, stiffness, and inflammation	H. Donepezil (Aricept)
____ 9. Prevention of meningitis in a high risk client	I. Filgrastim (Neupogen)
____ 10. Treatment of several foul-smelling episodes of diarrhea	J. Formoterol (Foradil)

Answer Key: 1. D; 2. G; 3. E; 4. J; 5. I; 6. H; 7. A; 8. F; 9. B; 10. C

References: Lehne, R. A. (2013). Pharmacology for nursing care (8th ed. pp. 205, 236, 479, 695, 820, 965-966). St. Louis, MO: Saunders.
Lewis, S. L, Dirksen, S. R., Heitkemper, M., M., & Bucher, L. (2014). Medical Surgical Nursing: Assessment and Management of Clinical Problems (9th ed. pp. 753, 776, 963, 1383, 1572). St. Louis, MO: Elsevier.

SECTION 3

Medications for the Cardiovascular System

ı Antihypertensives

Treatment for clients who have hypertension includes lifestyle modification and medications.

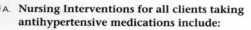

A. **Nursing Interventions for all clients taking antihypertensive medications include:**

1. Monitor weight, vital signs, and hydration status.
2. Monitor blood pressure in supine, sitting, and standing positions.
3. Monitor laboratory profiles: renal function, coagulation.
4. Administer medication at same time each day.
5. Clients should avoid hot tubs and saunas.
6. Do not discontinue medication abruptly.
7. Prevent orthostatic hypotension.

B. **Angiotensin-Converting Enzyme (ACE) Inhibitors and Angiotensin II Receptor Blockers (ARBs)**

1. **Action**

   a. ACE inhibitors: block the conversion of angiotensin I to angiotensin II

   b. ARBs: selectively block the binding of angiotensin II to AT_1 receptors found in tissues

ACE INHIBITORS

Captopril (Capoten)
Enalapril (Vasotec)
Enalaprilat (Vasotec IV)—intravenous route
Fosinopril (Monopril)
Lisinopril (Prinivil)

ARBs

Losartan (Cozaar)
Valsartan (Diovan)
Irbesartan (Avapro)

2. **Therapeutic use:** hypertension, heart failure, MI, diabetic nephropathy

3. **Precautions/Interactions**

   a. Use with caution if diuretic therapy is in place.

   b. Monitor potassium levels.

4. **Side/Adverse Effects**

   a. Persistent non-productive cough with ACE inhibitors

   b. Angioedema; hypotension

   c. Should not be used in second and third trimester of pregnancy

5. **Nursing Interventions and Client Education**

   a. Captopril should be taken 1 hr before meals.

   b. Monitor blood pressure.

   c. Monitor for angioedema and promptly administer epinephrine 0.5 mL of 1:1,000 solution subcutaneously.

C. **Calcium Channel Blockers**

1. **Action:** Slows movement of calcium into smooth-muscle cells, resulting in arterial dilation and decreased blood pressure

2. **Medications**
   a. Nifedipine (Adalat, Procardia)
   b. Verapamil (Calan)
   c. Diltiazem (Cardizem)
   d. Amlodipine (Norvasc)

3. **Therapeutic Use**
   a. Angina, hypertension
   b. Verapamil and diltiazem may be used for atrial fibrillation, atrial flutter, or SVT.

4. **Precautions/Interactions**
   a. Use cautiously in clients taking digoxin and beta blockers.
   b. Contraindicated for clients who have heart failure, heart block, or bradycardia.
   c. Clients should not consume grapefruit juice (toxic effects).

5. **Side/Adverse Effects**
   a. Constipation
   b. Reflex tachycardia
   c. Peripheral edema
   d. Toxicity

6. **Nursing Interventions and Client Education**
   a. Do not crush or chew sustained-release tablets.
   b. Slowly taper dose if discontinuing.
   c. Monitor heart rate and blood pressure.

D. **Alpha Adrenergic Blockers (Sympatholytics)**

1. **Action:** Selectively inhibit alpha$_1$ adrenergic receptors, resulting in peripheral arterial and venous dilation that lowers blood pressure

2. **Medications**
   a. Prazosin (Minipress)
   b. Doxazosin mesylate (Cardura)

3. **Therapeutic Use**
   a. Primary hypertension
   b. Cardura may be used in treatment of BPH.

4. **Precautions/Interactions**
   a. Increased risk of hypotension and syncope if given with other antihypertensives, beta blockers, or diuretics.
   b. NSAIDs can decrease the effect of prazosin.

5. **Side/Adverse Effects**
   a. Dizziness
   b. Fainting

6. **Nursing Interventions and Client Education**
   a. Monitor heart rate and blood pressure.
   b. Take medication at bedtime to minimize effects of hypotension.
   c. Advise to notify prescriber immediately about adverse reactions.
   d. Consult prescriber before taking any OTC medications.

E. **Centrally Acting Alpha$_2$ Agonists**

1. **Action:** Stimulate alpha-adrenergic receptors (alpha$_2$) in the brain to reduce peripheral vascular resistance, heart rate, and systolic and diastolic blood pressure

2. **Medications**
   a. Clonidine (Catapres)
   b. Guanfacine HCl (Tenex)
   c. Methyldopa (Aldomet)

3. **Therapeutic Use**
   a. Primary hypertension—may be used in combination with diuretics or other antihypertensives
   b. Hypertensive crisis
   c. Severe cancer pain (parenteral administration via epidural)

4. **Precautions/Interactions**
   a. Contraindicated with anticoagulant therapy, hepatic failure.
   b. Do not administer to clients taking MAOIs.
   c. Use cautiously in CVA, MI, diabetes mellitus, major depression, or chronic renal failure.
   d. Do not use during lactation.

5. **Side/Adverse Effects**
   a. Dry mouth
   b. Drowsiness and sedation (resolves over time)
   c. Rebound hypertension
   d. Black or sore tongue
   e. Leukopenia

6. **Nursing Interventions and Client Education**
   a. Monitor for adverse CNS effects.
   b. Monitor CBC, heart rate, and blood pressure.
   c. Monitor for weight gain or edema.
   d. Monitor closely for rebound hypertension when medication is discontinued (48 hr).
   e. Do not miss scheduled dose.
   f. Take at bedtime to minimize effects of hypotension.
   g. Notify prescriber of any involuntary jerky movements, prolonged dizziness, rash, yellowing of skin.

F. **Beta Adrenergic Blockers (Sympatholytics)**

1. **Action:** Inhibit stimulation of receptor sites, resulting in decreased cardiac excitability, cardiac output, myocardial oxygen demand; lower blood pressure by decreasing release of renin in the kidney

NOTE: Beta$_1$ receptors are primarily in the cardiac and renal tissues. Beta$_2$ receptors are found primarily in the lungs, gastrointestinal tract, liver, uterus, vascular smooth muscle, and skeletal muscle.

2. **Medications:** Can be selective or nonselective

  a. Cardioselective Beta$_1$ Medications

    1) Metoprolol (Lopressor)

    2) Atenolol (Tenormin)

    3) Metoprolol succinate (Toprol XL)

  b. Nonselective (Beta$_1$ and Beta$_2$) Medications

    1) Propranolol (Inderal)

    2) Nadolol (Corgard)

    3) Labetalol (Normodyne)

3. **Therapeutic Use**

  a. Primary hypertension

  b. Angina

  c. Tachydysrhythmias, heart failure, and MI

4. **Precautions/Interactions**

  a. Contraindicated in clients who have AV block and sinus bradycardia.

  b. Do not administer nonselective beta blockers to clients who have asthma, bronchospasm, or heart failure.

  c. Propranolol can mask effects of hypoglycemia in clients who have diabetes mellitus.

5. **Side/Adverse Effects**

  a. Bradycardia

  b. Nasal stuffiness

  c. AV block

  d. Rebound myocardium excitation if stopped abruptly

  e. Bronchospasm

 6. **Nursing Interventions and Client Education**

  a. Administer 1 to 2 times daily as prescribed.

  b. Do not discontinue without consulting provider.

  c. Do not crush (or chew) extended-release tablets.

  d. Hold medication and notify provider if systolic blood pressure less than 100 mm Hg or pulse less than 60/min.

  e. Monitor clients who have diabetes mellitus for indications of hypoglycemia.

G. **Vasodilators**

1. **Action:** Direct vasodilation of arteries and veins, resulting in rapid reduction of blood pressure (decreased preload and afterload)

2. **Medications**

  a. Nitroglycerin (Nitrostat IV)

  b. Enalaprilat (Vasotec IV)

  c. Nitroprusside (Nipride)

  d. Hydralazine (Apresoline)

3. **Therapeutic Use**

  a. Hypertensive emergencies

4. **Precautions/Interactions**

  a. Clients who have hepatic or renal disease

  b. Older adults

  c. Electrolyte imbalances

5. **Side/Adverse Effects**

  a. Dizziness

  b. Headache

  c. Profound hypotension

  d. Cyanide toxicity

  e. Thiocyanate poisoning

6. **Nursing Interventions and Client Education**

  a. Nitroprusside may not be mixed with any medication.

  b. Apply protective cover to container.

  c. Discard unused fluid after 24 hr.

  d. Provide continuous ECG and blood pressure monitoring.

ⅠⅠ Cardiac Glycosides

Used in the treatment of clients who have cardiac failure or ineffective pumping mechanism of the heart muscle.

A. **Action**

1. Increase the force and velocity of myocardial contractions to improve stroke volume and cardiac output.

2. Slow the conduction rate, allowing for increased ventricular filling.

B. **Medication**

1. Digoxin (Lanoxin, Lanoxicaps, Digitek)

C. **Therapeutic Uses**

1. Heart failure

2. Atrial fibrillation

D. **Precautions/Interactions**

1. Thiazide or loop diuretics increase risk of hypokalemia and precipitate digoxin toxicity.

2. ACE and ARBs increase risk of hyperkalemia.

3. Verapamil (Calan) increases risk of toxicity.

E. **Side/Adverse Effects**

1. Digoxin toxicity: GI effects (anorexia, nausea/vomiting, abdominal pain); CNS effects (fatigue, weakness, diplopia, blurred vision, yellow-green or white halos around objects)

F. **Nursing Interventions and Client Education**

1. Auscultate apical pulse for 1 min prior to administration.

2. Notify provider if HR less than 60/min (adult), less than 70/min (child), or less than 90/min (infant).

3. Monitor for signs of digoxin toxicity, hypokalemia, and hypomagnesemia.

4. Notify provider of any sudden increase in pulse rate that previously had been normal or low.

5. Maintain therapeutic digoxin level.

G. **Management of Digoxin Toxicity**

1. Discontinue digoxin and potassium-wasting medications.

2. Treat dysrhythmias with phenytoin (Dilantin) or lidocaine.

3. Treat bradycardia with atropine.

4. For excess overdose, administer Digibind to prevent absorption.

III Antianginal Medications

The use of organic nitrates, beta adrenergic-blocking agents, and calcium channel blockers to treat pain related to imbalances between myocardial oxygen supply and demand

A. **Organic Nitrates**

1. **Action**

   a. Relax peripheral vascular smooth muscles, resulting in dilation of arteries and veins, thus reducing venous blood return (reduced preload) to the heart, which leads to decreased oxygen demands on the heart.

   b. Increase myocardial oxygen supply by dilating large coronary arteries and redistributing blood flow.

2. **Medications**

   a. Nitrostat (sublingual)

   b. Nitrolingual (translingual spray)

   c. Nitro-Bid (topical ointment)

   d. Nitro-Dur (transderm patch)

B. **Therapeutic Use**

1. Acute angina attack

2. Prophylaxis of chronic stable or variant angina

C. **Precautions/Interactions**

1. Contraindicated in clients who have head injury

2. Hypotensive risk with antihypertensive medications

3. Erectile dysfunction medications—life-threatening hypotension

D. **Side/Adverse Effects**

1. Headache

2. Orthostatic hypotension

3. Reflex tachycardia

4. Tolerance

 E. **Nursing Interventions and Client Education**

1. Nitrostat/Nitrolingual

   a. Administer sublingual.

   b. Repeat in 5 min if no relief and call 911; may take up to three doses.

   c. Keep Nitrostat in original dark container.

   d. Nitrolingual may be used prophylactically 5 to 10 min before exercise.

   e. Do not shake Nitrolingual canister (forms bubbles).

   f. Replace NTG tablets every 6 months.

   g. Wear medical alert identification.

2. Nitro-Bid (topical ointment)

   a. Wear gloves for administration.

   b. Do not massage or rub area.

   c. Apply to area without hair (chest, flank, or upper arm preferable).

   d. Cover the area where the patch is placed with a clear plastic wrap, and tape in place.

   e. Gradually reduce the dose and frequency of application over 4 to 6 weeks.

3. Nitro-Dur (transderm patch)

   a. Skin irritation may alter medication absorption.

   b. Optimal locations for patch are upper chest or side; pelvis; and inner, upper arm.

   c. Rotate skin sites daily.

IV Antidysrhythmic Agents

A. **Action:** Antidysrhythmic agents are complex agents with multiple mechanisms of action. They are classified according to their effects on the electrical conduction system of the heart (Class I, II, III, IV).

B. **Medications**

1. Adenosine (Adenocard): slows conduction time through the AV node, interrupts AV node pathways to restore NSR

2. Amiodarone (Cordarone): prolongs repolarization, relaxes smooth muscles, decreases vascular resistance

3. Atropine: increases firing of the sinoatrial node (SA) and conduction through the atrioventricular node (AV) of the heart, opposes the actions of the vagus nerve by blocking acetylcholine receptor sites

C. **Precautions/Interactions**

1. Toxicity is a major concern due to additive effects.

2. Caution is needed when used with an AV block.

3. Caution is needed when using anticholinergic medications.

ANTIDYSRHYTHMIC MEDICATIONS

Adenosine

THERAPEUTIC USE	Convert SVT to sinus rhythm
SIDE/ADVERSE EFFECTS	Flushing, nausea Bronchospasm, prolonged asystole
NURSING INTERVENTIONS	Monitor for sinus bradycardia and chest discomfort.

Amiodarone

THERAPEUTIC USE	Ventricular fibrillation, unstable ventricular tachycardia
SIDE/ADVERSE EFFECTS	Bradycardia Cardiogenic shock Pulmonary disorders
NURSING INTERVENTIONS	Incompatible with heparin. May be given in PO maintenance dose. Monitor for respiratory complications.

Atropine

THERAPEUTIC USE	Bradycardia, known exposure to chemical nerve agent (AtroPEN)
SIDE/ADVERSE EFFECTS	When used for life-threatening emergency, has no contraindications
NURSING INTERVENTIONS	Monitor for dry mouth, blurred vision, photophobia, urinary retention, and constipation.

v Antilipemic Medications

A. **Action:** Aids in lowering low-density lipoprotein (LDL) levels and increases high-density lipoprotein (HDL) levels. Therapy includes diet, exercise, and weight control.

B. **Therapeutic Uses**
   1. Primary hypercholesterolemia
   2. Prevention of coronary events
   3. Protection against MI and stroke in clients who have diabetes

C. **Precautions/Interactions**
   1. Should be discontinued during pregnancy.
   2. Use with caution in renal dysfunction.

D. **Side/Adverse Effects**
   1. Muscle aches
   2. Hepatotoxicity
   3. Myopathy
   4. Rhabdomyolysis
   5. Peripheral neuropathy

E. **Nursing Interventions and Client Education**
   1. Take medication in the evening (cholesterol synthesis increases).
   2. Monitor liver and renal function laboratory profiles.
   3. Low-fat/high-fiber diet.
   4. Note dietary precautions with specific classes.

F. **Statin Medications**
   1. **Action:** Interfere with hepatic enzyme HMG-CoA to reduce formation of cholesterol precursors
   2. **Medications**
      a. Simvastatin (Zocor)
      b. Lovastatin (Mevacor)
      c. Pravastatin sodium (Pravachol)
      d. Rosuvastatin (Crestor)
      e. Fluvastatin (Lescol, Lescol XL)
   3. **Precautions/Interactions**
      a. Prolonged bleeding in clients taking warfarin (Coumadin)
      b. Multiple drug interactions: digoxin, warfarin, thyroid hormones, thiazide diuretics, phenobarbital, NSAIDs, tetracycline, beta-blocking agents, gemfibrozil, glipizide, glyburide, oral contraceptives, and phenytoin

   4. **Nursing Interventions and Client Education**
      a. Do not administer with grapefruit juice.

G. **Cholesterol Absorption Inhibitor**
   1. **Action:** Inhibits the absorption of cholesterol secreted in the bile and from food. Often used in combination with other antilipemic medications.
   2. **Medications**
      a. Ezetimibe (Zetia)

   3. **Nursing Interventions and Client Education**
      a. Take 1 hr before or 4 hr after other antilipemics.
      b. Risk of liver damage increased when combined with statins.

Medications for the Respiratory System

Medications used to treat chronic inflammatory conditions caused by asthma, bronchitis, and emphysema.

A. **Treatment for chronic respiratory disorders often includes multiple drug therapies.** When administered as inhalation therapies, the following guidelines should be implemented.
   1. Advise to take the beta$_2$ agonist before the inhaled glucocorticoid to increase steroid absorption.
   2. Instruct on procedures for inhalation:
      a. Remove the mouthpiece cap.
      b. If appropriate for medication, shake container.
      c. Stand or sit upright; exhale deeply.
      d. Place the mouthpiece between teeth, and close lips tightly around the inhaler.
      e. While breathing in, press down on the inhaler to activate and release the medication. Continue breathing in slowly for several more seconds (slow, long, steady inhalation is better than a quick short breaths).
      f. Hold breath for 5 to 10 seconds.
      g. Breathe in/out normally.
   3. Examine mouth for irritation.
   4. Perform frequent oral care.

i Beta$_2$ Adrenergic Agonists

A. **Action:** Promote bronchodilation by activating beta$_2$ receptors in bronchial smooth muscle

BETA$_2$ ADRENERGIC AGONISTS MEDICATIONS

Albuterol (Proventil, Ventolin)

ROUTE/ONSET	Inhaled (short-acting) Few minutes
USE	Acute bronchospasm

Formoterol (Foradil), salmeterol (Serevent)

ROUTE/ONSET	Inhaled (long-acting) 15 to 20 min, lasts 12 hr
USE	Long-term control of asthma

Terbutaline (Brethine)

ROUTE/ONSET	Oral (long-acting)
USE	Long-term control of asthma

B. **Precautions/Interactions**

1. Contraindicated for clients who have tachydysrhythmias.

2. Caution: diabetes mellitus, hyperthyroidism, heart disease, hypertension, angina.

3. Beta blockers will reduce effects.

4. MAOIs will increase effects.

C. **Side/Adverse Effects**

1. Tachycardia, palpitations

2. Tremors

 D. **Nursing Interventions and Client Education**

1. Caution against using salmeterol more frequently than every 12 hr.

II Methylxanthines

A. **Action:** Relaxation of bronchial smooth muscle, resulting in bronchodilation

B. **Medications**

1. Aminophylline (Truphylline)

2. Theophylline (Theolair, Theo-24)

C. **Therapeutic Uses**

1. Relief of bronchospasm

2. Long-term control of asthma

D. **Precautions/Interactions**

1. Contraindicated with active peptic ulcer disease.

2. Caution: diabetes mellitus, hyperthyroidism, heart disease, hypertension, angina.

3. Do not mix parenteral form with other medications.

4. Phenobarbital and phenytoin decrease theophylline levels.

5. Caffeine, furosemide, cimetidine, fluoroquinolones, acetaminophen, and phenylbutazone falsely elevate therapeutic levels.

E. **Side/Adverse Effects**

1. Irritability and restlessness

2. Toxic effects: tachycardia, tachypnea, seizures

F. **Nursing Interventions and Client Education**

1. Monitor therapeutic level.

2. Avoid caffeine intake.

3. Monitor for signs of toxicity.

4. Smoking will decrease effects.

5. Alcohol abuse will increase effects.

G. **Treatment of Toxicity**

1. Stop parenteral infusion.

2. Activated charcoal to decrease absorption in oral overdose.

3. Lidocaine for dysrhythmias.

4. Diazepam to control seizures.

III Inhaled Anticholinergics

A. **Action:** muscarinic receptor blocker resulting in bronchodilation

B. **Medications**

1. Ipratropium (Atrovent)

2. Tiotropium (Spiriva)

C. **Therapeutic Uses**

1. Prevent bronchospasm

2. Manage allergen- or exercise-induced asthma

3. COPD

D. **Precautions/Interactions**

1. Contraindicated for clients who have peanut allergy (contains soy lecithin).

2. Use extreme caution with narrow-angle glaucoma and BPH.

3. Do not use for treatment of acute bronchospasms.

E. **Side/Adverse Effects**

1. Dry mouth and eyes

2. Urinary retention

F. **Nursing Interventions and Client Education**

1. Reinforce teaching that maximum effects can take up to 2 weeks.

2. Shake inhaler well before administration.

3. When using two different inhaled medications, wait 5 min between.

4. If administered via nebulizer, use within 1 hr of reconstitution.

IV Glucocorticoids

A. **Action:** Prevent inflammatory response by suppression of airway mucus production, immune responses, and adrenal function

GLUCOCORTICOID MEDICATIONS

Oral	Inhalation	Intravenous
Prednisone	Beclomethasone dipropionate (QVAR)	Hydrocortisone sodium succinate (Solu-Cortef)
Prednisolone (Prelone)	Budesonide (Pulmicort Flexhaler)	Methylprednisolone sodium succinate (Solu-Medrol)
Betamethasone (Celestone)	Fluticasone propionate (Advair, Flovent)	Betamethasone sodium phosphate (Betnesol, Celestone Phosphate)
	Triamcinolone acetonide	

B. **Respiratory Therapeutic Uses**

1. Short-term

   a. IV agents: status asthmaticus

   b. Oral: treatment of symptoms following an acute asthma attack

2. Long-term

   a. Inhaled: prophylaxis of asthma

   b. Oral: treatment of chronic asthma

C. **Precautions/Interactions**

1. Clients who have diabetes mellitus can require higher doses.

2. Never stop medication abruptly.

D. **Side/Adverse Effects**

1. Euphoria, insomnia, psychotic behavior

2. Hyperglycemia

3. Peptic ulcer

4. Fluid retention (increased appetite)

5. Withdrawal symptoms

 E. **Nursing Interventions and Client Education**

1. Monitor client activity and behavior.

2. Administer medication with meals.

3. Reinforce teaching about symptoms to report.

4. Do not take with NSAIDs.

5. Medication dose will be gradually reduced to prevent Addisonian crisis.

v Leukotriene Modifiers

A. **Action:** Prevent effects of leukotriene resulting in decreased inflammation, bronchoconstriction, airway edema, and mucus production

B. **Medications**

1. Montelukast (Singulair)

2. Zileuton (Zyflo)

3. Zafirlukast (Accolate)

C. **Therapeutic Uses**

1. Long-term management of asthma in adults and children

2. Prevention of exercise-induced bronchospasm

D. **Precautions/Interactions**

1. Do not use for acute asthma attack.

2. Zileuton or zafirlukast: high risk of liver disease, increased warfarin effects, and theophylline toxicity.

3. Phenobarbital will decrease circulating levels of montelukast.

4. Chewable tablets contain phenylalanine.

E. **Side/Adverse Effects**

1. Elevated liver enzymes (zileuton or zafirlukast)

2. Warfarin and theophylline toxicity (zileuton or zafirlukast)

 F. **Nursing Interventions and Client Education**

1. Never abruptly substitute for corticosteroid therapy.

2. Administer medication daily

3. Do not decrease or stop taking other prescribed asthma drugs until instructed.

4. If using oral granules, pour directly into mouth or mix with cold soft foods (never liquids).

5. Use open packets within 15 min.

vi Antitussives, Expectorants, Mucolytics

DRUG ACTIONS AND THERAPEUTIC USE BY CLASS

Antitussives: hydrocodone, codeine

ACTION	Suppress cough through action in the CNS
THERAPEUTIC USE	Chronic nonproductive cough

Expectorants: guaifenesin (Mucinex)

ACTION	Promote increased mucous secretion to increase cough production
THERAPEUTIC USE	Often combined with other agents to manage respiratory disorders

Mucolytics: acetylcysteine (Mucomyst, Acetadote), hypertonic saline

ACTION	Enhance the flow of secretions in the respiratory tract
THERAPEUTIC USE	Acute and chronic pulmonary disorders with copious secretions
	Cystic fibrosis
	Antidote for acetaminophen poisoning

A. **Precautions/Interactions**

1. Only saline solutions should be used in children younger than 2 years.

2. Opioid antitussives have potential for abuse.

3. Caution with OTC medications—potentiate effects.

B. **Side/Adverse Effects**

1. Drowsiness

2. Dizziness

3. Aspiration and bronchospasm risk with mucolytics

4. Constipation

 C. **Nursing Interventions and Client Education**

1. Monitor cough frequency, effort, and ability to expectorate.

2. Monitor character, tenacity of secretions.

3. Auscultate for adventitious lung sounds.

4. Reinforce teaching to explain why multiple therapies are needed.

5. Promote fluid intake.

VII Decongestants, Antihistamines

DRUG ACTIONS AND THERAPEUTIC USE BY CLASS

Decongestants: phenylephrine (Sudafed), ephedrine (Pretz-D), naphazoline (Privine)

ACTION	Stimulate alpha₁ adrenergic receptors, causing reduced inflammation of nasal membranes
THERAPEUTIC USE	Allergic rhinitis
	Sinusitis
	Common cold

Antihistamines: diphenhydramine, loratadine (Claritin), cetirizine (Zyrtec), fexofenadine (Allegra), desloratadine (Clarinex)

ACTION	Decrease allergic response by competing for histamine receptor sites
THERAPEUTIC USE	Relieve/prevent hypersensitivity reactions

A. **Precautions/Interactions**

1. Use cautiously in clients who have HTN, glaucoma, peptic ulcer disease, and urinary retention.
2. Children can have symptoms of excitation, hallucinations, incoordination, and seizures.
3. Avoid alcohol intake.
4. Products containing pseudoephedrine should not be used longer than 7 days.

B. **Side/Adverse Effects**

1. Anticholinergic effects
2. Drowsiness

C. **Nursing Interventions and Client Education**

1. Monitor for hypokalemia.
2. Monitor blood pressure.
3. Reinforce teaching about how to manage anticholinergic effects.
4. Advise to take at night.

Medications for the Endocrine System

I Oral Hypoglycemics

Used in conjunction with diet and exercise to control glucose levels in clients who have type 2 diabetes mellitus

A. **Precautions/Interactions**

1. Caution in clients who have renal, hepatic, or cardiac disorders.
2. Generally avoided during pregnancy and lactation. Instruct client to discuss with prescriber.

ORAL HYPOGLYCEMIC MEDICATIONS

Alpha-glucosidase inhibitors: acarbose (Precose), miglitol (Glyset)

ACTION	Slows carbohydrate absorption and digestion
PRECAUTIONS/INDICATIONS	Contraindicated in clients who have intestinal disease due to increased gas formation

Biguanides: metformin (Glucophage)

ACTION	Reduces gluconeogenesis
	Increases uptake of glucose by muscles
PRECAUTIONS/INDICATIONS	Withhold 48 hr prior to and 48 hr after a test with contrast media
	Contraindicated in clients who have severe infection, shock, hypoxic conditions

Gliptins: sitagliptin (Januvia)

ACTION	Promotes release of insulin, lowers glucagon secretion and slows gastric emptying
PRECAUTIONS/INDICATIONS	Caution with impaired renal function—dose will be reduced

Meglitinides: repaglinide (Prandin), nateglinide (Starlix)

ACTION	Reduces production of glucose within the liver through suppression of gluconeogenesis
	Increases muscle uptake and use of glucose
PRECAUTIONS/INDICATIONS	Should not be used with NPH insulin due to risk of angina

Sulfonylureas: glipizide (Glucotrol), glyburide (DiaBeta)

ACTION	Promotes release of insulin from the pancreas
PRECAUTIONS/INDICATIONS	Extreme high risk of hypoglycemia in clients who have renal, hepatic, or adrenal disorders

Thiazolidinediones: rosiglitazone (Avandia), pioglitazone (Actos)

ACTION	Decreases insulin resistance
PRECAUTIONS/INDICATIONS	High risk of CHF due to fluid retention

B. **Nursing Interventions and Client Education**

1. Reinforce teaching to include signs and management for hypoglycemia, especially with sulfonylureas.

2. Encourage diet and exercise to follow American Diabetes Association recommendations.

3. Monitor glycosylated hemoglobin (HbA1C).

4. Collaborate with diabetic nurse educator.

II Insulin

Various forms of insulin are available to manage diabetes. The medications vary in onset, peak, and duration.

FORMS OF INSULIN

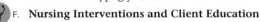

ONSET	PEAK	DURATION
Rapid-acting: Lispro (Humalog)		
Less than 15 min	0.5 to 1 hr	3 to 4 hr
Short-acting: Regular (Humulin R)		
0.5 to 1 hr	2 to 3 hr	5 to 7 hr
Intermediate: NPH (Humulin N)		
1 to 2 hr	4 to 12 hr	18 to 24 hr
Long-acting: Insulin glargine (Lantus)		
1 hr	None	10.5 to 24 hr

A. **Therapeutic Uses**

1. Glycemic control of diabetes mellitus (type 1, type 2, gestational) to prevent complications

2. Clients taking oral hypoglycemic agents can require insulin therapy when:

   a. Undergoing diagnostic tests

   b. Pregnant

   c. Severe kidney or liver disease is present

   d. Oral agents are inefficient

   e. Treatment of hyperkalemia

B. **Precautions/Interactions**

1. When mixing regular with NPH insulin, draw up regular first.

2. Do not mix other insulins with lispro, glargine, or combination 70/30.

3. Only regular insulin is given IV (only in normal saline).

4. Administer glargine at bedtime.

C. **Side/Adverse Effects**

1. Hypoglycemia/hyperglycemia

2. Lipodystrophy

D. **Nursing Interventions and Client Education**

1. Monitor serum glucose levels before meals and at bedtime or patterned schedule-specific to client.

2. Roll vial of insulin (except regular) to mix; do not shake.

3. Instruct client to rotate injection sites to prevent lipodystrophy.

4. Teach signs and management for hypo/hyperglycemia.

5. Encourage diet and exercise to follow ADA recommendations.

6. Monitor glycosylated hemoglobin (HbA1c).

7. Collaborate with diabetic nurse educator.

III Glycemic Agent

A. **Action:** Initiates regulatory processes to promote breakdown of glycogen to glucose in the liver, resulting in increased serum glucose levels

B. **Medications**

1. Glucagon (GlucaGen)

C. **Therapeutic Uses**

1. Emergency treatment of severe hypoglycemia

D. **Precautions/Interactions**

1. Do not mix with sodium chloride or dextrose solutions.

E. **Side/Adverse Effects**

1. Nausea and vomiting

2. Rebound hypoglycemia

F. **Nursing Interventions and Client Education**

1. Administer medication for unresponsive client.

2. Monitor blood glucose levels.

3. Reinforce teaching for recognizing and managing early signs of hypoglycemia.

4. Client should wear medical alert ID.

5. Reinforce teaching with family members related to medication administration.

6. Provide carbohydrates when client awakens from hypoglycemic reaction.

IV Thyroid Hormone

A. **Action:** Stimulates metabolism of all body systems by accelerating the rate of cellular oxygenation

B. **Medications**

1. Levothyroxine/T_4 (Synthroid)

C. **Therapeutic Uses**

1. Hypothyroidism

2. Emergency treatment of myxedema coma

D. **Precautions/Interactions**

1. Overmedication can result in signs of hyperthyroidism.

E. **Side/Adverse Effects**
   1. Tachycardia
   2. Restlessness
   3. Diarrhea
   4. Weight loss
   5. Decreased bone density
   6. Heat intolerance
   7. Insomnia

F. **Nursing Interventions and Client Education**
   1. Monitor cardiac system.
   2. Therapy initiated with low doses; advance to higher dosages while monitoring laboratory values.
   3. Monitor T_4 and TSH levels.
   4. Take in early morning.

V Thyroid Hormone Antagonist

A. **Action:** Inhibits synthesis of thyroid hormone
B. **Medication**
   1. Methimazole (Tapazole)
C. **Therapeutic Uses**
   1. Hyperthyroidism
   2. Preoperative thyroidectomy
   3. Thyrotoxic crisis
   4. Thyroid storm
D. **Precautions/Interactions**
   1. Administer with caution to clients who have bone marrow depression, hepatic disease, or bleeding disorders.
   2. Discontinue prior to radioactive iodine uptake testing.
   3. Contraindicated with breastfeeding.
E. **Side/Adverse Effects**
   1. Skin rash, pruritus
   2. Abnormal hair loss
   3. GI upset
   4. Paresthesias
   5. Periorbital edema
   6. Joint and muscle pain
   7. Jaundice
   8. Agranulocytosis
   9. Thrombocytopenia

F. **Nursing Interventions and Client Education**
   1. Administer with food at the same time each day.
   2. Increase fluids to 3 L/day.
   3. Client should avoid OTC products containing iodine.
   4. Client should take medication as prescribed.
   5. If discontinuing dose must be tapered off.
   6. Monitor client for therapeutic response: weight gain, decreased pulse, blood pressure, and T_4 levels.
   7. Monitor client for signs of overdose: periorbital edema, cold intolerance, mental depression.

VI Anterior Pituitary/Growth Hormones

A. **Action:** Increase production of insulin-like growth factor throughout the body
B. **Medications**
   1. Somatropin (Genotropin, Nutropin)
   2. Somatrem (Protropin)
C. **Therapeutic Use**
   1. Treat growth hormone deficiencies
   2. Turner's syndrome
D. **Precautions/Interactions**
   1. Contraindicated in clients who are severely obese.
   2. Therapy must be discontinued prior to epiphyseal closure.
   3. Avoid concurrent use of glucocorticoids.
E. **Side/Adverse Effects**
   1. Hyperglycemia
   2. Hypothyroidism

F. **Nursing Interventions and Client Education**
   1. Monitor growth patterns.
   2. Reconstitute medication. (Do not shake.)
   3. Administer subcutaneous per protocol.
   4. Dose is individualized.

VII Posterior Pituitary Hormones/Antidiuretic Hormones

A. **Action:** Promote reabsorption of water with the kidneys; vasoconstriction of vascular smooth muscle
B. **Medications**
   1. Desmopressin (DDAVP): oral, intranasal, subcutaneous, IV
   2. Vasopressin: intranasal, subcutaneous, IV
C. **Therapeutic Uses**
   1. Diabetes insipidus
   2. Cardiac arrest
   3. Nocturnal enuresis
D. **Precautions/Interactions**
   1. Contraindicated in clients who have chronic nephritis or high risk for myocardial infarction
E. **Side/Adverse Effects**
   1. Hyponatremia
   2. Seizures
   3. Coma

F. **Nursing Interventions and Client Education**
   1. Monitor urine specific gravity.
   2. Monitor blood pressure.
   3. Monitor urinary output.
   4. Prevent hyponatremia due to water intoxication.
   5. Reinforce teaching for use of nasal spray.

VIII Adrenal Hormone Replacement

A. **Action:** Anti-inflammatory suppresses immune response

B. **Medications**
   1. Dexamethasone
   2. Hydrocortisone (Solu-Cortef)
   3. Fludrocortisone acetate (Florinef)
   4. Prednisone

C. **Therapeutic Uses**
   1. Acute and chronic replacement for adrenocortical insufficiency (Addison's disease)
   2. Inflammation, allergic reactions, cancer

D. **Precautions/Interactions**
   1. Contraindicated in clients who have systemic fungal infection.
   2. Caution in clients who have hypertension, gastric ulcers, diabetes, osteoporosis.
   3. Requires higher doses in acute illness or extreme stress.

E. **Side/Adverse Effects**
   1. Adrenal suppression when administered for inflammation, allergic reactions
   2. Infection
   3. Hyperglycemia
   4. Osteoporosis
   5. GI bleeding
   6. Fluid retention

F. **Nursing Interventions and Client Education**
   1. Do not skip doses.
   2. Monitor blood pressure.
   3. Monitor fluid and electrolyte (F&E) balance, weight, and output.
   4. Monitor for signs of bleeding and GI discomfort.
   5. Client should take calcium supplements and maintain vitamin D levels.
   6. Give with food.
   7. Taper off dose regimen when discontinuing medication.
   8. Provide immunoprotection.

SECTION 6

Medications for the Hematologic System

I Blood and Blood Products

A. **Examples**
   1. Whole blood
   2. Packed red blood cells (RBCs)
   3. Platelet concentrations

ADMINISTRATION OF BLOOD PRODUCTS

Whole blood

TIME COMPLETED	2 to 4 hr	
ACTION/ THERAPEUTIC USE	Replace volume › Hemorrhage › Surgery	› Trauma › Burns › Shock
MONITOR FOR REACTION	Acute hemolytic Febrile Anaphylactic	Mild allergic Hypervolemia Sepsis

Packed RBCs

TIME COMPLETED	2 to 4 hr	
ACTION/ THERAPEUTIC USE	Increase available RBC Severe anemia Hemoglobinopathies	Hemolytic anemia Erythroblastosis fetalis
MONITOR FOR REACTION	Acute hemolytic Febrile Anaphylactic	Mild allergic Sepsis

Platelets

TIME COMPLETED	15 to 30 min	
ACTION/ THERAPEUTIC USE	Increase platelet count Active bleeding Thrombocytopenia	Aplastic anemia Bone marrow suppression
MONITOR FOR REACTION	Febrile	Sepsis

FFP

TIME COMPLETED	30 to 60 min	
ACTION/ THERAPEUTIC USE	Replace clotting factors › Hemorrhage › Burns › Shock	› Thrombotic thrombocytopenic purpura (TTP) › Reverse effects of warfarin
MONITOR FOR REACTION	Acute hemolytic Febrile Anaphylactic	Mild allergic Hypervolemia Sepsis

Pheresed granulocytes

TIME COMPLETED	45 to 60 min	
ACTION/ THERAPEUTIC USE	Severe neutropenia Neonatal sepsis	Neutrophil dysfunction
MONITOR FOR REACTION	Acute hemolytic Febrile Anaphylactic	Mild allergic Hypervolemia Sepsis

Albumin

TIME COMPLETED	5% (1 to 10 mL/min)	25% (4 mL/min)
ACTION/ THERAPEUTIC USE	Expand volume via oncotic changes Hypovolemia Hypoalbuminemia	Burns Severe nephrosis Hemolytic disease of the newborn
MONITOR FOR REACTION	Risk for hypervolemia and pulmonary edema	

B. **Nursing Interventions and Client Education**

1. Client ID, name, and blood type must be verified by two nurses.

2. Prior to administration, obtain baseline vital signs, including temperature.

3. IV access, 20-gauge or larger catheter, must be established.

4. Must have 0.9% sodium chloride primed tubing.

5. For the first 15 min, the RN must stay with the client and infuse slowly, monitoring for any reaction. If a reaction occurs, perform the following interventions.

   a. Stop blood immediately and take vital signs.

   b. Infuse 0.9% sodium chloride.

   c. Notify the provider.

   d. Follow facility policy (send urine sample, CBC, and bag and tubing to laboratory for analysis).

6. Complete infusion of product within 4 hr.

II Hematopoietic Growth Factors

A. **Action:** Stimulate the bone marrow to synthesize the specific blood cells

MEDICATIONS

Epoetin alfa (Procrit)

THERAPEUTIC USES	Stimulate RBC production Anemia related to: › CKD › Retrovir therapy › Chemotherapy
SIDE/ADVERSE EFFECTS	Hypertension
NURSING INTERVENTIONS	Subcutaneous or IV › Do not agitate vial › Monitor Hct

Filgrastim (Neupogen) injection
Pegfilgrastim (Neulasta) IV over 2 to 4 hr

THERAPEUTIC USES	Stimulate WBC production Neutropenia related to cancer
SIDE/ADVERSE EFFECTS	Bone pain Leukocytosis
NURSING INTERVENTIONS	Subcutaneous or IV Do not agitate vial Monitor CBC

Oprelvekin (Neumega)

THERAPEUTIC USES	Stimulate platelet production Thrombocytopenia related to cancer
SIDE/ADVERSE EFFECTS	Fluid retention Papilledema Cardiac dysrhythmia
NURSING INTERVENTIONS	Administer within 6 to 24 hr after chemotherapy Subcutaneous

III Iron Preparations

A. **Oral**

1. Dilute liquid preparations with juice or water and administer with a plastic straw or medication dosing syringe (avoid contact with teeth).

2. Encourage orange juice fortified with vitamin C (vitamin C facilitates absorption)

3. Avoid antacids, coffee, tea, dairy products, or whole grain breads concurrently and for 1 hr after administration due to decreased absorption.

4. Monitor the client for constipation and gastrointestinal upset.

B. **Intramuscular**

1. Use a large-bore needle (19- to 20-gauge, 3-inch).

2. Change needle after drawing up from vial.

3. Z-track (ventrogluteal preferable), never in deltoid muscle.

4. Do not massage injection site.

IV Anticoagulants

A. **Heparin Sodium and Enoxaparin (Lovenox) (Parenteral Medications)**

1. **Action**

   a. Modify or inhibit clotting factors or cellular properties to prevent clot formation

   b. Enoxaparin (Lovenox) prevents conversion of prothrombin to thrombin by inactivating coagulation enzymes.

2. **Therapeutic Uses**

   a. Evolving stroke

   b. Pulmonary embolism

   c. Massive deep-vein thrombosis

   d. Cardiac catheterization

   e. MI

   f. DIC

3. **Precautions/Interactions**

   a. Must be given subcutaneous or IV.

   b. Incompatible with many medications (any bicarbonate base).

   c. Avoid NSAIDs, aspirin, or medications containing salicylates.

4. **Side/Adverse Effects**

   a. Hemorrhage

   b. Heparin-induced thrombocytopenia

   c. Toxicity/overdose

5. **Nursing Interventions and Client Education**

   a. Clients receiving heparin: Monitor aPTT every 4 to 6 hr for IV administration.

   b. Monitor for signs of bleeding.

   c. Safety precautions to prevent bleeding.

   d. Administer subcutaneous heparin to abdomen, 2 inches from umbilicus (do not aspirate or massage).

   e. Rotate injection sites and observe for bleeding or hematoma.

   f. Administer protamine sulfate for heparin toxicity (1 mg neutralizes 100 units of heparin).

B. **Warfarin (Coumadin) (Oral Medication)**

1. **Action:** Prevents the synthesis of coagulation factors VII, IX, X, and prothrombin

2. **Therapeutic Uses**

   a. Venous thrombosis

   b. Thrombus prevention for clients who have atrial fibrillation or prosthetic heart valves

   c. Prevention of recurrent MI

   d. Transient ischemic attacks (TIAs)

3. **Precautions/Interactions**

   a. Not safe for use during pregnancy.

   b. Contraindications: thrombocytopenia, vitamin K deficiency, liver disease, alcohol use disorder.

   c. Decreased effects with phenobarbital, carbamazepine (Tegretol), phenytoin (Dilantin), oral contraceptives.

   d. Food sources high in vitamin K may decrease effects.

4. **Side/Adverse Effects**

   a. Hemorrhage

   b. Toxicity/overdose

5. **Nursing Interventions and Client Education**

   a. Administer once daily.

   b. Monitor INR or PT.

   c. Reinforce client teaching that bleeding risk remains up to 5 days after discontinued therapy.

   d. Client should avoid NSAIDs and medications with aspirin.

   e. Client should wear medical alert bracelet.

   f. Client may self-monitor for PT/INR.

   g. Reinforce teaching with client to prevent injury and bleeding.

   h. Administer vitamin K for warfarin toxicity.

   i. Garlic, ginger, gingko, and ginseng can increase risk of bleeding.

C. **Dabigatran (Pradaxa) (Oral Medication)**

1. **Action:** Prevents thrombus formation by directly inhibiting thrombin formation

2. **Therapeutic Use**

   a. Reduces the risk of stroke and embolism for clients who have nonvalvular atrial fibrillation

3. **Precautions/Interactions**

   a. Caution when client is making a change in medication if currently receiving warfarin. (Must discontinue warfarin and start dabigatran when INR is below 2.0)

   b. When possible, discontinue 1 to 2 days prior to surgical procedures.

4. Side Effects/Adverse Effects

   a. Bleeding

   b. GI discomfort

5. **Nursing Interventions and Client Education**

   a. Medication should be taken daily. Do not skip doses.

   b. If a dose is missed, it should not be taken within 6 hr of the next scheduled dose.

   c. Tablets should not be crushed, broken, or chewed.

   d. Clients should avoid NSAIDs and medications with aspirin.

   e. Reinforce client teaching to monitor for signs of GI bleeding.

v Antiplatelet Medications

A. **Action:** Prevent platelets from aggregating (clumping together) by inhibiting enzymes and factors that normally promote clotting

B. **Medications**

1. Aspirin (Ecotrin)

2. Abciximab (ReoPro)

3. Clopidogrel (Plavix)

4. Ticlopidine (Ticlid)

5. Pentoxifylline (Trental)

6. Dipyridamole (Persantine)

C. **Therapeutic Uses**

1. Prevention of acute myocardial infarction or acute coronary syndromes

2. Prevention of stroke

3. Intermittent claudication

D. **Precautions/Interactions**

1. Contraindicated in thrombocytopenia

2. Caution with peptic ulcer disease

E. **Side/Adverse Effects**

1. Prolonged bleeding

2. Gastric bleeding

3. Thrombocytopenia

F. **Nursing Interventions and Client Education**

1. Monitor for signs of prolonged bleeding.

2. Client should report tarry stool, ecchymosis.

vi Thrombolytic Medications

A. **Action:** Dissolve clots that have already formed by converting plasminogen to plasmin, which destroys fibrinogen and other clotting factors

B. **Medications**

1. Alteplase (Activase, tPA)

2. Tenecteplase (TNKase)

3. Reteplase (Retavase)

C. **Therapeutic Uses**

1. Acute myocardial infarction

2. Deep-vein thrombosis (DVT)

3. Massive pulmonary emboli (PE)

4. Ischemic stroke (alteplase)

D. **Precautions/Interactions**

1. Contraindicated for intracranial hemorrhage, active internal bleeding, aortic dissection, brain tumors.

2. Use caution when using in clients who have severe hypertension.

3. Concurrent use of anticoagulants or antiplatelet medications increases risk for bleeding.

E. **Side/Adverse Effects**

1. Serious bleeding risks from recent wounds, puncture sites, weakened vessels

2. Hypotension

3. Possible anaphylactic reaction

F. **Nursing Interventions and Client Education**

1. Administration must take place within 4 to 6 hr of symptom onset.

2. Continuous monitoring is required.

3. Clients will begin anticoagulant therapy to prevent repeated thrombotic event.

SECTION 7

Medications for the Gastrointestinal System

I Antacids

A. **Action:** Neutralize gastric acid and inactivate pepsin

MEDICATIONS

Aluminum hydroxide (Amphojel)

SIDE/ADVERSE EFFECTS	Constipation	Hypophosphatemia

Magnesium hydroxide (Milk of Magnesia)

SIDE/ADVERSE EFFECTS	Diarrhea	Hypermagnesemia
	Renal impairment	

Sodium bicarbonate

SIDE/ADVERSE EFFECTS	Constipation

B. **Therapeutic Uses**

1. Peptic ulcer disease

2. GERD

C. **Nursing Interventions and Client Education**

1. Do not administer to clients who have GI perforation or obstruction.

2. Clients who have renal impairment should only use aluminum-based preparations.

3. Other medications should be taken 1 hr before or after antacids.

4. Require repeated doses up to 7 times per day: 1 hr and 3 hr after meals and at bedtime.

II Antisecretory/Blocking Agents

A. **Action:** Prevent or block selected receptors within the stomach

B. **Therapeutic Uses**

1. Gastric and peptic ulcers

2. GERD

3. Zollinger-Ellison syndrome

C. **Medication Classifications**

1. **Proton Pump Inhibitors**

   a. **Medications**

      1) Omeprazole (Prilosec)

      2) Lansoprazole (Prevacid)

      3) Rabeprazole sodium (AcipHex)

      4) Esomeprazole (Nexium)

   b. **Precautions/Interactions**

      1) Omeprazole promotes increased risk for infection; use with caution in COPD.

      2) Digoxin levels can be increased with omeprazole.

      3) Long-term therapy has increased risk of gastric cancer and osteoporosis.

   c. **Side Effects/ Adverse Effects**

      1) Low incidence of diarrhea, nausea, and vomiting.

      2) Can increase the risk for fractures, pneumonia, and acid rebound.

   d. **Nursing Interventions and Client Education**

      1) Do not crush, chew, or break tablets.

      2) Notify prescriber of any sign of GI bleeding.

      3) Reinforce client teaching to take medication as scheduled.

2. **Histamine$_2$ Receptor Antagonists**

   a. **Medications**

      1) Ranitidine hydrochloride (Zantac)

      2) Cimetidine (Tagamet)

      3) Nizatidine (Axid)

      4) Famotidine (Pepcid)

   b. **Precautions/Interactions**

      1) Can cause toxicity for clients taking phenytoin, warfarin, theophylline, and lidocaine.

      2) Cimetidine promotes increased risk for infection; use with caution in COPD.

   c. **Side/Adverse Effects**

      1) Decreased libido/impotence

      2) Lethargy, depression, confusion

   d. **Nursing Interventions and Client Education**

      1) Clients should seek appropriate care (many take OTC preparations).

      2) Client should follow medication regimen.

      3) Ranitidine can be taken with or without food.

      4) Reinforce teaching with client to modify diet as prescribed.

III Mucosal Protectants

A. **Sucralfate (Carafate)**

1. **Action:** Adheres to injured gastric ulcers upon contact with gastric acids; protective action for up to 6 hr; has no systemic effects

2. **Therapeutic Use**

   a. Gastric and duodenal ulcers

   b. GERD

3. **Nursing Interventions and Client Education**

   a. Administer on an empty stomach at least 1 hr before meals.

   b. Do not administer within 30 min of antacids.

IV Antiemetics

A. **Action:** Multiple classifications of medications that affect the GI tract or the "vomiting center" of the brain to reduce nausea/vomiting

B. **Therapeutic Uses**

1. Postoperative

2. Chemotherapy

3. Nausea/vomiting associated with disease process

MEDICATIONS

Promethazine

SIDE/ADVERSE EFFECTS	Drowsiness	EPSs
	Anticholinergic effects	Potentiates effects when given with narcotics
NURSING INTERVENTIONS	Monitor vital signs Safety precautions	IM—large muscle

Metoclopramide (Reglan)

SIDE/ADVERSE EFFECTS	Drowsiness	EPSs
	Anticholinergic effects	Tardive dyskinesia
	Restlessness	
NURSING INTERVENTIONS	Instruct client about rapid GI emptying Discontinue with signs of EPSs	

Ondansetron (Zofran)

SIDE/ADVERSE EFFECTS	Headache	EPSs
NURSING INTERVENTIONS	Administer tablets 30 min prior to chemotherapy and 1 to 2 hr before radiation	

Scopolamine

SIDE/ADVERSE EFFECTS	Blurred vision	Anticholinergic effects
	Sedation	
NURSING INTERVENTIONS	Do not use with angle-closure glaucoma Apply transdermal patches behind ear Use lubricating eye drops	

V Antidiarrheals

A. **Action:** Activate opioid receptors in the GI tract to decrease intestinal motility and to increase the absorption of fluid and sodium in the intestine

B. **Medications**

1. Diphenoxylate plus atropine (Lomotil)

2. Loperamide (Imodium)

C. **Precautions/Interactions**

1. Increased risk of megacolon for clients who have IBS

2. May cause drowsiness or dizziness

D. **Nursing Interventions and Client Education**

1. Monitor F&E.

2. Avoid caffeine intake (increases GI motility).

VI Stool Softeners/Laxatives

MEDICATIONS

Psyllium (Metamucil)

THERAPEUTIC USES	Decrease diarrhea (bulk-forming)

Docusate sodium (Colace)

THERAPEUTIC USES	Relieve constipation (surfactant)

Bisacodyl (Dulcolax)

THERAPEUTIC USES	Preprocedure colon evacuation (stimulant)

Magnesium hydroxide (Milk of Magnesia)

THERAPEUTIC USES	Prevent painful elimination (low-dose osmotic) Promote rapid evacuation (high-dose osmotic)

A. **Nursing Interventions and Client Education**

1. Contraindicated with fecal impaction, bowel obstruction, and acute surgical abdomen.

2. Encourage regular exercise and promote regular bowel elimination.

3. Monitor for chronic laxative use/abuse.

4. Provide adequate fluid intake to avoid obstruction.

SECTION 8

Medications Affecting the Urinary System

I Diuretics

A. **Action:** Increase the amount of fluid excretion via the renal system

MEDICATIONS

Loop	Thiazide	Potassium Sparing
Furosemide (Lasix) Bumetanide (Bumex)	Hydrochlorothiazide (Microzide) Chlorothiazide (Diuril)	Spironolactone (Aldactone) Triamterene (Dyrenium)

B. **Therapeutic Use**

1. Pulmonary edema caused by heart failure

2. Edema unresponsive to other diuretics

C. **Precautions/Interactions**

1. Use cautiously in clients who have diabetes mellitus.

2. Contraindicated in pregnancy.

3. NSAIDs reduce diuretic effect.

D. **Side/Adverse Effects**

1. Loop and thiazide diuretics

   a. Hypovolemia

   b. Ototoxicity

   c. Hypokalemia

   d. Hyponatremia

   e. Hyperglycemia

   f. Digoxin toxicity

   g. Lithium toxicity

2. Potassium-sparing diuretics

   a. Hyperkalemia

   b. Endocrine effects (impotence, menstrual irregularities)

 E. **Nursing Interventions and Client Education**

1. Monitor I&O.

2. Monitor vital signs.

3. Monitor for F&E imbalances.

4. Administer early morning to prevent nocturia.

5. Clients taking loop/thiazide diuretics will need to increase intake of foods high in potassium.

6. Clients taking potassium-sparing diuretics should avoid salt substitutes.

II Osmotic Diuretics

A. **Action:** Pull fluid back into the vascular and extravascular space by increasing serum osmolality to promote osmotic changes

B. **Medication**

1. Mannitol (Osmitrol)

C. **Therapeutic Uses**

1. Prevent renal failure related to hypovolemia

2. Decrease intracranial pressure related to cerebral edema

3. Decrease intraocular pressure

D. **Precautions/Interactions**

1. Use with caution in heart failure.

2. Can increase digoxin levels due to hypokalemia.

E. **Side/Adverse Effects**

1. Pulmonary edema

2. F&E imbalances

3. Thirst, dry mouth

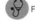 F. **Nursing Interventions and Client Education**

1. Monitor daily weight, I&O, and electrolytes.

2. Monitor for signs of hypovolemia.

3. Monitor neurological status.

III Alpha-Adrenergic Blockers for Urinary Hesitancy

A. **Tamsulosin (Flomax)**

1. **Action:** Inhibits smooth muscle contraction in the prostate, which improves the rate of urine flow for clients who have BPH

2. **Precautions/Interactions**

   a. Must rule out bladder cancer prior to administering tamsulosin.

   b. Combined use with cimetidine can facilitate toxicity.

B. **Bethanechol (Urecholine)**

1. **Action:** Increases detrusor muscle tone to allow strong start to voiding for clients who have postoperative urinary hesitancy

2. **Precautions/Interactions**

   a. Do not administer IV or IM.

   b. Contraindicated for clients who have hypotension or decreased cardiac output.

ALPHA-ADRENERGIC BLOCKERS

Tamsulosin (Flomax)

SIDE/ADVERSE EFFECTS	Can cause decreased libido, reduced ejaculate
NURSING INTERVENTIONS AND CLIENT EDUCATION	Take 30 min after meal at same time each day Clients should contact prescriber if greater than 4 doses are missed

Bethanechol (Urecholine)

SIDE/ADVERSE EFFECTS	Excessive salivation, tearing
NURSING INTERVENTIONS	Administer on empty stomach

IV Anticholinergic Medications for Overactive Bladder

A. **Action:** Antispasmodic actions to decrease detrusor muscle spasms and contractions

B. **Medications**

1. Oxybutynin (Ditropan, Gelnique)
2. Tolterodine (Detrol)
3. Darifenacin (Enablex)
4. Solifenacin (Vesicare)
5. Trospium (Sanctura)
6. Fesoterodine (Toviaz)

C. **Therapeutic Use**

1. Urinary incontinence
2. Urinary urgency and frequency

D. **Precautions/Interactions**

1. Do not use for clients who have intestinal obstruction.
2. Use with other anticholinergics can increase anticholinergic effects.

E. **Side/Adverse Effects**

1. Anticholinergic symptoms
2. Drowsiness
3. Dyspepsia

 F. **Nursing Interventions and Client Education**

1. Administer medication with a full glass of water.
2. Reinforce teaching with client:
   a. Full effects can take 1 to 2 months.
   b. How to manage side effects of anticholinergics.
   c. Report constipation lasting longer than 3 days.

V Sexual Dysfunction

A. **Action:** Enhances the effect of nitric oxide to promote relaxation of penile muscles, allowing increased blood flow to produce an erection

B. **Medications**

1. Sildenafil (Viagra)
2. Tadalafil (Cialis)
3. Vardenafil (Levitra)

C. **Therapeutic Uses**

1. Erectile dysfunction
2. Sexual dysfunction in women (unlabeled use)

D. **Precautions/Interactions**

1. Contraindicated for clients taking nitrate drugs, anticoagulants, alpha blockers for BPH, or antihypertensives.
2. Contraindicated for clients who have history of stroke, uncontrolled diabetes mellitus, hypo/hypertension, or heart failure.

E. **Side/Adverse Effects**

1. Headache
2. Heartburn
3. Diarrhea
4. Flushing
5. Nosebleeds
6. Difficulty falling asleep or staying asleep
7. Paresthesias
8. Muscle aches
9. Changes in color vision
10. Sensitivity to light

F. **Nursing Interventions and Client Education**

1. Administer 1 hr before sexual activity; do not use more than once daily.
2. Client should notify provider of all medications currently taken including herbal preparations.
3. Client should avoid intake of any organic nitrates.
4. Client should stop taking medication and notify prescriber immediately for any of the following: erection lasting longer than 4 hr, any loss of vision, and unusual bleeding problems.

Medications for the Immune System

I Immunizations

A. **Action:** Stimulate production of antibodies to prevent illness

CHILDHOOD IMMUNIZATIONS*

DTaP, Tdap

SIDE/ADVERSE EFFECTS**	Fever	Irritability	Seizures
CONTRAINDICATION	Occurrence of seizures within 3 days of vaccine		

Hib

SIDE/ADVERSE EFFECTS**	Low-grade fever
CONTRAINDICATION	Age younger than 6 weeks

Rotavirus

SIDE/ADVERSE EFFECTS**	Infant with diarrhea and vomiting Immunocompromised
CONTRAINDICATION	Allergy to "mycin" drugs

IPV

SIDE/ADVERSE EFFECTS**	Allergic reaction

MMR

SIDE/ADVERSE EFFECTS**	Joint pain	Anaphylaxis	Thrombocytopenia
CONTRAINDICATION	Allergy to gelatin and neomycin Immunocompromised		

CHILDHOOD IMMUNIZATIONS (CONTINUED)

Varicella

SIDE/ADVERSE EFFECTS**	Vesicles on skin Pruritus
CONTRAINDICATION	Pregnancy Allergy to gelatin and neomycin Immunocompromised

Seasonal influenza

SIDE/ADVERSE EFFECTS**	Fever
CONTRAINDICATION	Nasal spray contraindicated for child younger than 2 and adults older than 50 years History of Guillain-Barré

Hepatitis A, B

SIDE/ADVERSE EFFECTS**	Anaphylaxis	
CONTRAINDICATION	Hep A: pregnancy	Hep B: allergy to yeast

Meningococcal vaccine

CONTRAINDICATION	History of Guillain-Barré

HPV – up to age 26

CONTRAINDICATION	Pregnancy	Allergy to yeast

*Schedule is determined by the Centers for Disease Control and Prevention.
**Risk in Addition to Localized Inflammation

ADULT IMMUNIZATIONS (AGES 18 YEARS AND OLDER)*

TYPE	SCHEDULE
Tetanus booster	Every 10 years
MMR	One or two doses at ages 19 to 49
Varicella	Two doses if no history of disease
Pneumococcal (PPSV)	Once after age 65 Recommended for immunocompromised, COPD, living in long-term care facility
Hepatitis A	Two doses for high-risk clients
Hepatitis B	Three doses for high-risk clients
Seasonal influenza	Annually
Meningococcal vaccine	Students entering college Adults older than 56 years Repeat every 5 years for high-risk clients
Herpes zoster	Over age 60

*Schedule is determined by the Centers for Disease Control and Prevention.

B. **Nursing Interventions and Client Education**

1. Consult CDC guidelines for schedule of administration.

2. Reinforce teaching about the purpose of immunizations and keeping records.

3. Parents should avoid administration of aspirin for management of adverse effects in children.

4. Reinforce teaching with clients regarding side/adverse effects and management.

II Antimicrobials

A. **Action:** Inhibit growth, destroy or otherwise control replication of microbes

MULTIGENERATION ANTIBIOTICS

Aminoglycosides

MEDICATIONS	Amikacin (Amikin)	Gentamicin sulfate
		Streptomycin
THERAPEUTIC USE	Septicemia, meningitis, pneumonia	
PRECAUTIONS	High risk for ototoxicity, nephrotoxicity Monitor creatinine and BUN Peak and trough levels	

Cephalosporins

MEDICATIONS	Cephalexin (Keflex)	Cefotaxime (Claforan)
	Cefaclor (Ceclor)	
THERAPEUTIC USE	Upper respiratory, skin, urinary infections Used as prophylaxis for clients at risk	
PRECAUTIONS	Cross-sensitivity with penicillins Monitor for signs of *Clostridium difficile*	

Fluoroquinolones

MEDICATIONS	Ciprofloxacin (Cipro)	Levofloxacin (Levaquin)
THERAPEUTIC USE	Bronchitis, chlamydia, gonorrhea, PID, UTI Pneumonia, prostatitis, sinusitis	
PRECAUTIONS	Caution with hepatic, renal, or seizure disorders	

Macrolides

MEDICATIONS	Azithromycin (Zithromax)	Clarithromycin (Biaxin)
		Erythromycin (Erythrocin)
THERAPEUTIC USE	Upper respiratory infections, sinusitis, Legionnaires' disease, whooping cough, acute diphtheria, chlamydia	
PRECAUTIONS	Used for clients who have penicillin allergy Administer with meals	

Nitrofurantoin (Macrodantin)

THERAPEUTIC USE	UTI
PRECAUTIONS	Broad-spectrum Contraindicated in renal dysfunction Urine will have brown discoloration

Penicillins

MEDICATIONS	Amoxicillin (Amoxil)	Ampicillin (Omnipen)
THERAPEUTIC USE	Pneumonia, upper respiratory infections, septicemia, endocarditis, rheumatic fever, GYN infections	
PRECAUTIONS	Hypersensitivity with possible anaphylaxis	

Sulfonamides

MEDICATIONS	Trimethoprim/sulfamethoxazole (Bactrim, Septra)
THERAPEUTIC USE	UTI, bronchitis, otitis media
PRECAUTIONS	Consume at least 3 L/day of fluid Use backup contraceptives Avoid sun exposure

Tetracyclines

MEDICATIONS	Doxycycline calcium (Vibramycin) Tetracycline HCl (Sumycin)
THERAPEUTIC USE	Fungal, bacterial, protozoal, rickettsial infections
PRECAUTIONS	Consume at least 3 L/day of fluid Use backup contraceptives Avoid sun exposure Permanent tooth discoloration if given to children younger than 8 years

SPECIAL CLASSES

Antifungal

MEDICATIONS	Fluconazole (Diflucan)
THERAPEUTIC USE	Candidiasis infections
PRECAUTIONS	Monitor hepatic and renal function Refrigerate suspensions Increased risk of bleeding for clients taking anticoagulants

Antimalarials

MEDICATIONS	Hydroxychloroquine (Plaquenil) Quinine sulfate (Quinine)
THERAPEUTIC USE	Prevent malarial attacks, rheumatoid arthritis Systemic lupus
PRECAUTIONS	Increased risk of psoriasis Monitor for drug-induced retinopathy

Antiprotozoal

MEDICATIONS	Metronidazole (Flagyl)
THERAPEUTIC USE	Trichomoniasis and giardiasis, *Clostridium difficile*, amebic dysentery, PID, vaginosis
PRECAUTIONS	Take with food Do not consume alcohol during therapy or 48 hr after completion of regimen

Antituberculars

MEDICATIONS	Isoniazid (INH) Rifampin (Rifadin)
THERAPEUTIC USE	Prevention and treatment of TB Latent TB INH: 6 to 9 months Active TB: multiple therapy up to 24 months
PRECAUTIONS	Risk of neuropathies and hepatotoxicity Consume foods high in vitamin B_6 Avoid foods with tyramine (INH) Increased risk of phenytoin (Dilantin) toxicity (INH) Avoid alcohol Discoloration of urine, saliva, sweat, and tears (rifampin)

Antiretrovirals

MEDICATIONS	Acyclovir (Zovirax) Valacyclovir HCl (Valtrex) Zidovudine (AZT, Retrovir)
THERAPEUTIC USE	Genital herpes, shingles, HIV
PRECAUTIONS	Acyclovir and valacyclovir: administer with food Zidovudine: empty stomach Increase fluid intake Begin therapy with first onset of symptoms

 B. **Nursing Interventions and Client Education**

1. Collect data about history of medication allergies and treatment.

2. Monitor for signs of medication reaction.

3. Monitor for signs of secondary infections.

4. Administer medications at appropriate time intervals to maintain therapeutic effects.

5. If C&S is ordered, perform test before initiating therapy.

6. Client should complete entire medication regimen.

SECTION 10

Medications for the Musculoskeletal System

Bisphosphonates

A. **Action:** Decrease the number and action of osteoclasts, resulting in bone resorption

B. **Medications**

1. Alendronate (Fosamax): daily or weekly

2. Risedronate (Actonel): daily, weekly, monthly

3. Ibandronate (Boniva): monthly or every 3 months

4. Zoledronic acid (Reclast, Zometa): IV annually

C. **Therapeutic Use**

1. Prevention and treatment of osteoporosis

2. Paget's disease

3. Hypercalcemia related to malignancy

D. **Precautions/Interactions**

1. Contraindicated during lactation.

2. Clients who have esophageal stricture or difficulty swallowing may only use zoledronate.

3. Absorption is decreased when taken with calcium supplements, antacids, orange juice, and caffeine.

E. **Side/Adverse Effects**

1. Musculoskeletal pain

2. Esophagitis and GI discomfort

3. Jaw pain with zoledronate

 F. **Nursing Interventions and Client Education**

1. Administer medication in the morning on an empty stomach.

2. Clients should consume at least 8 oz water (not carbonated).

3. Client must remain upright (sitting or standing) for 30 min after taking medication.

4. Consume adequate amounts of vitamin D.

II Antirheumatics

A. **Action:** Provide symptomatic relief and delay in disease progression by inhibiting or modulating inflammatory processes

ANTIRHEUMATIC DRUG CATEGORIES

Disease-modifying antirheumatic drugs (DMARDs)

MEDICATIONS	Methotrexate (Rheumatrex)	Etanercept (Enbrel)
		Infliximab (Remicade)
	Hydroxychloroquine (Plaquenil)	Adalimumab (Humira)
ACTION	Interrupt complex immune responses, preventing disease progression	

Glucocorticoids

| MEDICATIONS | Prednisone | Prednisolone (Prelone) |
| ACTION | Decrease inflammation by suppressing leukocytes and fibroblasts, and reversing capillary permeability | |

NSAIDs

MEDICATIONS	Ibuprofen (Advil, Motrin)	Naproxen (Naprosyn)
	Diclofenac (Voltaren)	Celecoxib (Celebrex)
	Indomethacin (Indocin)	
ACTION	Inhibit prostaglandin synthesis resulting in decreased inflammatory responses	

III DMARDs

A. **Therapeutic Use**

1. Slow joint degeneration and progression of rheumatoid arthritis

B. **Precautions/Interactions**

1. Methotrexate: Contraindicated in pregnancy, kidney or liver failure, psoriasis, alcohol use disorder, or hematologic dyscrasias.

C. **Side/Adverse Effects**

1. Methotrexate: Increased risk of infection, bone marrow suppression, GI ulceration

2. Hydroxychloroquine: retinal damage (blindness)

 D. **Nursing Interventions and Client Education**

1. Reinforce teaching about measures to prevent infection.

2. Monitor liver function tests.

3. Reinforce teaching with client to use reliable contraception.

4. Reinforce teaching with client that initial effects may take 3 to 6 weeks, and full therapeutic effects make take several months.

5. Administer with food.

6. Clients taking hydroxychloroquine should have a retinal examination every 6 months.

IV Glucocorticoids

A. **Therapeutic Use**

1. Provide symptomatic relief of inflammation and pain.

B. **Precautions/Interactions**

1. Contraindicated in systemic fungal infection.

2. Do not administer live virus vaccines during therapy.

3. Should only be used for a short duration.

C. **Side/Adverse Effects**

1. Risk of infection

2. Osteoporosis

3. Adrenal suppression

4. Fluid retention

5. GI discomfort

6. Hyperglycemia

7. Hypokalemia

D. **Nursing Interventions and Client Education**

1. Do not skip doses.

2. Monitor blood pressure.

3. Monitor F&E balance and weight.

4. Monitor for signs of bleeding, GI discomforts.

5. Client should take calcium supplements and maintain vitamin D levels.

6. Give with food.

7. Never stop abruptly.

8. Provide immunoprotection.

v NSAIDs

A. **Therapeutic Use**

1. Provide rapid, symptomatic relief of inflammation and pain.

B. **Precautions/Interactions**

1. Hypersensitivity to aspirin or other NSAIDs.

2. Can increase the risk of MI and stroke.

C. **Side/Adverse Effects**

1. GI discomforts

2. GI ulceration

3. Renal impairment

4. Photosensitivity

D. **Nursing Interventions and Client Education**

1. Administer with food and full glass of water.

2. Avoid lying down for 30 min after administration.

3. Reinforce teaching with client to use only as needed for symptoms to reduce risk of GI ulceration.

4. Client should use sunscreen.

vi Antigout

MEDICATIONS

Allopurinol (Zyloprim)

ACTION	Inhibits uric acid production
THERAPEUTIC USE	Chronic gouty arthritis

Colchicine (Colcrys)

ACTION	Inhibits processes to prevent leukocytes from invading joints
THERAPEUTIC USE	Acute gouty arthritis

A. **Precautions/Interactions**

1. Use caution in clients who have renal, cardiac, or gastrointestinal dysfunction.

2. Should not be combined with theophylline (Theo-24).

B. **Side/Adverse Effects**

1. GI distress

2. Hepatitis

C. **Nursing Interventions and Client Education**

1. Instruct client to avoid foods high in purines to reduce uric acid.

2. Monitor CBC and uric acid levels.

3. Client should avoid aspirin.

4. Administer with meals.

Medications for the Nervous System

i Antianxiety Medications

A. **Action:** Increase the efficacy of GABA to reduce anxiety

B. **Medications**

1. Alprazolam (Xanax)

2. Buspirone

3. Chlordiazepoxide (Librium)

4. Clonazepam (Klonopin)

5. Diazepam (Valium)

6. Lorazepam (Ativan)

C. **Therapeutic Use**

1. Generalized anxiety disorder and panic disorder

2. Insomnia

3. Alcohol withdrawal

4. Induction of anesthesia

D. **Precautions/Interactions**

1. Diazepam and buspirone are used with caution in clients who have substance use disorder and liver disease.

2. Buspirone is contraindicated for clients taking MAOIs.

E. **Side/Adverse Effects**

1. CNS depression

2. Paradoxical response (insomnia, excitation, euphoria)

3. Withdrawal symptoms (not with buspirone)

4. Risk of abuse and potential for overdose

F. **Nursing Interventions and Client Education**

1. Monitor vital signs.

2. Reinforce teaching with client to never abruptly discontinue medication.

3. Monitor clients for side/adverse effects.

4. Reinforce teaching with client to avoid alcohol.

5. Treat overdose with flumazenil (Romazicon).

II Antidepressants

A. Action

1. SSRI inhibits serotonin reuptake.

2. Tricyclic blocks reuptake of norepinephrine and serotonin.

3. MAOI increases norepinephrine, dopamine, and serotonin by blocking MAO-A.

ANTIDEPRESSANT CLASSES

SSRI

MEDICATIONS	Citalopram (Celexa) Fluoxetine (Prozac) Escitalopram (Lexapro)	Fluvoxamine (Luvox) Paroxetine (Paxil, Pexeva) Sertraline (Zoloft)
PRECAUTIONS/INTERACTIONS	Avoid alcohol. Do not discontinue abruptly. Monitor for serotonin syndrome (agitation, confusion, hallucinations) within first 72 hr.	
SIDE/ADVERSE EFFECTS	Weight gain Sexual dysfunction	Fatigue Drowsiness

SNRI

MEDICATIONS	Duloxetine (Cymbalta)	Venlafaxine (Effexor)
PRECAUTIONS/INTERACTIONS	Do not administer with MAOI. Do not administer to clients who have uncontrolled narrow-angle glaucoma. Monitor for suicidal tendencies.	
SIDE/ADVERSE EFFECTS	Insomnia Nausea	Sexual dysfunction Seizures

Tricyclic

MEDICATIONS	Amitriptyline Clomipramine (Anafranil)	Doxepin (Sinequan) Imipramine (Tofranil)
PRECAUTIONS/INTERACTIONS	Do not administer with MAOIs or St. John's wort Must avoid alcohol. Contraindicated for clients who have seizure disorder.	
SIDE/ADVERSE EFFECTS	Anticholinergic effects Sedation	Toxicity Decreased seizure threshold

MAOI

MEDICATIONS	Isocarboxazid (Marplan) Tranylcypromine (Parnate) Phenelzine (Nardil)
PRECAUTIONS/INTERACTIONS	Avoid foods containing tyramine. Antihypertensives have additive hypotensive effect. Contraindicated with SSRIs, tricyclics, heart failure, CVA, renal insufficiency.
SIDE/ADVERSE EFFECTS	CNS stimulation Orthostatic hypotension Hypertensive crisis with intake of tyramine, SSRIs, and tricyclics

 B. Nursing Interventions and Client Education

1. Monitor and collect data about client's risk for suicide.

2. Client should take medication on daily basis and never miss a dose.

3. Reinforce teaching with client about therapeutic effects and time of onset.

4. Client must avoid discontinuing drug abruptly.

5. Reinforce teaching with client to take SSRIs in the morning to minimize sleep disturbances.

6. Provide clients taking MAOIs a list of foods containing tyramine.

7. Reinforce teaching with client to avoid taking other medications without consulting provider.

III Bipolar Disorder Medications

A. Action: Produce neurochemical changes in the brain to control acute mania, depression and incidence of suicide

B. Medication

1. Lithium carbonate (Lithobid)

C. Therapeutic Uses

1. Bipolar disorder

2. Alcohol use disorder

3. Bulimia

4. Schizophrenia

D. Precautions/Interactions

1. Use cautiously in clients who have renal dysfunction, heart disease, hyponatremia, and dehydration.

   a. NSAIDs will increase lithium levels.

   b. Monitor serum sodium levels.

E. Side/Adverse Effects

1. GI distress

2. Fine hand tremors

3. Polyuria

4. Weight gain

5. Renal toxicity

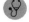 **F. Nursing Interventions and Client Education**

1. Monitor therapeutic levels.

2. Monitor serum sodium levels.

3. Reinforce teaching with clients that therapeutic effects begin in 7 to 14 days.

4. Doses must be administered 2 to 3 times daily per prescriber.

5. Reinforce teaching about nutrition and food sources containing sodium.

6. Administer with food to decrease GI distress.

IV Antipsychotic Medications

A. **Action:** Block dopamine, acetylcholine, histamine, and norepinephrine receptors in the brain and periphery

B. **Medications**

1. Conventional (Typical)

   a. Chlorpromazine

   b. Fluphenazine

   c. Haloperidol (Haldol)

   d. Thiothixene (Navane)

2. Atypical (less severe side/adverse effects)

   a. Aripiprazole (Abilify)

   b. Clozapine (Clozaril)

   c. Olanzapine (Zyprexa)

   d. Paliperidone (Invega)

   e. Quetiapine (Seroquel)

   f. Ziprasidone (Geodon)

C. **Therapeutic Use**

1. Acute and chronic psychosis

2. Schizophrenia

3. Manic phase of bipolar disorders

4. Tourette's syndrome

5. Delusional and schizoaffective disorders

6. Dementia

D. **Precautions/Interactions**

1. Contraindicated for clients who have severe depression, Parkinson's disease, prolactin-dependent cancer, and severe hypotension.

2. Use with caution in clients who have glaucoma, paralytic ileus, prostate enlargement, or seizure disorder.

E. **Side/Adverse Effects**

1. Sedation

2. Extrapyramidal effects (administer benzatropine)

3. Anticholinergic effects

4. Tardive dyskinesia

5. Agranulocytosis

6. Neuroleptic malignant syndrome

7. Seizures (can require increased dose of antiseizure medications)

 F. **Nursing Interventions and Client Education**

1. Monitor for side effects within 5 hr to 5 days of administration.

2. Reinforce teaching with client about potential side effects.

3. Monitor CBC.

4. Encourage fluids.

5. Medication must be discontinued if signs of neuroleptic malignant syndrome develop.

V Attention Deficit Hyperactive Disorder Medications

A. **Action:** Increase attention span; reduce impulsive behavior and hyperactivity

1. Stimulants increase levels of norepinephrine, serotonin, and dopamine into the CNS.

2. Nonstimulants increase levels of norepinephrine into the CNS.

ADHD CLASSES

Stimulants

MEDICATION	Dextroamphetamine and amphetamine (Adderall/Adderall XR)
	Methylphenidate (Daytrana—transdermal)
	Methylphenidate (Concerta, Ritalin)
SIDE EFFECTS	Mood changes Insomnia Anxiety
NURSING INTERVENTIONS AND CLIENT EDUCATION	Administer in early morning.
	Do not abruptly discontinue.
	Monitor for signs of abuse.
	Monitor for signs of agitation.

Nonstimulants

MEDICATION	Atomoxetine (Strattera)
	Guanfacine (Intuiv): may be used in treatment of Asperger's syndrome
SIDE EFFECTS	GI upset Constipation Fatigue
NURSING INTERVENTIONS AND CLIENT EDUCATION	Take medication daily.
	Do not crush or chew.
	Client should immediately report worsening of anxiety, agitation.
	Do not take with MAOIs.

VI Sedative/Hypnotic Medications

A. **Action:** Slow neuronal activity in the brain to induce sedation/sleep

B. **Medications**

1. Eszopiclone (Lunesta)

2. Temazepam (Restoril)

3. Zolpidem tartrate (Ambien)

C. **Therapeutic Use**

1. Short-term insomnia

2. Difficulty falling or staying asleep

D. **Precautions/Interactions**

1. Use cautiously in clients who have severe mental depression.

2. Avoid combined use with alcohol and medications that depress CNS function.

E. **Side/Adverse Effects**

1. Dry mouth

2. Decreased libido

3. Respiratory depression

 F. **Nursing Interventions and Client Education**

1. Client should take medication immediately before bedtime because it has abrupt onset of sleep.

2. Client should avoid alcohol.

3. Warn client and caregivers of potential for sleep activities without recall; notify prescriber immediately.

VII Abstinence Maintenance Medications

A. **Disulfiram (Antabuse)**

1. **Action:** Interferes with hepatic oxidation of alcohol, resulting in elevation of blood acetaldehyde levels

2. **Therapeutic Use**

   a. Adjunct to maintain sobriety in treatment of alcohol use disorder

3. **Precautions/Interactions**

   a. INH will increase risk of adverse CNS effects for clients taking disulfiram.

   b. Ingestion of large amounts of alcohol may cause respiratory depression, arrhythmias, and cardiac arrest.

   c. Adjust medication doses of warfarin and phenytoin.

4. **Side/Adverse Effects**

   a. Drowsiness

   b. Headache

   c. Metallic taste

 5. **Nursing Interventions and Client Education**

   a. Must wait 12 hr between time of last alcohol intake and starting medication.

   b. Reinforce teaching with client that consumption of alcohol while taking disulfiram will result in flushing, throbbing in head and neck, respiratory difficulty, nausea, copious vomiting, sweating, thirst, chest pain, palpitation, dyspnea, hyperventilation, tachycardia, hypotension, syncope, marked uneasiness, weakness, vertigo, blurred vision, and confusion.

   c. Reinforce teaching with client that:

   1) undesirable effects last 30 min to several hours when alcohol is consumed.

   2) effects of disulfiram can stay in the body for weeks after therapy is discontinued.

   3) therapy can last months to years.

B. **Methadone (Dolophine)**

1. **Action:** Binds with opiate receptors in CNS to produce analgesic and euphoric effects

2. **Therapeutic Use**

   a. Prevents withdrawal symptoms in clients who were addicted to opiate drugs

3. **Precautions/Interactions**

   a. Do not use in clients who have severe asthma, chronic respiratory disease, or history of head injury.

4. **Side/Adverse Effects**

   a. Sedation

   b. Respiratory depression

   c. Paradoxical CNS excitation

5. **Nursing Interventions and Client Education**

   a. Monitor clients for signs of drug tolerance and psychological dependence.

   b. Monitor pancreatic enzymes because medication may cause biliary spasms.

   c. Doses of methadone must be slowly reduced to produce detoxification.

   d. Client must be monitored through treatment center.

VIII Chronic Neurological Disorders

A. **Cholinesterase Inhibitors**

1. **Action:** Prevent cholinesterase from inactivating acetylcholine, resulting in improved transmission of nerve impulses

2. **Medications**

   a. Neostigmine (Prostigmin)

   b. Ambenonium (Mytelase)

   c. Edrophonium (Tensilon)

3. **Therapeutic Use**

   a. Myasthenia gravis

4. **Precautions/Interactions**

   a. Do not administer if systolic blood pressure less than 90 mm Hg.

5. **Side/Adverse Effects**

   a. Slow heart rate

   b. Chest pain, weak pulse, increased sweating, and dizziness

   c. Client feeling like he or she might pass out

   d. Weak or shallow breathing

   e. Urinating more than usual

   f. Seizures

   g. Trouble swallowing

6. **Nursing Interventions and Client Education**

   a. Dose must be individualized.

   b. Client should keep individual diary to record side effects.

   c. Client should wear medical alert bracelet.

   d. Monitor for cholinergic crisis.

B. **Anti-Parkinson's**

1. **Action:** Increase dopamine to minimize tremors and rigidity

2. **Medications**
   a. Benzatropine (Cogentin)
   b. Carbidopa/levodopa (Sinemet, Parcopa)

3. **Therapeutic Use**
   a. Parkinson's disease

4. **Precautions/Interactions**
   a. Do not use levodopa within 2 weeks of MAOI use.
   b. Pyridoxine (vitamin B_6) decreases effects of levodopa.
   c. Benzatropine is contraindicated in clients who have narrow-angle glaucoma.
   d. Must discontinue 6 to 8 hr before anesthesia.

5. **Side/Adverse Effects**
   a. Muscle twitching (especially eyelid spasms)
   b. Headache
   c. Dizziness
   d. Dark urine
   e. Agitation

6. **Nursing Interventions and Client Education**
   a. Reinforce teaching with family members to assist with medication regimen.
   b. Client should notify prescriber if sudden loss of the medication effects occurs.
   c. Reinforce teaching with client that maximum therapeutic effects may take 4 to 6 weeks.
   d. Monitor closely for signs of adverse reactions.
   e. Client should avoid high-protein meals and snacks.
   f. Keep medication away from heat, light, and moisture. If pills become darkened, they have lost potency and must be discarded.

C. **Antiseizure**

1. **Action:** Slows rates of neuronal activity in the brain by blocking specific channels responsible for neuron firing, which results in an elevation of the seizure threshold

2. **Medications**
   a. Carbamazepine (Tegretol)
   b. Gabapentin (Neurontin)
   c. Phenobarbital (Luminal)
   d. Phenytoin (Dilantin)
   e. Valproic acid (Depakote)

3. **Therapeutic Use**
   a. Prevent and/or control seizure activity

ANTISEIZURE MEDICATIONS

Carbamazepine (Tegretol)

PRECAUTIONS/ INTERACTIONS	Contraindicated in clients who have bone marrow suppression or bleeding disorders
	Warfarin therapy decreases effectiveness
SIDE/ADVERSE EFFECTS	Anemia, leukopenia, Stevens-Johnson syndrome

Gabapentin (Neurontin)

| PRECAUTIONS/ INTERACTIONS | Do not abruptly discontinue |
| SIDE/ADVERSE EFFECTS | Dizziness, ataxia, somnolence, hypertension, bruising |

Phenobarbital (Luminal)

| PRECAUTIONS/ INTERACTIONS | Contraindicated in history of substance use disorder |
| SIDE/ADVERSE EFFECTS | Drowsiness, hypotension, respiratory depression |

Phenytoin (Dilantin)

| PRECAUTIONS/ INTERACTIONS | Causes increased excretion of digoxin, warfarin, oral contraceptives |
| SIDE/ADVERSE EFFECTS | Gingival hypertrophy, diplopia, drowsiness, hirsutism |

Valproic acid (Depakote)

| PRECAUTIONS/ INTERACTIONS | Contraindicated in liver disease, pregnancy |
| SIDE/ADVERSE EFFECTS | Hepatotoxicity, teratogenic effects, pancreatitis |

4. **Nursing Interventions and Client Education**
   a. Monitor for therapeutic effects.
   b. Monitor clients taking phenytoin for toxic effects, including serum levels for toxicity.
   c. Reinforce teaching with client regarding the importance of compliance; medication is treatment, not a cure.
   d. Individualize treatment regimen.
   e. Reinforce teaching with client regarding side/adverse effects.
   f. Medication therapy for status epilepticus: IV phenytoin and diazepam.

D. **Cognitive Disorders**

1. **Therapeutic Use:** Delay progression of symptoms related to Alzheimer's disease

2. **Medications**
   a. Cholinesterase inhibitor
      1) Donepezil (Aricept)
      2) Galantamine (Razadyne)
   b. NMDA receptor antagonist
      1) Mematine (Namenda)

3. **Precautions/Interactions**
   a. Do not increase or abruptly decrease

4. **Side/Adverse Effects**
   a. Anorexia
   b. Diarrhea
   c. Incontinence
5. Generally well tolerated with minimal side effects

E. **Nursing Interventions/Client Education**
   1. Administer between meals.
   2. Monitor blood pressure.
   3. Monitor behavioral changes.
   4. Reinforce teaching that medication relieves symptoms and is not a cure.

F. **Ophthalmologic Medications (Antiglaucoma)**
   1. **Action:** Reduction of aqueous humor
   2. **Medications**
      a. Levobunolol (Betagan)
      b. Pilocarpine HCl (Pilocar)
      c. Timolol maleate (Timoptic)
   3. **Precautions/Interactions**
      a. Use caution in clients taking oral beta blocker or calcium channel blocker
   4. **Side/Adverse Effects**
      a. Blurred vision
      b. Photophobia
      c. Dry eyes
      d. May have systemic effects of beta blockade
   5. **Nursing Interventions and Client Education**
      a. Sterile technique should be used when handling applicator portion of the container.
      b. Hold gentle pressure on the nasolacrimal duct for 30 to 60 seconds immediately after instilling drops.
      c. Monitor pulse rate/rhythm for clients taking oral beta or calcium channel blocker.

SECTION 12

Medications for Pain and Inflammation

I NSAIDs

See "Medications for the Musculoskeletal System" on page 50.

II Acetaminophen

A. **Action:** Slows production of prostaglandins in the CNS
B. **Therapeutic Use**
   1. Analgesic
   2. Antipyretic
C. **Precautions/Interactions**
   1. Use caution in clients who consume three or more alcoholic beverages per day.
   2. Concurrent use of rifampin, INH, carbamazepine, and barbiturates may increase hepatotoxic effects.
   3. Slows the metabolism of warfarin.

D. **Side/Adverse Effects**
   1. Nausea and vomiting
   2. Long-term therapy: hemolytic anemia, leukopenia, neutropenia, and thrombocytopenia

E. **Nursing Interventions and Client Education**
   1. Monitor liver function.
   2. Monitor kidney function.
   3. The recommended dosage is 325 to 650 mg every 4 to 6 hr. Clients should not exceed 4,000 mg/day.
   4. Reinforce teaching with client about risk of hepatotoxicity.
   5. Administration to children should be based on age, not to exceed five doses per day (read labels carefully).
   6. Treat acetaminophen overdose with acetylcysteine (Mucomyst).

III Opioid Analgesics

A. **Action:** Bind with opiate receptors in the CNS to alter the perception of and emotional response to pain
B. **Medications**
   1. Fentanyl (Sublimaze, Duragesic)
   2. Hydromorphone (Dilaudid)
   3. Morphine sulfate
   4. Meperidine (Demerol)
   5. Codeine, oxycodone (OxyContin)
C. **Therapeutic Use**
   1. Relief of moderate to severe pain
   2. Sedation
D. **Precautions/Interactions**
   1. Morphine is contraindicated after biliary tract surgery.
   2. Meperidine is contraindicated in clients who have kidney failure.
   3. Monitor for potentiate effects when given with barbiturates, benzodiazepines, phenothiazines, hypnotics, and sedatives.
E. **Side/Adverse Effects**
   1. Orthostatic hypotension
   2. Constipation
   3. Urinary retention
   4. Blurred vision
   5. Respiratory depression
   6. Abstinence syndrome
F. **Nursing Interventions and Client Education**
   1. Monitor vital signs.
   2. Monitor for respiratory depression.
   3. Reinforce teaching with client regarding administration with PCA pump.
   4. Administer naloxone (Narcan) for clients who have respiratory depression.

PHARMACOLOGICAL PAIN MANAGEMENT

Identify important teaching points a PN should reinforce for a client receiving each of the following pain control modalities.

1. Epidural: _____

_____

2. Patient-controlled analgesia: _____

_____

3. Peripheral nerve catheter: _____

_____

Answer Key: 1. Notify the provider for signs of infection, such as back pain, paresthesia, or fever. Notify the provider for signs of systemic infection, such as a metallic taste, tinnitus, vomiting, blurred vision, nausea, and confusion. Notify provider of any changes in sensation and movement of lower extremities. 2. Self-administer before pain becomes severe. Administer prophylactically prior to activities that can cause pain. Reassure clients of safeguards that prevent excessive doses. 3. Notify provider of signs of systemic infection, such as metallic taste, tinnitus, vomiting, blurred vision, nausea, and confusion. Notify provider for signs of infection, such as fever, swelling, redness, increase in pain or severe headache, sudden weakness to lower extremities, or decrease in bowel or bladder control. Protect area of numbness from injury.

References: ATI PN Pharmacology module. (pp. 293; 437-438).
Lehne, R. A. (2013). Pharmacology for nursing care. (8th ed. pp. 130). St. Louis, MO: Saunders.

Medications for the Reproductive System

Contraception

A. **Consider the following when providing client education and support regarding contraception.** Factors that influence choice of a contraceptive include:

1. Age and health status, including risk for STI
2. Religion and culture
3. Plans for future conception
4. Frequency of intercourse
5. Number of sexual partners
6. Personal concerns about availability, spontaneity, ease of use

CONTRACEPTION METHODS

Rhythm method

CONSIDERATIONS FOR USE	Develop "fertile awareness" by noting › Cervical mucus changes › Menstrual cycle pattern › Basal temperature
CLIENT EDUCATION	Do not have sexual intercourse during "fertile periods." Low reliability for preventing pregnancy.

Oral contraceptives

CONSIDERATIONS FOR USE	Pill is taken daily. Adverse effects: breast tenderness, bleeding, nausea/vomiting.
CLIENT EDUCATION	Antibiotic therapy reduces effectiveness. Avoid smoking.

CONTRACEPTION METHODS (CONTINUED)

Ethinyl estradiol and norelgestromin (Ortho Evra) contraceptive patch

CONSIDERATIONS FOR USE	Replace patch each week for 3 weeks.
CLIENT EDUCATION	Apply patch to buttocks, abdomen, upper torso, upper/outer arm. Period will begin on week 4 (no patch).

Medroxyprogesterone (Depo-Provera)

CONSIDERATIONS FOR USE	Injection is administered every 3 months during menstrual cycle.
CLIENT EDUCATION	Use backup form of birth control for 7 days after first injection. Fertility returns approximately 1 year after stopping.

Emergency contraception

CONSIDERATIONS FOR USE	A larger-than-normal dose of oral contraceptive.. Taken no later than 72 hr after unprotected sex. Second dose is repeated 12 hr later. Antiemetics can be needed.
CLIENT EDUCATION	Should discuss options with provider. Should never be used as the primary method of birth control.

Etonogestrel, ethinyl estradiol vaginal ring (NuvaRing)

CONSIDERATIONS FOR USE	Placed deep into the vagina once every 3 weeks.
CLIENT EDUCATION	One size fits most women. If falls out, rinse in warm water and replace within 5 hr. Remove ring during week 4; menses should begin.

CONTRACEPTION METHODS (CONTINUED)

Intrauterine device (IUD)

CONSIDERATIONS FOR USE	Contraindicated for women with diabetes or history of PID High risk of infection Can have cramping and heavier periods
CLIENT EDUCATION	Hormonal IUD effective for up to 7 years. Copper IUD effective for up to 12 years. Must monitor for signs of infection. Verify string is present.

Cervical cap

CONSIDERATIONS FOR USE	Use with spermicide. Fit by prescriber. Pap smear every 3 months. Increased risk of vaginal infections.
CLIENT EDUCATION	Leave in place 6 hr after intercourse but not longer than 48 hr.

Cervical diaphragm

CONSIDERATIONS FOR USE	Use with spermicide. Fit by prescriber. Refitted after childbirth or weight gain/loss.
CLIENT EDUCATION	Leave in place 6 hr after intercourse. Refit size with 10 lb or more weight change.

Condom

CONSIDERATIONS FOR USE	Use with spermicide.
CLIENT EDUCATION	Protects against STDs. Apply and remove correctly. Use only water-soluble lubricants.

Spermicides

CONSIDERATIONS FOR USE	Available as › Cream › Foam	› Gel › Suppository › Film
CLIENT EDUCATION	Should use with barrier method. Can insert up to 1 hr before intercourse.	

B. Nursing Interventions and Client Education

1. Discuss conception and contraceptive plans with client to include reliability, benefits, and risks.
2. Client should maintain regular health screening visits.
3. Reinforce teaching with client about measures to prevent PID, STIs.
4. Reinforce teaching about contraceptive decisions changing over the life span.
5. Reinforce teaching about unreliable forms of birth control including coitus interruptus (withdrawal), douching, and breastfeeding.

II Oxytocic

A. Cervical "Ripening"

1. **Action:** Prostaglandins cause cervical softening in preparation for cervical dilation and effacement

2. **Medication**
   a. Dinoprostone cervical gel (Cervidil)

3. **Precautions/Interactions**
   a. Contraindicated in clients who have genital herpes, ruptured membranes, or placenta previa.

4. **Side/Adverse Effects**
   a. Nausea
   b. Stomach pain
   c. Back pain
   d. Feeling of warmth in the vaginal area

5. **Nursing Interventions and Client Education**
   a. Maintain client on bed rest for 1 to 2 hr after insertion.
   b. Monitor and record maternal vital signs and fetal heart rate.
   c. Monitor for uterine contractions.
   d. Remove by gently pulling the netted string and discard.
   e. Oxytocin augmentation may be initiated as needed.

B. Oxytocin (Pitocin)

1. **Action:** Stimulates uterine contractions for the purpose of induction or augmentation of labor

2. **Therapeutic Use**
   a. Antepartum for contraction stress test (CST)
   b. Intrapartum for induction or augmentation of labor
   c. Postpartum to promote uterine involution

3. **Precautions/Interactions**
   a. Contraindicated with placental insufficiency.
   b. Bishop Score of 6 and greater when planning induction.

4. **Side/Adverse Effects**
   a. Intense uterine contractions
   b. Uterine hyperstimulation (contraction longer than 90 seconds)
   c. Uterine rupture

5. **Nursing Interventions and Client Education**
   a. Administer as secondary infusion via infusion pump for induction or augmentation.
   b. Continuously monitor uterine contractions and fetal heart rate.
   c. Discontinue oxytocin with any signs of uterine hyperstimulation.
   d. Administer oxygen via face mask 10 L for signs of hyperstimulation.
   e. When used in postpartum, monitor client for uterine bleeding.

III Methylergonovine (Methergine)

A. **Action:** Acts directly on the uterine muscle to stimulate forceful contractions

B. **Therapeutic Use**
1. Postpartum hemorrhage

C. **Precautions/Interactions**
1. Use with extreme caution in clients who have hypertension, preeclampsia, heart disease, venoatrial shunts, mitral valve stenosis, sepsis, or hepatic or renal impairment.

D. **Side/Adverse Effects**
1. Potent vasoconstriction
2. Hypertension
3. Headache

 E. **Nursing Interventions and Client Education**
1. Continuously monitor blood pressure.
2. Monitor uterine bleeding and uterine tone.

IV Tocolytics

A. **Action:** Act on uterine muscle to cease contractions

B. **Therapeutic Use**
1. Stop preterm labor

MEDICATIONS

Terbutaline sulfate (Brethine)

SIDE/ADVERSE EFFECTS	Nervousness	Hyperglycemia
	Tremulousness	Severe palpitations
	Headache	Chest pain
	Nausea and vomiting	Pulmonary edema
NURSING INTERVENTIONS	Monitor contractions and FHT. Monitor vital signs. Do not administer if pulse rate greater than 130/min or client has chest pain. Administer beta blocking agent as antidote.	

Nifedipine (Procardia)

SIDE/ADVERSE EFFECTS	Hypotension	Flushing
	Fatigue	Uteroplacental perfusion complications
	Nausea	
NURSING INTERVENTIONS	Monitor BP. Avoid concurrent use with magnesium sulfate.	Monitor contractions and FHT. Prevent complication with hypotension.

Magnesium sulfate

SIDE/ADVERSE EFFECTS	Warmth	Diminished DTRs
	Flushing	Decreased urine output
	Respiratory depression	Pulmonary edema
NURSING INTERVENTIONS	Monitor vital signs and DTRs. Monitor magnesium levels (therapeutic range 4 to 8 mg/dL). Administer via infusion pump in diluted form.	Use indwelling catheter to monitor urinary elimination. Administer calcium gluconate 10% if available for signs of toxicity.

V Antenatal Steroids — Betamethasone (Celestone)

A. **Action:** Stimulate production of surfactant in fetus between 24 and 34 weeks gestation

B. **Therapeutic Use**
1. Promote fetal lung maturity in preterm labor when delivery is likely

C. **Side/Adverse Effects**
1. Fluid retention
2. Elevated blood pressure

 D. **Nursing Interventions and Client Education**
1. Administer two doses (usually IM) 24 hr apart (repeat doses not recommended).
2. Provide emotional support to family.

VI Medications for the Postpartum Client

A. **Rho(D) Immune Globulin (Rhogam)**
1. **Action:** Suppresses the stimulation of active immunity by Rh-positive foreign red blood cells that enter the maternal circulation at the time of delivery
2. **Therapeutic Use**
   a. Rh factor incompatibility to prevent sensitization for subsequent pregnancies
3. **Precautions**
   a. Confirm that the mother is Rh-negative.
   b. Never administer the IGIM full-dose or microdose products intravenously.
   c. Never administer to a neonate.

 4. **Nursing Interventions and Client Education**
   a. Rhogam is administered as an injection after any event where fetal cells can mix with maternal blood.
      1) Miscarriage
      2) Ectopic pregnancy
      3) Induced abortion
      4) Amniocentesis
      5) Chorionic villus sampling (CVS)
      6) Abdominal trauma

B. **Varicella Vaccine**
1. Women who are not immune to varicella should be immunized in the postpartum period.
2. Instruct client to use reliable form of contraception and avoid pregnancy for 3 months.

Complementary and Alternative Therapies

I Safety and Efficacy

A. **The Dietary Supplement Health and Education Act limits the U.S. Food and Drug Administration's (FDA) control over dietary supplements.**

1. Many herbal drug companies make claims based on their own studies, indicating health benefits from using herbal drugs.

   a. These studies are not approved by the FDA.

   b. Labels on the herbal medications must include a disclaimer, stating that the FDA has not approved the product for safety and effectiveness.

2. Herbal medications may interact with other medicines and produce serious side effects.

II Saw palmetto (Serenoa repens)

A. **Purported Use**

1. Treats and prevents benign prostatic hypertrophy (BPH)

B. **Side/Adverse Effects**

1. Prolonged bleeding time

2. Altered platelet function

C. **Herb/Medication Interactions**

1. Additive effect with anticoagulants

D. **Studies**

1. Several well-conducted studies support the use of saw palmetto for reducing symptoms of BPH.

E. **Nursing Considerations**

1. Allow 4 to 6 weeks to see effects.

2. Discontinue use prior to surgery.

III Valerian root

A. **Purported Uses**

1. Insomnia

2. Migraines

3. Menstrual cramps

B. **Side/Adverse Effects**

1. Drowsiness

2. Anxiety

3. Hepatotoxicity (long-term use)

C. **Herb/Medication Interactions**

1. Additive effect with barbiturates and benzodiazepines

D. **Studies**

1. Several studies support the use of valerian for mild to moderate sleep disorders and mild anxiety.

E. **Nursing Considerations**

1. Client should not drive or operate machinery

2. Reinforce teaching with client against long-term use.

3. Discontinue valerian at least 1 week prior to surgery.

IV St. John's wort (Hypericum perforatum)

A. **Purported Uses**

1. Depression

2. Seasonal affective disorder

3. Anxiety

B. **Side/Adverse Effects**

1. Headache

2. Sleep disturbances

3. Hepatotoxicity (long-term use)

4. Constipation

C. **Herb/Medication Interactions**

1. May reduce the effects of many medications

   a. Theophylline (Theo-24)

   b. HIV protease inhibitors and non-nucleoside reverse transcriptase inhibitors

   c. Cyclosporine (Neoral)

   d. Diltiazem (Cardizem) and nifedipine (Procardia)

D. **Studies**

1. Several well-conducted studies support the use of St. John's wort for mild to moderate depression

E. **Nursing Considerations**

1. St. John's wort has many medication interactions and should not be taken with other medications.

2. Should not be used to treat severe depression.

3. Should only be used with medical guidance.

V Echinacea (Echinacea purpurea)

A. **Purported Uses**

1. Prevents and treats the common cold

2. Stimulates the immune system

3. Promotes wound healing

B. **Side/Adverse Effects**

1. Headache

2. Epigastric pain

3. Constipation

C. **Herb/Medication Interactions**

1. Can reduce the effects of immunosuppressants

2. Can increase serum levels of alprazolam (Xanax), calcium-channel blockers, and protease inhibitors

D. **Studies**

1. Well-conducted studies have conflicted as to the effectiveness of echinacea in the treatment of the common cold.

E. **Nursing Considerations**

1. Long-term use can cause immunosuppression.

VI Ginkgo (Gingko biloba)

A. **Purported Uses**

   1. Improves cerebral circulation to treat dementia and memory loss

B. **Side/Adverse Effects**

   1. Dizziness

   2. Palpitations

C. **Herb/Medication Interactions**

   1. Can increase the effects of MAOIs, anticoagulants, and antiplatelet aggregates

   2. Can reduce the effectiveness of insulin

D. **Studies**

   1. Studies conflict as to the effectiveness of gingko in all purported uses

E. **Nursing Considerations**

   1. Discontinue 2 weeks prior to surgery.

   2. Can cause seizures with overdose.

   3. Keep out of the reach of children.

VII Ginseng (Panax quinquefolius)

A. **Purported Uses**

   1. Improves strength and stamina

   2. Prevents and treats cancer and diabetes mellitus

B. **Side/Adverse Effects**

   1. Insomnia

   2. Nervousness

C. **Herb/Medication Interactions**

   1. Can decrease effectiveness of anticoagulants and antiplatelet aggregates

   2. Can increase effectiveness of antidiabetic agents and insulin

D. **Studies**

   1. Conflict as to the effectiveness of ginseng in all purported uses

E. **Nursing Considerations**

   1. Contraindicated for women who are pregnant and/or lactating.

VIII Glucosamine (2-Amino-2-deoxyglucose)

A. **Purported Uses**

   1. Relieves osteoarthritis

   2. Promotes joint health

B. **Side/Adverse Effects**

   1. Itching

   2. Edema

   3. Headache

C. **Herb/Medication Interactions**

   1. Can increase resistance to antidiabetic agents and insulin

D. **Studies**

   1. Several studies support the use of glucosamine in reducing the symptoms of osteoarthritis in the knees.

E. **Nursing Considerations**

   1. Use glucosamine with caution in clients who have a shellfish allergy.

   2. Monitor glucose frequently in clients who have diabetes mellitus.

   3. Allow extended time to see the effects of glucosamine.

   4. Used often in combination with chondroitin.

IX Chondroitin sulfate

A. **Purported Use**

   1. Relieves osteoarthritis

B. **Side/Adverse Effects**

   1. Headache

   2. Hives

   3. Photosensitivity

   4. Hypertension

   5. Constipation

C. **Herb/Medication Interactions**

   1. Can increase the effects of anticoagulants

D. **Studies**

   1. Several studies support the use of chondroitin sulfate in reducing the symptoms of osteoarthritis in the knees

E. **Nursing Considerations**

   1. Do not administer chondroitin sulfate to women who are pregnant or breastfeeding.

   2. Often used in combination with glucosamine.

   3. Allow extended time to see effects.

X Omega-3 fatty acids

A. **Purported Uses**

   1. Improves hypertriglyceridemia

   2. Helps maintain cardiac health

B. **Side/Adverse Effects**

   1. Nausea

   2. Diarrhea

   3. Hypotension

C. **Herb/Medication Interactions**

   1. Can increase risk of vitamin A or D overdose

D. **Studies**

   1. Several well-conducted studies support the use of omega-3 fatty acids in reducing blood triglyceride levels, preventing cardiovascular disease in clients who have a history of a heart attack, and slightly reducing blood pressure.

E. **Nursing Considerations**

   1. Omega-3 fatty acids are found in fish oils, nuts, and vegetable oils.

   2. Some fish contain methylmercury and polychlorinated biphenyls (PCBs) that can be harmful in large amounts, especially in women who are pregnant or nursing.

XI Melatonin

A. **Purported Use**

  1. Treats insomnia and jet lag

B. **Side/Adverse Effects**

  1. Morning grogginess

  2. Lower body temperature

  3. Vivid dreams

C. **Herb/Medication Interactions**

  1. Beta blockers

  2. Warfarin

  3. Steroids

D. **Studies**

  1. Several studies support antioxidant effects.

E. **Nursing Considerations**

  1. Pregnant or nursing women should not take melatonin.

HERBS AND PURPORTED USES

Match the following herbs with their purported use.

1. Treat and prevent benign prostatic hypertrophy
2. Manage migraines, insomnia, and menstrual cramps
3. Treat depression, seasonal affective disorder, and anxiety
4. Prevent and treat the common cold, stimulate immune system
5. Improve cerebral circulation
6. Relieve osteoarthritis and promote joint health
7. Improve hypertriglyceridemia and maintain cardiac health
8. Manage insomnia and jet lag
9. Improve strength and stamina

A. Glucosamine
B. Echinacea
C. Ginkgo
D. Omega-3 fatty acids
E. Ginseng
F. Saw palmetto
G. St. John's wort
H. Valerian root
I. Melatonin

Answer Key: 1. F; 2. H; 3. G; 4. B; 5. C; 6. A; 7. D; 8. I; 9. E

Reference: Lehne, R.A. (2013). *Pharmacology for Nursing Care.* (8th ed.). St. Louis, MO: Saunders. (p. 1264-1271).

XII Nursing Assessments for Herbal Medications

A. **Ask the client specifically about herbal medications, vitamins, or other supplements during the client interview.**

B. **Over-the-counter medications are often not considered medications by the client.**

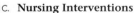 C. **Nursing Interventions**

  1. Reinforce teaching with client that herbal medications and supplements are not regulated by the FDA, often interact with other medications, and may cause serious adverse effects.

  2. Reinforce teaching with client that herbal medications and supplements should be used cautiously and under medical supervision.

  3. Use in pregnant and nursing mothers, infants, young children, and older adults who have cardiovascular or liver disease is discouraged.

Fundamentals for Nursing

Client Safety

I Falls

A significant number of reported facility accidents are related to falls. The nurse is accountable for implementation of essential actions to reduce the risk associated with falls.

A. **Contributing Factors**

1. Identify characteristics that increase risk for falls:
   a. Older age
   b. Impaired mobility
   c. Cognitive and/or sensory impairment
   d. Bowel and bladder dysfunction
   e. Side effects of medications
   f. History of falls

B. **Nursing Interventions**

1. Collaborate with health care team to complete a fall risk assessment upon admission and update as needed. See the worksheet at the end of the Fundamentals section to complete a fall risk assessment.
2. Communicate identified risks with the health care team.
3. Assign clients at risk for falls to a room close to the nurses' station and assess frequently.
4. Provide the client with nonskid footwear.
5. Keep the floor free of clutter and maintain an unobstructed path to the bathroom.
6. Orient the client to the setting (grab bars, call light), including how to use and locate all necessary items.
7. Maintain the bed in low position.
8. Verify clients who are unsteady know how to use the call light for assistance before ambulating.
9. Answer call lights promptly to prevent clients who are at risk from trying to ambulate independently.
10. Provide adequate lighting (a nightlight for necessary trips to the bathroom).
11. Determine the client's ability to use assistive devices (walkers, canes, etc.). Keep all items within reach.
12. Use chair or bed sensors for clients who are at risk.
13. Lock wheels on beds, wheelchairs, and gurneys to prevent rolling during transfers or stops.
14. Report and document all incidents per the facility's policy.

II Restraints

A. **Current client safety standards focus on reducing the need for client restraints.** The type or technique of restraint or seclusion used must be the least restrictive intervention that will be effective to protect the client, staff members, or others from harm.

B. **Definition:** Restraints include human, mechanical, chemical, or physical devices that restrict freedom of movement or diminish the client's access to parts of the body.

C. **Nursing Interventions**

1. Implement nonpharmacologic measures such as distraction, frequent observation, or diversion activities.
2. Prior to application, review manufacturer's instructions for correct application. Apply devices correctly.
3. Notify the provider immediately when restraints are implemented.
4. Remove the restraints and check client every 2 hr.
5. Monitor and document neurovascular and neurosensory status every 2 hr.
6. Leave the restraint loose enough to prevent injury.
7. Always tie the restraint to the bed frame (using loose knots that are easily removed).
8. Collaborate with the health care team to determine need for continued use.
9. Document:
   a. Behaviors making restraint necessary.
   b. Alternatives attempted and the client's response.
   c. Type and location of the restraint and time applied.
   d. Frequency and type of assessments.
10. Restraints should **never**:
    a. Interfere with treatment.
    b. Be used because of short-staffing or staff convenience.

III Seizure Precautions

Seizures may have a sudden onset and include loss of consciousness, violent tonic-clonic movements, or risk of injury to the client (head injury, aspiration, and falls).

A. **Nursing Interventions**

1. Collect data about seizure history, noting frequency, presence of auras, and sequence of events.
2. Identify precipitating factors that may exacerbate or lead to seizures.
3. Review medication history. If routine lab work is required (e.g., Dilantin), when was last level drawn?
4. Place rescue equipment at the client's bedside, including oxygen, an oral airway, and suction equipment.
5. High-risk clients should have IV or saline lock access.
6. Inspect the client's environment for items that may cause injury in the event of a seizure. Remove any unnecessary items from the immediate environment.
7. At the onset of a seizure, position the client for safety, and remain with the client.
8. If sitting or standing, ease the client to the floor. Protect the client's head. If the client is in bed, raise the side rails and pad for safety.
9. Roll the client to the side with the head flexed slightly forward.
10. Do not put anything in the client's mouth.
11. Loosen restrictive clothing.
12. Accurately document the event, including timing, precipitating behaviors or events, and a description of the event (movements, loss of consciousness, loss of continence, injuries, mention of aura, postictal state).
13. Report the seizure to the provider.

SECTION 2

Environmental Safety

ı Fire

All staff must be instructed in fire response procedures.

A. **Nursing Interventions**

1. Know the facility's fire drill and evacuation plan.

2. Keep emergency numbers near or on the phone at all times.

3. Know the location of all fire alarms, extinguishers, and exits, including oxygen shut-off valves.

4. Follow the fire response sequence in the facility (**RACE**):

    a. **R – Rescue:** Protect and evacuate clients in immediate danger.

    b. **A – Alarm:** Activate the alarm and report the fire.

    c. **C – Contain:** Close doors or windows.

    d. **E – Extinguish:** Use correct fire extinguisher to eliminate the fire.

        1) **Class A:** paper, wood, cloth, or trash

        2) **Class B:** flammable liquids and gases

        3) **Class C:** electrical fires

5. Extinguish properly (**PASS**):

    a. **P – Pull**

    b. **A – Aim**

    c. **S – Squeeze**

    d. **S – Sweep**

6. Considerations for home health setting

    a. Post "No Smoking" signs.

    b. Identify risk (oxygen therapy, smoking, electrical equipment).

    c. Client should develop a plan of action in the event of a fire, including a route of exit and a location where family members will meet.

    d. Client should keep fire extinguisher accessible.

    e. Review "Stop, Drop, and Roll."

ıı Equipment

All staff should be alert for potential safety hazards.

A. **Nursing Interventions**

1. Electrical equipment must be grounded.

2. Do not overcrowd outlets.

3. The use of extension cords is not permitted in any client care areas.

4. Only use equipment for its intended purpose.

5. Regularly inspect equipment for frayed cords.

6. Disconnect all equipment prior to cleaning.

ııı Chemical Agents and Radiation

Nurses must review institutional guidelines and follow all safety guidelines.

A. **Nursing Interventions**

1. Determine type and amount of radiation used.

2. Place a sign on door: "Caution Radioactive Material."

3. Wear monitoring badge to record amount of exposure.

4. Wear appropriate protective equipment.

5. Dispose of items removed from the room in appropriate containers.

6. Never handle any type of radioactive agent with bare hands.

SECTION 3

Ergonomics and Client Positioning

ı Lifting and Transfer of Clients

Implement safe care using proper body mechanics when lifting, positioning, transporting, or assisting a client to reduce the risk of injury. Obtain proper training before using any mechanical lift device, and always follow manufacturers' recommendations for use.

A. **Nursing Interventions**

1. Assess mobility and strength.

2. Client should assist when possible.

3. Use mechanical lift and assistive devices.

4. Avoid twisting the thoracic spine or bending at the waist.

5. Use major muscle groups, and tighten abdominal muscles.

ıı Client Transfer and Positioning

Maintain safe practices with patient transfer and ensure proper positioning of clients to maintain good body alignment.

A. **Nursing Interventions**

1. Transferring clients from bed to chair or chair to bed

    a. Verify client's functional ability.

    b. Encourage client to assist when possible.

    c. Lower the bed to the lowest setting.

    d. Position the bed or chair so that the client is moving toward the strong side.

    e. Assist the client to stand, then pivot.

2. Repositioning clients in bed

    a. Raise the bed to waist level.

    b. Lower side rails.

    c. Use slide boards or draw sheets.

    d. Have the client fold his arms across his chest while lifting the head.

    e. Proceed in one smooth movement.

    f. Collaborate with other staff members for assistance.

POSITIONING CLIENTS

Position: Semi-Fowler's

DESCRIPTION	Head of bed elevated to 30°
INDICATIONS	Gastric feedings, head injury, postoperative cranial surgery, respiratory illness with dyspnea, postoperative cataract removal, increased intracranial pressure

Position: Fowler's

DESCRIPTION	Head of bed elevated to 45°
INDICATIONS	Head injury, postoperative cranial surgery, postoperative abdominal surgery, respiratory illness or cardiac problems with dyspnea, bleeding esophageal varices, postoperative thyroidectomy or cataract removal, increased intracranial pressure

Position: High-Fowler's

DESCRIPTION	Head of bed elevated to 90°
INDICATIONS	Respiratory illness with dyspnea: emphysema, status asthmaticus, pneumothorax, cardiac problems with dyspnea, feeding, meal times, hiatal hernia, during and after meals

Position: Supine

DESCRIPTION	Lying on back, head, and shoulders; slightly elevated with a small pillow
INDICATIONS	Spinal cord injury (no pillow)

Position: Prone

DESCRIPTION	Lying on abdomen, legs extended, and head turned to the side
INDICATIONS	Client who is immobilized or unconscious, post lumbar puncture 6 to 12 hr, post myelogram 12 to 24 hr (oil-based dye), postoperative tonsillectomy and adenoidectomy

Position: Lateral (side-lying)

DESCRIPTION	Lying on side with most of the body weight borne by the lateral aspect of the lower ilium
INDICATIONS	Post abdominal surgery, client who is unconscious, seizures (head to side), postoperative tonsillectomy and adenoidectomy, postoperative pyloric stenosis of the lower scapula and the lateral (right side), post liver biopsy (right side), rectal irrigations

Position: Sims' (semi-prone)

DESCRIPTION	Lying on left side with most of the body weight borne by the anterior aspect of the ilium, humerus, and clavicle
INDICATIONS	Client who is unconscious, enemas

Position: Lithotomy

DESCRIPTION	Lying on the back with hips and knees flexed at right angles and feet in stirrups
INDICATIONS	Perineal, rectal, and vaginal procedures

POSITIONING CLIENTS (CONTINUED)

Position: Trendelenburg

DESCRIPTION	Head and body lowered while feet are elevated
INDICATIONS	Some surgeries; during labor if umbilical cord pressure is trying to be relieved

Position: Modified Trendelenburg

DESCRIPTION	Supine with the legs elevated
INDICATIONS	Shock

Position: Reverse Trendelenburg

DESCRIPTION	Head elevated while feet are lowered
INDICATIONS	Cervical traction; to feed clients restricted to supine position, such as post cardiac catheterization

Position: Elevate one or more extremities

DESCRIPTION	Elevate legs/feet or arms/hands by adjusting or supporting with pillows
INDICATIONS	Thrombophlebitis, application of cast, edema, postoperative surgical procedure on extremity

Position: Dorsal Recumbent

DESCRIPTION	Supine with knees flexed
INDICATIONS	Urinary catheterization of female, abdominal assessment, abdominal wound evisceration

---

SECTION 4

Assistive Devices for Ambulation

Definition: Used to provide an extension of the upper extremities to help transmit body weight and provide support for the client (e.g., canes, crutches, walkers)

A. **Collaborative Care**

1. Nursing Interventions

   a. Determine mobility status and ability to bear weight per provider's order.

   b. Identify the need of a safety belt.

   c. Client should wear shoes with nonslip soles.

   d. Identify risk of orthostatic hypotension.

   e. Provide safe environment free of clutter.

B. **Client Education and Referral**

1. Avoid rapid position changes to prevent orthostatic hypotension.

2. Inspect rubber tips on the device for wear and replace as needed.

3. Physical therapy consult.

C. **Crutches**

1. Verify correct fit of crutches: 2 to 3 finger widths between the axilla and top of the crutch.

2. Position hands on crutch pads with elbows flexed. (Do not bear weight on axilla.)

D. **Crutches: Non-weight bearing**

1. Begin in the tripod position, maintain weight on the "unaffected" (weight-bearing) extremity.

2. Advance both crutches and the affected extremity.

3. Move the unaffected weight-bearing foot/leg forward (beyond the crutches).

4. Advance both crutches, and then the affected extremity.

5. Continue sequence making steps of equal length.

E. **Crutches: Weight bearing**

1. Move crutches forward about one step's length.

2. Move "affected" leg forward; level with the crutch tips.

3. Move the "unaffected" leg forward.

4. Continue sequence making steps of equal length.

BASIC TRIPOD POSITION.

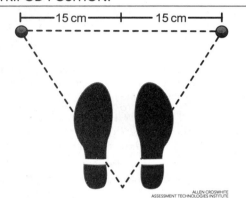

ALLEN CROSWHITE
ASSESSMENT TECHNOLOGIES INSTITUTE

A. FOUR-POINT ALTERNATING GATE	B. THREE-POINT GAIT	C. TWO-POINT GAIT
Order of foot/crutch movement is shown with solid foot and crutch tips.	Unaffected leg bears weight. Weight-bearing indicated with solid foot and crutch tips.	Weight partially distributed on each foot. Weight-bearing indicated with solid foot and crutch tips.

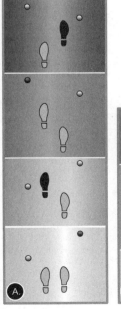
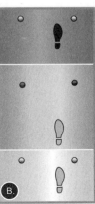
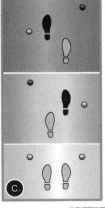

ALLEN CROSWHITE
ASSESSMENT TECHNOLOGIES INSTITUTE

F. **Walking up stairs**

1. Hold onto rail with one hand and crutches with the other hand.

2. Push down on the stair rail and the crutches and step up with the unaffected leg.

3. If not allowed to place weight on the affected leg, hop up with the unaffected leg.

4. Bring the affected leg and the crutches up beside the unaffected leg.

5. Remember, the unaffected leg goes up first and the crutches move with the affected leg.

G. **Walking down stairs**

1. Place the affected leg and the crutches down on the step below; support weight by leaning on the crutches and the stair rail.

2. Bring the unaffected leg down.

3. Remember the affected leg goes down first and the crutches move with the affected leg.

H. **Cane**

1. For correct size, have the client wear shoes. The correct length is measured from the wrist to the floor.

2. Cane is used on the unaffected side to provide support to the opposite lower limb.

3. In initial gait assistance, having the client move the affected leg forward (after balance is achieved) is optimal. This should only be done with personnel present to assist if a fall occurs, and a gait belt should be worn.

4. As the client gains strength, PT should instruct the client to move the affected extremity and cane at the same time, as this reduces contact pressure by at least 50% and continues to aid in balance.

5. Long-term cane use should involve the client moving the affected extremity and cane at the same time to improve muscle function.

I. **Walker**

1. For correct size, have the client wear shoes. The client's wrists are even with the hand grips on the walker when arms are dangling downward.

2. Advance the walker approximately 12 inches.

3. Advance with the affected lower limb.

4. Move unaffected limb forward.

5. Identify appropriateness of a rolling walker if walker is being used for support due to overall weakness. A rolling walker is not appropriate for a client with Parkinson's disease due to shuffling gait.

Infection Control

All members of the health care team are accountable for adhering to measures to reduce the growth and transmission of infectious agents. According the Centers for Disease Control and Prevention (CDC), hand hygiene is the single most important practice in preventing health care associated infections (HAIs).

CHAIN OF INFECTION

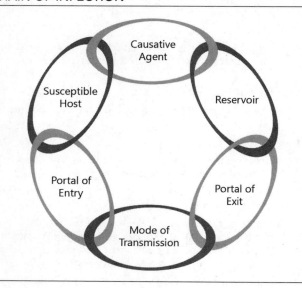

I Medical Asepsis (Clean Technique)

Precise practices to reduce the number, growth, and spread of microorganisms

 A. **Nursing Interventions**

1. Perform hand hygiene frequently.
2. Use personal protective equipment (PPE) as indicated.
3. Do not place items on the floor of client's room.
4. Do not shake linens.
5. Clean least soiled area first.
6. Place moist items in plastic bags.
7. Reinforce education with client and caregivers.

II Surgical Asepsis (Sterile Technique)

Precise practices to eliminate all microorganisms from an object or area (surgical technique)

 A. **Nursing Interventions**

1. Avoid coughing, sneezing, and talking directly over field.
2. Only dry sterile items touch the field (1-inch border is nonsterile).
3. Keep all objects above the waist.
4. Wash hands and don sterile gloves to perform procedure.

III Isolation Guidelines

A group of actions that include hand hygiene and the use of standard precautions intended to reduce the transmission of infectious organisms

IV Standard Precautions (Tier One)

Applies to all body fluids, nonintact skin, and mucous membranes

A. **PPE:** As needed to prevent contact with body fluids: gloves, mask, gown, and goggles.

 B. **Nursing Interventions**

1. Implement standard precautions for all clients.
2. Determine need for client-specific, disease-specific precautions.
3. Provide education to health care team, clients, and visitors.
4. Report communicable diseases per CDC policy.
5. Handle all blood and body fluids as if contaminated.
6. Use PPE to reduce risk of transmission.
   a. Gown and gloves when touching blood or body fluids, nonintact skin, mucous membranes, or contaminated materials.
   b. Masks and face and eye protection when anticipating splashing of body fluids.
   c. PPE is disposed of in the client's room.
7. Consider room placement for client safety.
   a. Private room (only transport client outside of the room as medically necessary)
   b. Cohort (patient must have same organism)
      1) Avoid placing clients on contact precautions in the same room with patients who are immunocompromised, have open wounds, or have anticipated prolonged lengths of stay.
      2) Ensure clients are located more than 3 feet from each other. (Use privacy curtain between beds to minimize opportunities for direct contact.)
      3) Change protective attire and perform hand hygiene between contact with clients in the same room, regardless of disease status.
8. Clean equipment according to facility policy.
9. Discard all needles and sharps in the appropriate containers; do not recap.
10. Place contaminated linens in the appropriate receptacle per the facility's policy.
11. Clean spills with a solution of bleach and water (1:10 dilution).

v Transmission-Based Precautions (Tier Two)

Transmission-based precautions are used in addition to standard precautions for clients who are known or suspected to be infected or colonized with infectious organisms.

A. **Airborne Precautions**

1. Diseases known to be transmitted by air for infectious agents smaller than 5 mcg (measles, varicella, pulmonary or laryngeal tuberculosis)

2. **PPE: Mask** (N95 respirator for known or suspected TB)

   a. **Nursing Interventions** (in addition to standard precautions)

      1) Provide private room with monitored negative airflow (air exchange and air discharge through HEPA filter).

      2) Keep door closed.

      3) Respiratory protection:

         a) The nurse must be FIT tested for N95 respirator.

         b) Apply a small, particulate mask to that client if leaving room for medical necessity.

B. **Droplet Precautions**

1. Prevent the transmission of pathogens spread through close contact with mucous membranes or respiratory secretions.

2. Protect against droplets larger than 5 mcg (streptococcal pharyngitis, pneumonia, scarlet fever, rubella, pertussis, mumps, mycoplasma pneumonia, meningococcal pneumonia/sepsis, pneumonic plague).

3. **PPE: Mask**

   a. **Nursing Interventions** (in addition to standard precautions)

      1) Private room preferred, may cohort with client who has infection with same organism.

      2) Keep door closed.

      3) Mask is required when working within 3 feet of the client.

C. **Contact Precautions** (includes enteric precautions)

1. Prevent transmission of infectious agents that are spread by direct or indirect contact with the client or the client's environment. These precautions are applied in the presence of wound drainage, fecal incontinence, or other bodily discharges that suggest an increased potential for environmental contamination and risk of transmission.

2. **PPE: Gloves, gown; as-needed use of mask and goggles**

   a. **Nursing Interventions** (in addition to standard precautions)

      1) Private room preferred; may cohort with client who has infection with same organism

      2) Gloves and gown worn by caregivers and visitors

      3) Disposal of infectious dressing material into nonporous bag

      4) Dedicated equipment for the patient or disinfect after each use

      5) Client to leave room only for essential clinical reasons

3. Protective Isolation

   a. Used to protect clients who have an increased susceptibility to infections, are receiving chemotherapy, or are immunosuppressed or neutropenic

   b. **Nursing Interventions**

      1) Follow standard precautions.

      2) Institute maximum protection, which may include the use of sterile linens, food, and other supplies.

      3) Minimize exposure to microorganisms found on the outer layers of fresh flowers, fruits, and vegetables.

      4) Wear sterile gloves and gown/mask when in contact with client.

      5) Maximum protection will require ventilated/positive pressure room.

ORDER OF PPE APPLICATION

Gown: Cover body from the bottom of the neck to the knees and wrists. Fasten securely behind the neck and at waist.

Mask: Secure with ties or elastic. Pinch the flexible bridge to secure at nose. Must extend below and under the chin.

Goggles/face shield: Verify fit is secure to prevent slipping.

Gloves: Use correct size for a snug fit. Must extend upward to completely cover the wrist portion of the gown.

ORDER OF PPE REMOVAL

Gloves: Extend arms and slowly peel one glove downward, turning it inside out. With the ungloved hand, slide a finger under the inside portion of the remaining glove, turning inside out, and discard.

Goggles/face shield: Grasp the ear pieces or headband only to remove.

Gown: Unfasten neck, then waist ties; pull gown forward away from the body, folding it inside out and rolling it into a bundle for disposal.

Mask: Remove by only touching ties. Take care not to touch the front of the mask.

PRECAUTIONS REQUIRED FOR SPECIFIC DISEASE PROCESS

AIDS/HIV

PRECAUTIONS	Standard
DURATION OF PRECAUTIONS	Duration of illness
RESERVOIR	Blood and body fluids including breast milk
NURSING CONSIDERATIONS	Hand hygiene; PPE if in contact with potentially contaminated materials

Chickenpox (varicella)

PRECAUTIONS	Standard/airborne/contact
DURATION OF PRECAUTIONS	Until lesions crust over
RESERVOIR	Lesions, respiratory secretions
NURSING CONSIDERATIONS	Persons who are pregnant or have not had chickenpox or the vaccine should not care for the client

Clostridium difficile

PRECAUTIONS	Standard/contact
DURATION OF PRECAUTIONS	Duration of illness
RESERVOIR	Feces
NURSING CONSIDERATIONS	Hand hygiene; PPE (enteric precautions) if in contact with potentially contaminated materials

Hepatitis A

PRECAUTIONS	Standard/contact if client has fecal incontinence
DURATION OF PRECAUTIONS	Until 7 days after onset of jaundice
RESERVOIR	Feces
NURSING CONSIDERATIONS	Contact precautions used, particularly for clients wearing diapers or who are incontinent; minimum of 1 week, depending on client's age

Hepatitis B (continued)

PRECAUTIONS	Standard
DURATION OF PRECAUTIONS	Duration of illness
RESERVOIR	Blood and body fluids
NURSING CONSIDERATIONS	Contact precautions for blood and body fluids; hand hygiene

Hepatitis C

PRECAUTIONS	Standard – Additional precautions specific to hemodialysis unit
DURATION OF PRECAUTIONS	Duration of illness
RESERVOIR	Blood and body fluids
NURSING CONSIDERATIONS	Contact precautions for blood and body fluids; hand hygiene

Herpes simplex (recurrent oral, skin, genital)

PRECAUTIONS	Standard/contact
DURATION OF PRECAUTIONS	Until lesions crust over
RESERVOIR	Fluid from lesions
NURSING CONSIDERATIONS	Horizontal transmission from contact with skin and secretions; vertical transmission from mother to child in utero or childbirth

Carbapenem-resistant enterobacteriaceae (CRE)

PRECAUTIONS	Standard/contact
DURATION OF PRECAUTIONS	Per CDC: No recommendation can be made for discontinuing contact precautions due to high mortality rate
RESERVOIR	Blood and body fluids, feces
NURSING CONSIDERATIONS	Hand hygiene, contact precautions

Herpes zoster (shingles) – disseminated or localized in clients who are immunocompromised

PRECAUTIONS	Standard/airborne/contact
DURATION OF PRECAUTIONS	Duration of illness or with visible lesions
RESERVOIR	Lesions
NURSING CONSIDERATIONS	Persons who have not had chickenpox or the vaccine should not provide care

Measles (Rubeola virus)

PRECAUTIONS	Standard/airborne
DURATION OF PRECAUTIONS	Duration of illness
RESERVOIR	Respiratory secretions
NURSING CONSIDERATIONS	Virus can live on infected surfaces for up to 2 hr

Meningococcal disease

PRECAUTIONS	Standard/droplet
DURATION OF PRECAUTIONS	Until 24 hr therapy continuous
RESERVOIR	Respiratory secretions
NURSING CONSIDERATIONS	Postexposure prophylaxis is recommended to control outbreaks

Methicillin-resistant *Staphylococcus aureus* (MRSA)

PRECAUTIONS	Standard/contact
DURATION OF PRECAUTIONS	Duration of illness
RESERVOIR	Body fluids and sites contaminated with MRSA
NURSING CONSIDERATIONS	Gloves; PPE including a gown/mask if in contact with site of infection

Pneumonia

PRECAUTIONS	Standard/droplet
DURATION OF PRECAUTIONS	Until culture is negative
RESERVOIR	Respiratory secretions
NURSING CONSIDERATIONS	Consider organism-specific precautions as indicated

Respiratory syncytial virus

PRECAUTIONS	Standard/contact/droplet
DURATION OF PRECAUTIONS	Duration of illness
RESERVOIR	Respiratory secretions
NURSING CONSIDERATIONS	Contact/droplet precautions; follow established guidelines for administration of ribavirin

Rotavirus

PRECAUTIONS	Standard/contact
DURATION OF PRECAUTIONS	Duration of illness
RESERVOIR	Feces
NURSING CONSIDERATIONS	Contact precautions used, particularly for children who are wearing diapers or incontinent

PRECAUTIONS REQUIRED FOR SPECIFIC DISEASE PROCESS (CONTINUED)

Rubella

PRECAUTIONS	Standard/droplet
DURATION OF PRECAUTIONS	7 days after onset of rash
RESERVOIR	Respiratory secretions
NURSING CONSIDERATIONS	Nonimmune pregnant women should not care for these clients

Salmonella

PRECAUTIONS	Standard/contact precautions
DURATION OF PRECAUTIONS	Duration of illness
RESERVOIR	Feces
NURSING CONSIDERATIONS	Contact precautions used, particularly for children who are wearing diapers or incontinent

Shigellosis (dysentery)

PRECAUTIONS	Standard/contact precautions
DURATION OF PRECAUTIONS	Duration of illness
RESERVOIR	Feces
NURSING CONSIDERATIONS	Contact precautions used, particularly for children who are wearing diapers or incontinent

Staphylococcus aureus (infection or colonization)

PRECAUTIONS	Standard/contact precautions
DURATION OF PRECAUTIONS	Duration of illness
RESERVOIR	Body fluids and sites contaminated with MRSA
NURSING CONSIDERATIONS	Gloves; PPE including gown/mask if in contact with site of infection

Tuberculosis (TB) (pulmonary)

PRECAUTIONS	Standard/airborne precautions
DURATION OF PRECAUTIONS	Until three sputum smears are negative on consecutive days or TB is ruled out
RESERVOIR	Airborne respiratory droplet nuclei
NURSING CONSIDERATIONS	N95 mask; client wears surgical mask when transported outside of negative-airflow room

Vancomycin-resistant enterococci (VRE) (infection or colonization)

PRECAUTIONS	Standard/contact precautions
DURATION OF PRECAUTIONS	Until three negative cultures from infectious site (1 week apart)
RESERVOIR	Stool, body sites from which VRE is isolated
NURSING CONSIDERATIONS	Hand hygiene and gloves; gowns if in contact with contaminated material

Health Promotion and Disease Prevention

Nurses contribute greatly to the health of clients and population groups using health promotion and disease prevention strategies. Nursing care of the client incorporates knowledge of early detection of disease and actions to promote optimal health.

I Health Promotion

Includes client education, health risk assessment, wellness assessment, lifestyle and behavior changes, and environmental control programs

HEALTH PROMOTION AND DISEASE PREVENTION

PREVENTIVE CARE	EXAMPLES OF PREVENTION ACTIVITIES
Primary prevention: Focus is on promoting health and preventing disease.	Immunization programs Child car seat education Nutrition and fitness activities Health education programs
Secondary prevention: Focus is on early identification of illness, providing treatment, and conducting activities geared to prevent a worsening health status.	Communicable disease screening and case finding Early detection and treatment of hypertension Exercise programs for older adults who are frail
Tertiary prevention: Focus is on preventing long-term consequences of chronic illness or disability and supporting optimal functioning.	Prevention of pressure ulcers as a complication of spinal cord injury Promoting independence for a client following stroke

II Disease Prevention

 A. **Nursing Interventions**

1. Conduct a risk factor assessment.
2. Reinforce teaching with clients to follow standards for recommended screenings.
3. Identify lifestyle risk behaviors requiring modification.
4. Encourage client to continue health-promoting behaviors.
5. Reinforce teaching with client about preventive immunizations.

SCREENING GUIDELINES*

TEST	FEMALE	MALE
Routine physical	Begin age 18 Annually	Begin age 18 Every 2 years Annually at age 40
Dental assessments	Every 6 months	Every 6 months
Blood pressure	Begin age 20 Minimum every 2 years Annually if higher than 120/80 mm Hg	Begin age 20 Minimum every 2 years Annually if higher than 120/80 mm Hg
Body mass index (BMI)	Begin age 20 Each health care visit	Begin age 20 Each health care visit
Blood cholesterol	Begin age 20 Minimum every 5 years (if no risk factors)	Begin age 20 Minimum every 5 years (if no risk factors)
Blood glucose	Begin age 45 Minimum every 3 years	Begin age 45 Minimum every 3 years
Colorectal screening	Fecal occult blood annually begin age 50 AND Flexible sigmoidoscopy every 5 years*, or Colonoscopy every 10 years, or Double-contrast barium enema every 5 years*, or CT colonography (virtual colonoscopy) every 5 years **NOTE:** Frequency may increase based upon results.	Fecal occult blood annually begin age 50 AND Flexible sigmoidoscopy every 5 years*, or Colonoscopy every 10 years, or Double-contrast barium enema every 5 years*, or CT colonography (virtual colonoscopy) every 5 years **NOTE:** Frequency may increase based upon results.
Pap test	Every 3 years starting at age 21 (not recommended prior to age 21)	n/a
Clinical breast exam	Begin age 20, every 3 years Begin age 40, yearly	n/a
Mammogram	Begin age 40, yearly	n/a
Prostate-specific antigen test and digital rectal exam	n/a	American Cancer Society recommends men be able to make an informed decision about prostate cancer screening. Starting at age 50, talk with provider about need for testing. If African American or if father or brother positive for prostate cancer before age 65, talk with provider at age 45. If screened, PSA test with or without a rectal exam. Future testing depends on results of PSA.

*American Diabetes Association, American Heart Association, American Cancer Society, and National Institutes of Health, CDC

FALL RISK ASSESSMENT ACTIVITY

An LPN is completing a fall risk determination on a 70-year-old resident of an assisted living facility who sustained a fall while attempting to ambulate to the restroom. Three months ago, the client had a CVA that resulted in right-sided hemiparesis requiring physical therapy and use of a walker. History reveals 36 pack-year history of smoking (stopped after MI), IDDM for 22 years, MI with CABG x three 2 years ago, and HTN. Current medications: Humulin N, Plavix, Lopressor, Lasix, Klor-Con, Ambien, and Vicodin PRN. **Based on the scenario, perform a fall assessment using the Morse Fall Scale below.**

Morse Fall Scale

		SCORE
1. History of falling; immediate or within 3 months	No = 0 Yes = 25	
2. Secondary diagnosis	No = 0 Yes = 15	
3. Ambulatory aid	None, bed rest, nurse = 0 Crutches, cane, walker = 15 Furniture = 30	
4. IV/heparin Lock	No = 0 Yes = 20	
5. Gait/transferring	Normal, bed rest, immobile = 0 Weak = 10 Impaired = 20	
6. Mental status	Oriented to own ability = 0 Forgets limitations = 15	
	TOTAL:	

http://cf.networkofcare.org/

Risk Level:

According to the score, look at the risk level on chart below. Before viewing the interventions as instructed on the chart, identify five nursing actions you should implement for the client to minimize risk of falls.

1. _____

2. _____

3. _____

4. _____

5. _____

Answer key on next page.

RISK LEVEL	MFS SCORE	ACTION
No Risk	0 to 24	None
Low Risk	25 to 50	See *Standard Fall Prevention Interventions on following page*
High Risk	51 or greater	See *High-Risk Fall Prevention Interventions on following page*
www.patientsafety.va.gov		

STANDARD FALL PREVENTION INTERVENTIONS

Clients who are scored "low-risk" on the **Morse Fall Scale** (score of 25 to 50) will have the following interventions implemented by the nursing staff.

› **Direct Care**
  » Assess fall risk upon admission, change in status, transfer to another unit and discharge.
  » Assign the client to a bed that enables the client to exit the bed toward the client's stronger side whenever possible.
  » Assess coordination and balance before assisting with transfer and mobility activities.
  » Implement bowel and bladder programs to decrease urgency and incontinence.
  » Use treaded socks for all clients.

› **All Staff**
  » Approach client towards unaffected side to maximize participation in care.
  » Transfer client towards stronger side.

› **Education**
  » Actively engage client and family in all aspects of fall prevention program.
  » Instruct client in all activities prior to initiating assistive devices.
  » Teach client use of grab bars.
  » Instruct client in medication time/dose, side/adverse effects, and interactions with food/medications.

› **Equipment**
  » Lock all moveable equipment before transferring clients.
  » Individualize equipment specific to client needs.

› **Environment**
  » Place client care articles within reach.
  » Provide physically safe environment (eliminate spills, clutter, electrical cords, and unnecessary equipment).
  » Provide adequate lighting.

www.patientsafety.va.gov

Answers to Fall Assessment Activity Answers
1. 25; 2. 15; 3. 15; 4. 0; 5. 20; Total: 75

Morse Fall Scale
www.patientsafety.va.gov

HIGH-RISK FALL PREVENTION INTERVENTIONS

These interventions are designed to be implemented for clients with multiple fall risk factors and those who have fallen. These interventions are designed to reduce severity of injuries due to falls as well as to prevent falls from reoccurring, supplementing standard fall prevention interventions.

› **Equipment**
  » Bed and/or chair alarms
  » Alarms at exits
  » Nurse call and communication systems
  » Low beds
  » Raised edge mattress
  » Video camera surveillance
  » Nonskid floor mat

› **Environment**
  » Clear client environment of all hazards

› **Education**
  » Exercise
  » Nutrition
  » Home safety
  » Plan for emergency fall notification procedure.

Risk Level: How Risk (answers may be any of the below)
1. Call light in reach.
2. Bed in low position.
3. Use non-skid bath mats.
4. Use non-skid footwear.
5. Use of pendant call alarm.
6. Assist client with transfers/ambulation.
7. Adequate lighting, including nightlights.
8. Promptly enter to assist client when called .
9. Determine if properly using ambulation devices.
10. Monitor blood glucose before meals and at bedtime.
11. Monitor for possible orthostatic hypotension related to diuretics.
12. Check sensations in lower extremities due to impaired circulation.
13. Encourage strengthening exercises identified by physical therapy.
14. Eliminate throw rugs and other environmental hazards in living space.

UNIT SIX

Adult Medical-Surgical Nursing

Fluids and Electrolytes

I Fluids and Electrolytes

Nurses should review the client's health history and laboratory data and perform clinical assessment. Many health problems can cause changes in balance of fluids and electrolytes. The nurse is prepared to manage the client with imbalances.

A. **Body Fluids**

1. Adults: 50% to 60% total body weight is water
2. Infants: 75% to 80% of total body weight is water
3. Two-thirds of body fluid is intracellular (ICF)
4. One-third of body fluid is extracellular (ECF)

NOTE: 1 kg (2.2 lb) of body weight is approximate to 1 L of fluid.

II Fluid Imbalance

A. **Fluid Volume Deficit (FVD)**

1. Fluid intake is less than needed to meet body requirements. The most common type is isotonic dehydration.
2. Contributing Factors
   a. Excess GI loss
   b. Diaphoresis
   c. Fever
   d. Excess renal loss
   e. Hemorrhage
   f. Insufficient intake
   g. Burns
   h. Diuretic therapy
   i. Aging: Older adults have less body water and decreased thirst sensation
3. Manifestations
   a. Weight loss
   b. Dry mucus membranes
   c. Increased heart rate and respirations
   d. Thready pulse
   e. Capillary refill less than 3 seconds
   f. Weakness, fatigue
   g. Orthostatic hypotension
   h. Poor skin turgor
   i. Late signs: Oliguria, decreased CVP, flattened neck veins
4. Diagnostic Procedures
   a. Serum electrolytes, BUN, creatinine, Hct
      1) Hct can be high due to hemoconcentration.
   b. Urine: specific gravity and osmolarity

5. Collaborative Care and **Nursing Interventions**
   a. Monitor vital signs.
   b. Monitor skin turgor. In older adults, check skin over sternum or forehead.
   c. Maintain strict I&O. Output should be at least 0.5 mL/kg/hr.
   d. Weigh client daily.
   e. Monitor laboratory data.
   f. Fluid replacement
      1) Increase oral fluid intake; initiate oral rehydration solution
      2) IV fluids for severe dehydration/maintain as ordered
   g. Initiate fall precautions
6. Medications
   a. Electrolyte replacement
   b. Intravenous fluids

INTRAVENOUS FLUIDS

Isotonic

INDICATION	Treatment of vascular system fluid deficit
CHARACTERISTICS	Concentration equal to plasma Prevent fluid shift between compartments
SOLUTIONS	Normal saline (0.9% NS) Lactated Ringer's (LR) 5% dextrose in water (D_5W)

Hypotonic

INDICATION	Treatment of intracellular dehydration
CHARACTERISTICS	Lower osmolality than the ECF Shift fluid from ECF to ICF
SOLUTIONS	0.45% normal saline (0.45% NS) 2.5% dextrose in 0.45% saline ($D_{2.5}$ 45% NS)

Hypertonic

INDICATION	Used only when serum osmolality is critically low
CHARACTERISTICS	Osmolality higher than the ECF Shift fluid from ICF to ECF
SOLUTIONS	10% dextrose in water ($D_{10}W$) 50% dextrose in water ($D_{50}W$) 5% dextrose in 0.9% saline (D_5NS) 5% dextrose in 0.45% saline (D_5W in 0.45% NaCl) 5% dextrose in lactated Ringer's (D_5LR)

B. **Fluid Volume Excess (FVE)**

1. Fluid intake or retention is greater than the body's needs.
2. Contributing Factors
   a. Kidney failure
   b. Heart failure
   c. Cirrhosis
   d. Interstitial to plasma fluid shifts (hypertonic fluids, burns)
   e. Excessive water intake

3. Manifestations
   a. Cough, dyspnea, crackles
   b. Increased blood pressure
   c. Tachypnea and tachycardia
   d. Bounding pulse
   e. Weight gain (1 L water = 1 kg weight)
   f. Increased urine output
   g. Increased central venous pressure
   h. Edema
4. Diagnostic Procedures (can be decreased due to hemodilution)
   a. Serum: electrolytes, BUN, creatinine, Hct
   b. Urine: specific gravity and osmolarity
   c. Chest x-ray if respiratory complications present
5. Collaborative Care and **Nursing Interventions**
   a. Monitor respiratory rate, symmetry, and effort.
   b. Monitor breath sounds.
   c. Monitor for edema. Measure pitting edema on scale of 1+ (minimal) to 4+ (severe). Monitor dependent edema by measuring circumference of extremities.
   d. Monitor for ascites, and measure abdominal girth.
   e. Weigh the client daily.
   f. Maintain strict I&O.
   g. Monitor vital signs.

h. Administer diuretics (osmotic, loop) as prescribed.
i. Limit fluid intake.
j. Provide frequent skin care.
k. Use semi-Fowler's position. Reposition every 2 hr.
l. Restrict sodium intake.

III Electrolyte Imbalances

A. **Major Intracellular Electrolytes**
   1. Potassium
   2. Phosphorus
   3. Magnesium
B. **Major Extracellular Electrolytes**
   1. Sodium
   2. Calcium
   3. Chloride
   4. Bicarbonate
C. **Function**
   1. Maintain homeostasis.
   2. Promote neuromuscular excitability.
   3. Maintain fluid volume.
   4. Distribute water between fluid compartments.
   5. Maintain cardiac stability.
   6. Regulate acid-base balance.

MAJOR ELECTROLYTES: IMBALANCE/INTERVENTIONS

Potassium (K⁺): Hypokalemia

RISK FACTORS	Adverse effects of medications › Corticosteroids › Diuretics › Digitalis › Laxatives (abuse of)	Body fluid loss › Vomiting › Diarrhea › Wound drainage › NG suction	Excessive diaphoresis Kidney disease Dietary deficiency Alkalosis
MANIFESTATIONS	Muscle weakness, cramping Fatigue Nausea, vomiting	Irritability, confusion Decreased bowel motility Paresthesia	Dysrhythmias Flat and/or inverted T waves (ECG)
INTERVENTIONS	Monitor respiratory status. Initiate fall precautions. Initiate and monitor potassium replacement (oral, IV).	Monitor ECG. Monitor I&O. Monitor arterial HCO_3 and pH.	Provide client education. Dietary sources Medications
	NOTE: NEVER give K⁺ IV bolus; MUST dilute. NOTE: "No P = No K." If the client is not urinating, do NOT administer potassium.		

Potassium (K⁺): Hyperkalemia

RISK FACTORS	Kidney failure Adrenal insufficiency	Acidosis Excessive potassium intake	Medications › Potassium-sparing diuretics › ACE inhibitors
MANIFESTATIONS	Peaked T waves (ECG) Ventricular dysrhythmias	Muscle twitching and paresthesia (early) Ascending muscle weakness (late)	Increased bowel motility
INTERVENTIONS	Monitor ECG. Monitor bowel sounds. Initiate dialysis. Dietary restriction and teaching.	Administer medications. › Kayexalate (monitor bowel sounds) › 50% glucose with insulin › Calcium gluconate	› Bicarbonate › Loop diuretics

Sodium (Na⁺): Hyponatremia

RISK FACTORS	GI loss SIADH Adrenal insufficiency	Water intoxication Excessive diaphoresis	Medications › Diuretics › Anti-convulsants › SSRIs › Lithium
MANIFESTATIONS	Weakness Lethargy Confusion Seizures	Headache Anorexia, nausea, vomiting Muscle cramps, twitching Hypotension	Tachycardia Weight gain, edema
INTERVENTIONS	Sodium replacement (oral, GI tube, IV) Restrict oral fluid intake	Daily weight I&O	Medication: conivaptan hydrochloride (Vaprisol)
	NOTE: Risk with hypertonic solutions—cerebral edema		

Sodium (Na⁺): Hypernatremia

RISK FACTORS	Water deficit GI loss	Hypertonic tube feedings Diabetes insipidus	Burns Heatstroke
MANIFESTATIONS	Fever Swollen, dry tongue Sticky mucous membranes Hallucinations	Lethargy, restlessness, irritability Seizures Tachycardia Hypertension	Hyperreflexia, twitching Pulmonary edema
INTERVENTIONS	Daily weight I&O Seizure precautions	IV infusion of hypotonic or isotonic fluid Diuretics	Dietary sodium restriction and education Increased oral fluid intake

Calcium (Ca⁺⁺): Hypocalcemia

RISK FACTORS	Hypoparathyroidism Hypomagnesemia Kidney failure	Vitamin D deficiency Inadequate intake	Disease process › Celiac disease › Lactose intolerance › Crohn's disease › Alcohol use disorder
MANIFESTATIONS	Tetany, cramps Paresthesias Dysrhythmias	Trousseau's sign Chvostek's sign Seizures	Hyperreflexia Impaired clotting time
INTERVENTIONS	Seizure precautions IV calcium replacement	Daily calcium supplements Vitamin D therapy	Monitor for orthostatic hypotension Dietary increase and education
	NOTE: IV calcium must be administered slowly and the site monitored for extravasation. It is diluted in D₅W, NEVER in NS.		

Calcium has an inverse relationship with phosphorus.

Calcium (Ca⁺⁺): Hypercalcemia

RISK FACTORS	Hyperparathyroidism Malignant disease Prolonged immobilization	Vitamin D excess Thiazide diuretics Lithium	Digoxin toxicity Overuse of calcium supplements
MANIFESTATIONS	Muscle weakness Hypercalciuria/kidney stones Dysrhythmias Lethargy/coma	Hyporeflexia Pathologic fractures Flank pain Deep bone pain	Polyuria, polydipsia, dehydration Hypertension Nausea, vomiting
INTERVENTIONS	Increase mobility Isotonic IVF Medications	Furosemide › Calcitonin › Glucocorticoids › Biphosphonates › Calcium chelators	Dialysis Cardiac monitoring

Calcium has an inverse relationship with phosphorus.

MAJOR ELECTROLYTES: IMBALANCE/INTERVENTIONS (CONTINUED)

Magnesium (Mg⁺⁺): Hypomagnesemia

RISK FACTORS	GI loss Alcohol use disorder Hypocalcemia Hypokalemia DKA	Hyperparathyroidism Malabsorption TPN Laxative abuse Acute MI	Medications › Gentamicin › Cysplatin › Cyclosporine
MANIFESTATIONS	Paresthesias Dysrhythmias Trousseau's sign Chvostek's sign	Agitation, confusion Hyperreflexia Hypertension	Insomnia, irritability Anorexia, nausea, vomiting Dysphagia
INTERVENTIONS	Seizure precautions Monitor swallowing Dietary measures and education	Administer medications › IV magnesium sulfate › PO magnesium salts	Monitor urine output Monitor respirations

NOTE: Monitor for signs of magnesium toxicity with IV replacement, and treat with calcium gluconate.

Magnesium (Mg⁺⁺): Hypermagnesemia

RISK FACTORS	Renal failure Excessive Mg⁺⁺ therapy	Adrenal insufficiency Laxative overuse	Lithium toxicity Extensive soft tissue injury or necrosis
MANIFESTATIONS	Hypotension Drowsiness Bradycardia	Bradypnea Coma Cardiac arrest	Hyporeflexia Nausea, vomiting Facial flushing
INTERVENTIONS	Mechanical ventilation IV fluids: lactated Ringer's or NS	Administer medications › IV calcium gluconate › Loop diuretics	Monitor respirations and blood pressure Monitor deep-tendon reflexes

NOTE: Magnesium should not be administered to clients in renal failure.

Phosphorus: Hypophosphatemia

RISK FACTORS	Vitamin D deficiency Refeeding after starvation Alcohol withdrawal DKA Alkalosis	Hypomagnesemia Hypokalemia Excessive loss of body fluids: sweat, diarrhea, vomiting, hyperventilation Burns	TPN Overuse of antacids
MANIFESTATIONS	Paresthesia Muscle weakness Bone pain and deformities	Chest pain Confusion	Seizures Nystagmus
INTERVENTIONS	Oral phosphate replacement Careful IV administration of phosphorus (for severe cases)	Gradual introduction of solution for clients on TPN Protect from infection	Dietary management and education Seizure precautions

Phosphorus has an inverse relationship with calcium.

Phosphorus: Hyperphosphatemia

RISK FACTORS	Kidney failure Chemotherapy	High vitamin D High phosphorus intake	Excessive enema use Acidosis
MANIFESTATIONS	Tetany, cramps Paresthesias Dysrhythmias	Trousseau's sign Chvostek's sign Hyperreflexia	Anorexia, nausea, vomiting Soft tissue calcifications
INTERVENTIONS	Medications › Vitamin D › Aluminum hydroxide (Amphogel) › Diuretics	IV NS Dialysis Dietary management and education	

Phosphorus has an inverse relationship with calcium.

IV Acid-Base Balance

A. **Definition:** Acid-base imbalances range from simple to complex. The four basic imbalances include the following.

ACID-BASE IMBALANCES

	PH	PCO$_2$	HCO$_3$
Normal value	7.35 to 7.45	35 to 45 mm Hg	21 to 28 mEq/L
Metabolic acidosis	↓	Normal	↓
Metabolic alkalosis	↑	Normal	↑
Respiratory acidosis	↓	↑	Normal
Respiratory alkalosis	↑	↓	Normal

B. **ROME:** "Respiratory Opposite, Metabolic Equal"

ROME

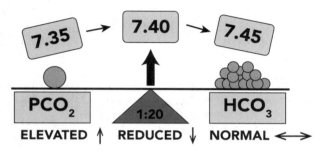

1. Remember the normal

pH	7.35 to 7.45
PCO$_2$	35 to 45
HCO$_3$	21 to 28

2. Remember the possibilities

Normal
Abnormal (uncompensated)
Partially compensated
Fully compensated

3. Use arrows

Normal
Elevated
Reduced

Abnormals

Respiratory acidosis	Metabolic acidosis
Respiratory alkalosis	Metabolic alkalosis

C. **Regulation of acid-base balance is primarily controlled by:**
1. Lungs (regulate carbonic acid through respiration)
2. Kidneys (regulate bicarbonate by retention or excretion)

ACID-BASED IMBALANCE INTERVENTIONS

Metabolic Acidosis

RISK FACTORS	Diarrhea	Overdose: salicylates or ethanol
	Fever	Kidney failure
	Hypoxia	DKA
	Starvation	Dehydration
	Seizure	
MANIFESTATIONS	Vital signs: bradycardia, weak pulses, hypotension, tachypnea	Hyporeflexia
		Lethargy
		Warm, flushed, dry skin
	Flaccid paralysis	Kussmaul's respirations
	Confusion	
INTERVENTIONS	Treat underlying cause	
	Administer fluids, electrolytes	

Metabolic Alkalosis

RISK FACTORS	Ingestion of antacids	TPN
	GI suction	Blood transfusion
	Hypokalemia	Prolonged vomiting
MANIFESTATIONS	Dizziness	Hypertonic muscles
	Paresthesias	Decreased respirations
INTERVENTIONS	Treat underlying cause	
	Administer fluids, electrolytes	

Respiratory Acidosis

RISK FACTORS	Respiratory depression	Airway obstruction
	Pneumothorax	Inadequate ventilation
MANIFESTATIONS	Dizziness	Muscle twitching
	Palpitations	Convulsions
INTERVENTIONS	Maintain patent airway	Regulation ventilation therapy
	Reversal agents for narcotics	Bronchodilators
		Mucolytics

Respiratory Alkalosis

RISK FACTORS	Hyperventilation	Asphyxiation
	Hypoxemia	Asthma
	Altitude sickness	Pneumonia
MANIFESTATIONS	Tachypnea	Palpitations
	Anxiety, tetany	Chest pain
	Paresthesias	
INTERVENTIONS	Regulate oxygen therapy	
	Reduce anxiety	
	Rebreathing techniques	

ACID-BASE WORKSHEET

	PH	CO$_2$	HCO$_3$	ACID-BASE IMBALANCE
1.	7.24	83	24	
2.	7.58	48	36	
3.	7.47	29	22	
4.	7.30	59	29	
5.	7.48	39	32	
6.	7.27	37	16	

Answer Key: 1. Respiratory acidosis; 2. Metabolic alkalosis; 3. Respiratory alkalosis; 4. Respiratory acidosis; 5. Metabolic alkalosis; 6. Metabolic acidosis

SECTION 2

Respiratory System Alterations

The respiratory system includes upper airways, lungs, lower airways, and alveolar air sacs (base of lungs). The lungs aid the body in oxygenation and tissue perfusion.

I Diagnostic Tests for Respiratory Disorders

A. **Noninvasive Procedures**

1. Chest x-ray (CXR): Use lead shield for adults of childbearing age.
2. Pulse oximetry
3. Pulmonary function tests
4. Sputum culture
5. Computed tomography (CT)
6. Magnetic resonance imaging (MRI)

B. **Invasive Procedures**

1. **Arterial blood gas** (ABGs via arterial puncture or arterial line): allows the most accurate method of assessing respiratory function

   a. Perform Allen test if no arterial line.

   b. Sample is drawn into heparinized syringe.

   c. Keep on ice and transport to laboratory immediately.

   d. Document amount and method of oxygen delivered for accurate results.

   e. Apply direct pressure to puncture site at least 5 min (longer for clients at risk for bleeding).

   f. Monitor for hematoma.

2. **Bronchoscopy**: visualize larynx, trachea, bronchi; obtain tissue biopsy; foreign body removal

   a. Obtain informed consent.

   b. Maintain NPO 8 to 12 hr.

   c. Provide local anesthetic throat spray.

   d. Position upright.

   e. Administer medications as prescribed, such as atropine (to reduce oral secretions), sedation, and antianxiety.

   f. Label specimens.

   g. Observe postprocedure.

      1) Gag reflex

      2) Bleeding

      3) Respiratory status, vital signs, and level of consciousness

3. **Mantoux test**: Positive test indicates exposure to tuberculosis. Diagnosis must be confirmed with sputum culture for presence of acid-fast bacillus (AFB).

   a. Administer 0.1 mL of purified protein derivation intradermal to upper half inner surface of forearm (insert needle bevel up).

   b. Monitor for reaction in 48 to 72 hr following injection; induration (hardening) of 10 mm or greater is considered a positive test; 5 mm may be considered significant if immunocompromised.

4. **QuantiFERON-TB Gold test (QFT-G) and T-SPOT.TB**: Identify the presence of *Mycobacterium tuberculosis* infection by measuring the immune response to the TB bacteria in whole blood.

5. **Thoracentesis**: Surgical perforation of the pleural space to obtain specimen, to remove fluid or air, or to instill medication.

   a. Informed consent.

   b. Reinforce teaching with client: remain still, feeling of pressure, positioning.

   c. Position upright.

   d. Monitor respiratory status and vital signs.

   e. Label specimens.

   f. Document client response, amount, color and viscosity of fluid (maximum amount of fluid to be removed at one time is 1 L).

   g. Chest tube at bedside.

   h. Obtain CXR before and after procedure.

II Disorders of the Respiratory System: Airflow Problems

A. **Asthma**: Chronic inflammatory disorder of the airways resulting in intermittent and reversible airflow obstruction of the bronchioles

1. Contributing Factors

   a. Extrinsic: antigen-antibody reaction triggered by food, medications, or inhaled substances

   b. Intrinsic: pathophysiological abnormalities within the respiratory tract

   c. Older clients: beta receptors are less responsive to agonist and trigger bronchospasms

2. Manifestations

   a. Sudden, severe dyspnea with use of accessory muscles

   b. Sitting up, leaning forward

   c. Diaphoresis and anxiety

   d. Wheezing, gasping

e. Coughing

f. Cyanosis (late sign)

g. Barrel chest

3. Diagnostic Procedures

a. ABGs

b. Sputum cultures

c. Pulmonary function tests

4. Collaborative Care

a. **Nursing Interventions**

1) Remain with the client during the attack.

2) Position in high-Fowler's.

3) Monitor lung sounds and pulse oximetry.

4) Administer oxygen therapy.

5) Maintain IV access.

b. Medications

1) Bronchodilators

a) Short-acting inhaled: albuterol (Proventil, Ventolin) for rapid relief

b) Methylxanthines: theophylline (Theo-24); monitor therapeutic range for toxicity

2) Anti-inflammatory

a) Corticosteroids: fluticasone (Flovent) and prednisone

b) Leukotriene antagonists: montelukast (Singulair)

3) Combination agents

a) Ipratropium and albuterol

b) Fluticasone and salmeterol (Advair)

NOTE: With inhaled agents, administer bronchodilators BEFORE anti-inflammatory medication.

c. Therapeutic Measures

1) Respiratory treatments

2) Oxygen administration

d. Client Education and Referral

1) Avoidance of allergens and triggers

2) Proper use of inhaler and peak flow monitoring

B. **Status Asthmaticus** is life-threatening episode of airway obstruction that is often unresponsive to treatment.

1. Manifestations

a. Extreme wheezing

b. Labored breathing

c. Use of accessory muscles

d. Distended neck veins

e. High risk for cardiac and/or respiratory arrest

2. **Nursing Interventions**

a. Place in high-Fowler's.

b. Prepare for emergency intubation.

c. Client will require oxygen, epinephrine, and systemic steroid therapy.

d. Provide emotional support.

C. **Chronic Obstructive Pulmonary Disease (COPD)** encompasses pulmonary emphysema and chronic bronchitis. COPD is not reversible.

1. **Pulmonary emphysema**: destruction of alveoli, narrowing of bronchioles, and trapping of air resulting in loss of lung elasticity

a. Contributing Factors

1) Cigarette smoking (main causative factor); passive smoke inhalation

2) Advanced age

3) Exposure to air pollution

4) Alpha-antitrypsin deficiency (inability to break down pollutants)

5) Occupational dust and chemical exposure

b. Manifestations

1) Dyspnea with productive cough

2) Difficult exhalation, use of pursed-lip breathing

3) Wheezing, crackles

4) Barrel chest

5) Shallow, rapid respirations

6) Respiratory acidosis with hypoxia

7) Weight loss

8) Clubbed fingernails

9) Fatigue

2. **Chronic bronchitis**: inflammation and hypersecretion of mucus in the bronchi and bronchioles caused by chronic exposure to irritants

a. Contributing Factors

1) Cigarette smoking (main causative factor)

2) Exposure to air pollution and other environmental irritants

b. Manifestations

1) Productive cough

2) Thick, tenacious sputum

3) Hypoxemia

4) Respiratory acidosis

c. Diagnostic Procedures for COPD

1) Chest x-ray

2) Pulmonary function tests: air remains trapped in lungs

3) Pulse oximetry: often less than 90%

4) ABGs: chronic respiratory acidosis

5) Computed tomography (CT)

d. Collaborative Care

1) **Nursing Interventions**

a) Monitor respiratory status.

b) Monitor cardiac status for signs of right-sided failure.

c) Position upright and leaning forward.

d) Schedule activities to allow for frequent rest periods.

e) Administer oxygen therapy as prescribed.

f) Use incentive spirometry.

g) Encourage fluids 2 to 3 L per day unless contraindicated.

h) Encourage high-calorie diet.

i) Provide emotional support.

2) Medications

a) Bronchodilators

b) Methylxanthines

c) Anti-inflammatory agents

d) Mucolytic agents

3) Therapeutic Measures

a) Chest physiotherapy/pulmonary drainage

b) Lung reduction surgery

4) Client Education and Referral

a) Breathing techniques

b) Oxygen therapy

c) Medications

d) Nutrition

e) Promote smoking cessation

f) Infection prevention measures

g) Encourage immunizations for pneumonia and influenza

h) Pulmonary rehabilitation

i) Activity pacing

3. Complications of COPD

a. Cor pulmonale: right-sided heart failure caused by pulmonary disease

1) Manifestations

a) Hypoxia and hypoxemia

b) Extreme dyspnea

c) Cyanotic lips

d) JVD

e) Dependent edema

f) Hepatomegaly

g) Pulmonary hypertension

2) Collaborative Care

a) **Nursing Interventions**

(1) Monitor respiratory status.

(2) Monitor cardiac status and for indications of right-sided heart failure.

(3) Administer oxygen therapy as prescribed.

(4) Ensure adequate rest periods.

(5) Encourage low-sodium diet.

(6) Maintain fluid balance; possible fluid restriction.

(7) Administer medications as prescribed.

b) Medications

(1) Diuretics

(2) Digoxin

c) Therapeutic Measures

(1) Mechanical ventilation

D. **Carbon Dioxide Toxicity:** Stuporous secondary to increased CO_2 retention

1. Contributing Factors

a. Carbon dioxide retention

b. Excessive oxygen delivery

2. Manifestations

a. Alteration in level of consciousness

b. Tachypnea

c. Increased blood pressure

d. Tachycardia with dysrhythmias

3. Collaborative Care

a. Monitor pulse oximetry and ABGs.

b. Avoid excessive concentrations of oxygen.

c. Provide pulmonary hygiene.

d. Provide ventilatory support with CPAP, BiPAP, or mechanical ventilation.

E. **Pneumonia** is an inflammatory process in the lungs that produces excess fluid and exudate that fill the alveoli; classified as bacterial, viral, fungal, or chemical.

1. Contributing Factors

a. Advanced age

b. Chronic lung disease

c. Immunocompromise

d. Mechanical ventilation

e. Postoperative

f. Sedation and opioid use

g. Prolonged immobility

h. Tobacco use

i. Enteral tube feeding

2. Manifestations

a. Tachypnea and tachycardia

b. Sudden onset of chills, fever, flushing, diaphoresis

c. Productive cough

d. Dyspnea with pleuritic pain

e. Crackles

f. Elevated WBC

g. Decreased O_2 saturation

3. Diagnostic Procedures

a. Chest x-ray

b. Pulse oximetry

c. Sputum culture and sensitivity

4. Collaborative Care

a. **Nursing Interventions**

1) Monitor respiratory status.

2) Administer oxygen.

3) Monitor sputum.

4) Monitor vital signs.

5) Encourage 3 L of fluid per day.

6) Provide pulmonary hygiene.

7) Encourage mouth care.

8) Promote nutrition.

b. Medications

1) Anti-infectives

2) Antipyretics

3) Bronchodilators

4) Anti-inflammatories

c. Client Education

1) Medication administration

2) Preventive measures

3) Pneumonia and influenza vaccine

F. **Tuberculosis** is an infectious disease caused by *Mycobacterium tuberculosis* and transmitted through aerosolization (airborne route).

1. Contributing Factors

a. Older and homeless populations

b. Lower socioeconomic status

c. Foreign immigrants

d. Those in frequent contact with untreated persons

e. Overcrowded living conditions

2. Manifestations

a. Cough, hemoptysis

b. Positive sputum culture for acid-fast bacillus (AFB)

c. Low-grade fever with night sweats

d. Anorexia, weight loss

e. Malaise, fatigue

3. Diagnostic Procedures

a. Mantoux

b. Sputum culture and smear for AFB to confirm diagnosis

c. Serum analysis, QFT-G

d. Chest x-ray

4. Collaborative Care

a. **Nursing Interventions**

1) Maintain airborne isolation precautions.

2) Obtain sputum sample before administering medications.

3) Maintain adequate nutritional status.

4) Reinforce teaching with client to avoid foods containing tyramine when taking INH.

5) Inform the client that rifampin can alter the metabolism of certain other medications.

6) Monitor laboratory findings for liver and kidney function.

b. Medications: Combination drug therapy

1) Administer medications on an empty stomach at the same time every day.

2) Medications should be taken for 6 to 12 months, as directed.

3) Reinforce teaching with client to recognize manifestations of hepatotoxicity, nephrotoxicity, and visual changes, and to notify a provider if any of these are noted.

4) Medications to treat TB

a) Isoniazid (INH)

b) Rifampin

c) Pyrazinamide

d) Streptomycin

e) Ethambutol

c. Client Education and Referral

1) Encourage the client to practice good hand hygiene and to always cover her nose and mouth when sneezing or coughing.

2) Ensure medication compliance and follow-up care.

5. Cases of diagnosed TB are reported to local or state health department.

a. Refer all high-risk clients to local health department for testing and prophylactic treatment regimen.

G. **Laryngeal Cancer**: Malignant cells occurring in the mucosal tissue of the larynx; more common in men ages 55 to 70.

1. Contributing Factors

a. Smoking

b. Radiation exposure

c. Chronic laryngitis and/or straining of vocal cords

2. Manifestations

a. Hoarseness extending longer than 2 weeks

b. Dysphagia

c. Dyspnea

d. Cough

e. Persistent sore throat

f. Hard, immobile lymph nodes in neck

g. Weight loss, anorexia

3. Diagnostic Procedures

a. MRI

b. Direct laryngoscopy with biopsy

c. X-ray and CT

d. Bone scan and positron emission tomography (PET) scan

4. Collaborative Care

a. **Nursing Interventions**

1) Maintain patent airway.

2) Maintain swallowing precautions.

3) Provide emotional support.

4) Nutrition.

5) Provide pain management.

6) Administer medications as elixir when possible.

b. Therapeutic Measures

1) Partial or total laryngectomy

2) Radiation therapy

c. Client Education and Referral

1) Communication method

2) Stoma care

3) Swallowing maneuvers

4) Speech therapy

H. **Lung Cancer:** Leading cause of cancer-related deaths for men and women in the U.S.; primary or metastatic disease; most commonly occurs between ages 45 and 70 years.

1. Contributing Factors

   a. Smoking (first- and secondhand smoke)

   b. Radiation exposure

   c. Chronic exposure to inhaled irritants

   d. Older adult

2. Manifestations

   a. Chronic cough

   b. Chronic dyspnea

   c. Hemoptysis

   d. Hoarseness

   e. Fatigue, weight loss, anorexia

   f. Clubbing of fingers

   g. Chest wall pain

3. Diagnostic Procedures

   a. Chest x-ray and CT scan

   b. CT guided needle aspiration

   c. Bronchoscopy with biopsy

   d. TNM system for staging

      1) T – Tumor

      2) N – Nodes

      3) M – Metastasis

4. Collaborative Care

   a. **Nursing Interventions**

      1) Maintain patent airway.

      2) Suction as indicated by assessment.

      3) Monitor vital signs and pulse oximetry.

      4) Monitor nutritional status.

      5) Position in high-Fowler's.

      6) Provide emotional support.

      7) Manage and treat stomatitis.

      8) Ensure protection for immunocompromised client.

   b. Medications

      1) Chemotherapeutic agents

      2) Opioid narcotics

   c. Therapeutic Measures

      1) Palliative care

         a) Medication

      2) Thoracentesis Surgical

         a) Tumor excision

         b) Pneumonectomy, lobectomy, wedge resection

         c) Radiation

   d. Client Education and Referral

      1) Medications

      2) Constipation prevention and management

      3) Mouth and skin care

      4) Nutrition

5. Respiratory services

6. Radiology

7. Rehabilitation

8. Nutrition

9. Hospice

III Respiratory Emergencies

A. **Pulmonary Embolism:** A life-threatening hypoxic condition caused by a collection of particulate matter (solid, gas, or liquid) that enters venous circulation and lodges in the pulmonary vessels causing pulmonary blood flow obstruction

1. Contributing Factors

   a. Chronic atrial fibrillation

   b. Hypercoagulability

   c. Long bone fracture

   d. Long-term immobility

   e. Oral contraceptive or estrogen therapy

   f. Obesity

   g. Postoperative

   h. PVD, DVT

   i. Sickle cell anemia

2. Manifestations

   a. Dyspnea, tachypnea

   b. Chest pain   — hemoptysis

   c. Tachycardia

   d. Anxiety

   e. Diaphoresis

   f. Decreased SaO_2

   g. Pleural effusion

   h. Crackles and cough

NOTE: Petechial rash is present with fat embolus.

3. Diagnostic Procedures

   a. ABGs

   b. D-dimer

   c. Chest x-ray

   d. V/Q scan

   e. Pulmonary angiography

4. Collaborative Care

   a. **Nursing interventions**

      1) Monitor respiratory status and vital signs.

      2) Provide respiratory support.

      3) Provide oxygen therapy.

      4) Position in high-Fowler's.

      5) Initiate IV access.

      6) Provide emotional support.

   b. Medications

      1) Thrombolytics

      2) Anticoagulants

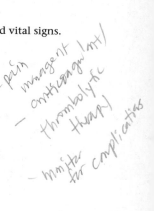

— pain management (antl)
anticoagulant
— thrombolytic therapy
— monitor for complications

c. Therapeutic Measures

   1) Embolectomy

   2) Vena cava filter

d. Client Education and Referral

   1) Preventive measures

   2) Dietary precautions with vitamin K

   3) Follow-up for PT or INR

   4) Bleeding precautions

5. Cardiology and pulmonary services

  a. Respiratory care

B. **Pneumothorax:** A collection of air or gas in the chest or pleural space that causes part or all of a lung to collapse due to a loss of negative pressure

C. **Tension Pneumothorax:** Occurs when air enters the pleural space during inspiration through a one-way valve and is not able to exit upon expiration. The trapped air causes pressure on the heart and the lung. As a result, the increase in pressure compresses blood vessels and limits venous return, leading to a decrease in cardiac output. Death can result if not treated immediately.

D. **Hemothorax:** Accumulation of blood in the pleural cavity

1. Contributing Factors

  a. Blunt chest trauma

  b. COPD

  c. Closed/occluded chest tube

  d. Advanced age

  e. Penetrating chest wounds

2. Manifestations

  a. Respiratory distress

  b. Tracheal deviation to unaffected side (tension pneumothorax)

  c. Reduced or absent breath sounds (affected side)

  d. Asymmetrical chest wall movement

  e. Hyperresonance on percussion due to trapped air (pneumothorax)

  f. Subcutaneous emphysema

  g. Chest pain

3. Diagnostic Procedures

  a. Chest x-ray

  b. Thoracentesis (hemothorax)

4. Collaborative Care

  a. **Nursing Interventions**

   1) Monitor respiratory status.

   2) Administer oxygen.

   3) Position in high-Fowler's.

   4) Monitor chest tube and dressing.

   5) Provide emotional support.

   6) Recognize and report changes in client's condition.

b. Therapeutic Measures

   1) Chest tube insertion

    a) Chest tube: inserted to pleural space for draining fluid, blood, or air; reestablishes a negative pressure; facilitates lung expansion

     (1) Position supine or semi-Fowler's.

     (2) Verify informed consent is signed.

     (3) Prepare chest drainage system prior to insertion.

     (4) Administer pain and sedation medication as ordered.

     (5) Assist provider as needed during insertion.

     (6) Apply dressing to insertion site.

     (7) Maintain chest tube system.

     (8) Monitor respiratory status, pulse oximetry, vital signs, and client response.

     (9) Monitor for complications.

CHEST TUBE COMPLICATIONS

COMPLICATION	NURSING INTERVENTIONS
Air leak (continuous rapid bubbling in the water seal chamber)	Start at the chest and move down tubing to locate leak; tighten connection or replace drainage system. Keep connection taped securely.
No tidaling in water seal chamber	Check for kinks in the tubing. Check breath sounds (lungs re-expanded).
No bubbling in suction control chamber	Verify tubing is attached. Verify water is filled to prescribed level. Check wall suction regulator.
Chest tube is disconnected from system	Insert open end of the chest tube into sterile water until system can be replaced.
Chest tube accidentally pulled from client	Cover insertion site with sterile dressing, taped on three sides. Contact provider. Prepare for reinsertion.

IV Airway Management

A. **Oxygen Therapy** is used in many acute and chronic respiratory problems to improve cellular oxygenation and prevent hypoxia or hypoxemia.

1. Clinical Manifestations

CLINICAL MANIFESTATIONS OF HYPOXIA AND HYPOXEMIA

EARLY	LATE
Tachypnea	Bradypnea
Tachycardia	Bradycardia
Restlessness	Confusion and stupor
Pale skin and mucous membranes	Cyanotic skin and mucous membranes
Elevated blood pressure	Hypotension
Use of accessory muscles, nasal flaring, adventitious lung sounds	Cardiac dysrhythmias

2. Collaborative Care

OXYGEN DELIVERY DEVICES

DEVICE	FIO₂/FLOW RATE
Nasal cannula	24% to 44% at 1 to 6 L/min
Simple face mask	40% to 60% at 6 to 8 L/min
Partial rebreather mask	50% to 75% at 8 to 11 L/min
Nonrebreather mask	80% to 100% at 12 L/min
Venturi mask	24% to 40% at 4 to 8 L/min
Aerosol mask, face tent	30% to 100% at 8 to 10 L/min
T-piece	30% to 100% at 8 to 10 L/min

3. Client Education

 a. Observe setting to identify electrical hazards.

 b. Post "oxygen in use" sign.

 c. Wear cotton gown.

 d. No smoking.

B. **Suctioning**: Use of a suction machine and catheter to remove secretions from the airway

 1. Clinical Manifestations (indicating a need for suctioning)

 a. Restlessness

 b. Tachypnea

 c. Tachycardia

 d. Decreased SaO₂

 e. Adventitious breath sounds

 f. Visualization of secretions

 g. Absence of spontaneous cough

 2. Collaborative Care

 a. Perform hand hygiene.

 b. Explain procedure.

 c. Don required PPE.

 d. Position client to semi- or high-Fowler's.

 e. Obtain baseline breath sounds, vital signs, and SaO₂.

 f. Use medical aseptic technique (oral suction).

 g. Use surgical aseptic technique for all other types.

 h. Hyperoxygenate client.

 i. Suction 10 to 15 seconds (rotating motion). Limit to 2 to 3 attempts.

 j. Allow recovery between attempts (20 to 30 seconds).

 k. Document amount, color, and consistency of secretions as well as client response.

C. **Tracheostomy Care**: Care of a tracheostomy to maintain a patent airway and optimal ventilation

 1. Collaborative Care

 a. Explain the procedure.

 b. Position client in semi- or high-Fowler's.

 c. At all times, keep two extra tracheostomy tubes (one the client's size and one a smaller size) at the bedside in the event of accidental decannulation.

 d. Suction client only as clinically indicated (never on routine schedule). Surgical asepsis is used for tracheal suctioning.

 e. Monitor for respiratory distress.

 f. Provide tracheostomy care every 8 hr and as needed.

 g. Change tracheostomy tubes as prescribed.

 2. Client Education and Referral

 a. Tracheostomy care

 b. Prevention of respiratory infections

 c. Nutrition

 d. Home health care agency

 e. Community support group

D. **Mechanical Ventilation** provides respiratory support through the controlled delivery of ventilation and oxygenation via an endotracheal tube, tracheostomy tube, or noninvasive ventilation via mask through continuous positive airway pressure (CPAP) or bi-level positive airway pressure (BiPAP).

 1. Indication

 a. During surgery

 b. Acute respiratory distress

 c. Respiratory failure

 2. Nursing Interventions

 a. Explain procedure to client

 b. Establish means of communication, such as asking yes/no questions, providing writing materials, using a dry-erase or picture communication board, or lip reading.

 c. Maintain patent airway

 1) Ensure advanced airway device is secured (endotracheal tube or tracheostomy tube).

 2) Monitor position and placement of tube. Document in centimeters at the client's lips or teeth.

 3) Prevent accidental extubation. Wrist restraints can be required.

 4) Suction oral and tracheal secretions as indicated by assessment.

 5) Monitor respiratory status every 1 to 2 hr and as needed.

6) Monitor ventilator settings and alarms. Never turn off ventilator alarms. If the cause of an alarm cannot be identified and corrected, and the client's respiratory status begins to decline, the nurse should ventilate the client using a manual resuscitation bag until the issue is resolved.

   a) Low-pressure alarm—indicates low volume and is usually associated with tube disconnection, cuff leak, or tube dislodgement

   b) High-pressure alarm—indicates increased pressure which may be caused by secretions, kinking of tube, pulmonary edema, or the client coughing or biting the tube

   c) Apnea alarm—indicates there has been no spontaneous breath within a preset time period.

7) Clients may receive the following medications while on a ventilator. The nurse should recognize and report changes in client status.

   a) Analgesics

   b) Sedation

   c) Neuromuscular blocking agents

8) The endotracheal tube should be repositioned every 24 hr by the RN or respiratory therapist.

d. Prevent complications

1) Pneumonia

   a) Hand hygiene

   b) Elevate head of bed

   c) Oral hygiene

2) Pneumothorax

   a) Caused by high ventilation pressures

   b) Auscultate lung sounds frequently

   c) Consider if sudden respiratory distress

   d) Requires immediate action (chest tube)

RESPIRATORY END-OF-SECTION REVIEW

1. An early sign of hypoxia is _____ and a late sign of hypoxia is _____.

2. The oxygen delivery system that provides the highest concentration of oxygen is the _____ mask.

3. The LPN notes the client is experiencing dyspnea. The initial action, unless contraindicated, should be to _____ the client's head of bed.

4. Health care team members providing care for a client who has TB should maintain _____ precautions.

5. It is important to provide adequate _____ nursing care for a client who has COPD.

6. A client has returned to the room following a bronchoscopy and requests a drink of water. It is important to ensure the _____ is present.

7. To prevent aspiration, it is important to maintain _____ precautions for a client who had a laryngectomy.

8. The client who has pneumonia is coughing up thick secretions. The LPN would encourage the client to increase _____.

9. The LPN is caring for a client with a chest tube. It would be acceptable to have bubbling in the _____ chamber.

10. _____ should be maintained when performing tracheal suctioning.

WORD BANK

Airborne

Clean technique

Confusion

Droplet

Elevate

Fluid intake

Gag reflex

Lower

Non-rebreather

Rest periods

Restlessness

Simple face

Suction

Surgical asepsis

Swallowing

Water seal

Answer Key: 1. Restlessness, Confusion; 2. Non-rebreather; 3. Elevate; 4. Airborne; 5. Rest periods; 6. Gag reflex; 7. Swallowing; 8. Fluid intake; 9. Suction; 10. Surgical asepsis

Perioperative Care

A. **Preoperative Phase:** Procedures or teaching completed prior to a surgical procedure reduce potential complications and postoperative discomfort, relieve anxiety, and increase participation in care.

1. Care of the client before surgery

   a. **Nursing Interventions**
      1) Review client history.
      2) Identify risk factors: infants, older adults, poor health, respiratory conditions, obesity, emergent procedures.
      3) Check for informed consent (a nurse may witness only).
      4) Verify baseline assessment is complete.
      5) Collect data about allergies.
      6) Verify NPO status.

   b. Medications
      1) Anesthesia
         a) Inhalation
         b) Intravenous
         c) Regional
         d) Topical
      2) Antibiotics
      3) Anticholinergics
      4) Narcotics
      5) Sedatives

   c. Diagnostic Tests
      1) Laboratory profile
      2) Chest x-ray
      3) ECG
      4) Pregnancy test for females

   d. Client Education
      1) Fears and anxiety
      2) Medications
         a) Hold anticoagulants for 7 to 10 days prior to surgery (e.g., warfarin [Coumadin] or aspirin)
      3) Invasive procedures
      4) Incentive spirometry
      5) Turn, position, and perform early ambulation, including leg exercises
      6) Analgesics and pain control methods
      7) Routine and expected postoperative care
      8) Pre-, intra-, and postoperative routines (frequent vital signs, monitoring, positioning)

B. **Intraoperative Phase:** Begins when client enters the surgical suite and ends with transfer to postanesthesia recovery area. Nursing focus is on safety, client advocacy, and health team collaboration.

1. The Universal Protocol (safety initiative from Joint Commission)
   a. Conduct a preprocedure verification process.
   b. Mark the procedure site.
   c. Perform a "time out" before starting the procedure.

2. Collaborative Care
   a. Perioperative Nursing Staff
      1) Holding area
      2) Circulator
      3) Scrub
      4) Specialty

   b. **Nursing Interventions**
      1) Implement role according to established standards.
      2) Maintain safe environment.
      3) Ensure strict asepsis.
      4) Apply grounding devices.
      5) Ensure correct sponge, needle, and instrument count.
      6) Position client.
      7) Remain alert to complications.
      8) Communicate with surgical team.

   c. Therapeutic Measures
      1) Blood transfusion
      2) Radiology
      3) Biopsy
      4) Laboratory profiles

C. **Postoperative Phase:** Begins when client enters the postanesthesia recovery area and continues until discharge from the health care facility.

1. Collaborative Care
   a. **Nursing Interventions:** Immediate recovery period
      1) Ongoing assessment
         a) Pulmonary
            (1) Verify airway and check gag reflex.
            (2) Check for bilateral breath sounds.
            (3) Encourage coughing and deep breathing.
         b) Circulatory
            (1) Compare vital signs to baseline.
            (2) Monitor tissue perfusion.
         c) Neurological
            (1) Evaluate the level of consciousness.
            (2) Monitor reflexes and movement.
         d) Genitourinary
            (1) Monitor I&O.
            (2) Monitor urinary output (color, clarity, and amount).
         e) Gastrointestinal
            (1) Monitor for bowel sounds.
            (2) Monitor for abdominal distention.

f) Integument
   (1) Monitor color.
   (2) Monitor wound.
   (3) Monitor drainage insertion sites.
g) Nursing Actions
   (1) Verify IV fluid type, rate, and site.
   (2) Monitor dressings for type and amount of drainage.
   (3) Identify drainage including color and amount
   (4) If NG tube, determine type and amount of suction ordered.
   (5) Position in semi-Fowler's to facilitate maximum oxygenation.
   (6) Monitor O_2 saturation.
   (7) Ensure thermoregulation.
   (8) Provide pain management.
   (9) Maintain NPO until the client is alert and a gag reflex returns.
   (10) Prevent complications (see table).
   (11) Transfer or discharge client to unit or home.

COMMON POSTOPERATIVE COMPLICATIONS

Atelectasis

OCCURRENCE	First 48 hr	
MANIFESTATIONS	Tachycardia Tachypnea	Shallow respirations
INTERVENTIONS	Incentive spirometer T,C,DB q 2 hr Early ambulation	Hydration Monitor respiratory rate and rhythm

Hypostatic pneumonia

OCCURRENCE	After 48 hr	
MANIFESTATIONS	Febrile Tachycardia	Tachypnea Crackles, rhonchi
INTERVENTIONS	Incentive spirometer T,C,DB q 2 hr Early ambulation	Hydration Mucolytics

Respiratory depression

OCCURRENCE	Immediate to 48 hr	
MANIFESTATIONS	Bradypnea Shallow respirations	Decreased LOC
INTERVENTIONS	Monitor respiratory rate and rhythm Monitor LOC Regulate narcotics	Oxygen therapy Narcotic antagonist: naloxone

Hypoxia

OCCURRENCE	Immediate to 48 hr	
MANIFESTATIONS	Confusion Increased BP, pulse	Tachypnea
INTERVENTIONS	Monitor vital signs Oxygen therapy	Resolve underlying problem

COMMON POSTOPERATIVE COMPLICATIONS (CONTINUED)

Nausea

OCCURRENCE	Immediate to 48 hr	
MANIFESTATIONS	Nausea	
INTERVENTIONS	Comfort measures Relaxation Mouth care	Antiemetic NG tube to decompress stomach

Shock

OCCURRENCE	Immediate to 48 hr	
MANIFESTATIONS	Decreased BP, pulse, urinary output Cold, clammy, pale skin	Lethargy Stupor
INTERVENTIONS	Monitor vital signs Replace fluids Position in modified Trendelenburg	I&O Monitor LOC Administer vasopressors as prescribed

Urinary retention/hesitancy

OCCURRENCE	Immediate to 3 days	
MANIFESTATIONS	Inability to void Bladder distention	Restlessness Increased BP
INTERVENTIONS	Privacy Bladder scan	Offer bedpan I&O

Decreased peristalsis/Paralytic ileus

OCCURRENCE	2 to 4 days
MANIFESTATIONS	Hypoactive/absent bowel sounds No flatus
INTERVENTIONS	NG to decompress stomach Limit narcotics Ambulation Prokinetic agents: metoclopramide (Reglan) as prescribed

Wound hemorrhage

OCCURRENCE	Immediate to discharge
MANIFESTATIONS	Bleeding from drainage tubes or surgical site Signs of shock
INTERVENTIONS	Monitor site Identify early signs Monitor drainage device, keep patent Avoid tension at surgical site

Thrombophlebitis

OCCURRENCE	7 to 14 days
MANIFESTATIONS	Redness, warmth, calf tenderness/pain, edema at site
INTERVENTIONS	Early ambulation Apply antiembolic stockings or sequential compression devices as prescribed Avoid actions that decrease venous flow Anticoagulant prophylaxis

COMMON POSTOPERATIVE COMPLICATIONS (CONTINUED)

Delayed wound healing

OCCURRENCE	5 to 6 days
MANIFESTATIONS	Edema, redness, pallor, separation at edges, absence of granulation tissue
INTERVENTIONS	Splint incision as needed Use incision support devices (abdominal binder) Promote high-protein diet

Wound infection

OCCURRENCE	3 to 5 days
MANIFESTATIONS	Signs of delayed healing with purulent/discolored drainage, pain in incisional area
INTERVENTIONS	Promote healthy diet, adequate fluid intake, adequate rest and exercise Wound care Antibiotics as prescribed

Wound dehiscence/evisceration

OCCURRENCE	4 to 15 days
MANIFESTATIONS	Open wound revealing underlying tissue (dehiscence) or organs (evisceration)
INTERVENTIONS	Position client to decrease tension at suture line Apply sterile saline-soaked gauze Immediately notify surgeon Client should not cough or strain Provide emotional support

Urinary tract infection

OCCURRENCE	5 to 8 days
MANIFESTATIONS	Frequency, urgency, dysuria Malodorous, cloudy urine
INTERVENTIONS	Wipe front to back after urination Limit use of indwelling catheters Encourage voiding Increase fluids 3 L/day Cranberry juice Antibiotics as prescribed Uroanalgesics as prescribed

Gastrointestinal, Hepatic, and Pancreatic Disorders

A. **Impaired function of the GI tract, pancreas, and liver result from structural, mechanical, motility, infection, or cancerous conditions**

B. **Contributing Factors**

1. History of autoimmune disorder
2. Alcohol use disorder
3. Dietary patterns
4. NSAID use
5. Age
6. Family history
7. Previous abdominal surgery
8. Allergies
9. Musculoskeletal impairment (e.g., CVA, MS)
10. Obesity
11. Smoking
12. Sedentary lifestyle
13. Stress

Diagnostic Procedures

A. **Laboratory Profiles: Gastric Aspirate**

1. Hydrochloric acid and pepsin (evaluate for Zollinger-Ellison syndrome)

   a. NPO 12 hr.

   b. Avoid alcohol, tobacco, and medications that change gastric pH for 24 hr.

   c. Insert NG tube.

   d. Aspirate gastric contents.

   e. Obtain pH.

POSTOPERATIVE CARE MATCHING EXERCISE

Match the postoperative complication in the left column with the appropriate nursing interventions in the right column.

1. Delayed wound healing	A.	Wipe front to back. Increase fluids. Encourage voiding.
2. Atelectasis	B.	Monitor respiratory rate, depth, effort, and LOC. Regulate narcotics. Oxygen therapy.
3. Decreased peristalsis	C.	Monitor vital signs. Modified Trendelenburg. IV fluids.
4. Nausea	D.	Incentive spirometer. TCDB q 2 hr. Hydration.
5. Respiratory depression	E.	Early ambulation. Antiembolic stockings. Anticoagulant prophylaxis.
6. Urinary tract infection	F.	Splint incision. Use abdominal binder. Promote high-protein diet.
7. Thrombophlebitis	G.	Position to decrease tension at suture line. Apply saline-soaked gauze.
8. Wound dehiscence/evisceration	H.	Ambulation. Limit narcotics. Metoclopramide.
9. Urinary retention/hesitancy	I.	Antiemetics. Mouth care. Comfort measures.
10 Shock	J.	Privacy for voiding. Bladder scan. Monitor I&O.

Answer Key: 1. F; 2. D; 3. H; 4. I; 5. B; 6. A; 7. E; 8. G; 9. J; 10. C

B. **Laboratory Profiles: Hepatic or Pancreatic Disease**

1. Albumin
2. Ammonia: liver's ability to break down protein by-products
3. Bilirubin: measured directly in the blood
4. Cholesterol
5. Liver enzymes (AST, ALT, ALP)
6. Pancreatic enzymes (amylase, lipase)

C. **Laboratory Profiles: GI Parasites, Bacteria, or Bleeding**

1. Stool sample
   a. Inspect for color, consistency
   b. Tests
      1) Ova and parasites
      2) *Clostridium difficile* (*C. diff*)
      3) Urobilinogen
      4) Fecal fat (steatorrhea)
      5) Fecal nitrogen
      6) Food residues
      7) Cytotoxic assay (preferred over stool culture)

KEY POINT: When obtaining a stool sample, have the client defecate into a bedpan or bedside commode. Use an approved specimen container. The sample must be uncontaminated by urine or toilet paper and sent promptly to the lab.

2. Fecal screening tests (may be obtained at home and mailed in)
   a. Fecal occult blood test
      1) Recommended annually to detect colon cancer.
      2) Instruct to avoid red meat, aspirin, turnips, and horseradish for at least 72 hr prior to testing to avoid false positive results. Ingestion of vitamin C-rich foods or supplements can result in a false negative.
      3) NSAIDs and anticoagulants should be discontinued 7 days prior to testing.
   b. Fecal immunochemical test (Hemosure, Hematest II SENSA, HemoQuant)
   c. Stool DNA

D. **Breath Tests**

1. Hydrogen breath test
   a. To evaluate carbohydrate absorption
   b. Aids in detection of bacterial overgrowth in intestine
2. Urea breath test
   a. To detect presence of *H. pylori*
   b. Instruct to avoid antibiotics and bismuth subsalicylate (Pepto-Bismol) 1 month before the test; proton pump inhibitors and sucralfate (Carafate) 1 week before testing; and H_2 inhibitors for 24 hr before testing.

E. **Endoscopy:** Allows direct visualization of tissues, cavities, and organs using a flexible fiber-optic tube

1. Colonoscopy: exam of the entire large intestine
   a. Bowel prep to clear fecal contents (1 to 3 day prep)
   b. Clear liquid diet 12 to 24 hr before procedure
   c. NPO except water 6 to 8 hr before procedure
   d. IV sedation
   e. Monitor postprocedure for excessive bleeding or severe pain
2. Virtual colonoscopy
   a. Bowel prep as for traditional colonoscopy
   b. Performed using MRI or CT
   c. Small tube is placed in the rectum
   d. Images viewed on screen
3. Sigmoidoscopy: exam of rectum and sigmoid colon
   a. Clear liquid diet 24 hr before procedure
   b. Laxative the evening before the procedure
   c. Enema the morning of the procedure
   d. Sedation is not required
   e. Tissue biopsy may be performed
   f. Report excessive bleeding
4. Small bowel capsule endoscopy: video exam of small bowel, including distal ileum
   a. Only water is allowed 8 to 10 hr before test.
   b. NPO 2 hr before test.
   c. Client's abdomen is marked for location of placement for sensors.
   d. Client wears abdominal belt housing data recorder.
   e. Administer video capsule with full glass of water.
   f. Resume normal diet 4 hr after swallowing pill.
   g. Return to the facility with capsule equipment for download of data.
   h. Procedure takes approximately 8 hr.
   i. Capsule will be excreted via stool (might not be seen); no action needed.
5. Esophagogastroduodenoscopy (EGD): exam of esophagus, stomach, and duodenum (identify bleeding, Crohn's disease, colitis)
   a. NPO 6 to 8 hr before procedure.
   b. Avoid anticoagulants, aspirin, or NSAIDs for several days before test.
   c. IV sedation.
   d. Atropine to dry secretions.
   e. Local anesthetic is sprayed to inactivate gag reflex.
   f. Prevent aspiration.
   g. Monitor for signs of perforation, pain, bleeding, or fever.
   h. Comfort measures for hoarseness or sore throat (several days).

6. Endoscopic retrograde cholangiopancreatography (ERCP): exam of liver, gallbladder, bile ducts, and pancreas

   a. NPO 6 to 8 hr before procedure.

   b. Avoid anticoagulants, aspirin, or NSAIDs for several days before test.

   c. Collect data about allergies to x-ray dye.

   d. IV sedation.

   e. May have colicky abdominal discomfort.

   f. Monitor for severe pain, fever, nausea, or vomiting (indicates perforation).

F. **Radiographic Studies** (with or without contrast)

   1. Barium series: x-ray visualization from the mouth to the duodenojejunal junction; can include a small bowel follow through

      a. NPO 8 hr before procedure.

      b. Avoid opioid analgesics and anticholinergic medications for 24 hr before the test.

      c. Have client drink 16 oz barium liquid.

      d. Client will assume multiple positions during the x-ray exam.

      e. Client should include additional fiber and fluids to promote barium elimination.

      f. Visualize stool for barium contents next 24 to 72 hr (will be chalky white).

      g. Brown stool should return when barium is evacuated.

      h. Mild laxative or stool softener as needed to promote bowel elimination.

G. **Liver Biopsy:** Needle inserted through abdominal wall to obtain sample for biopsy or tissue examination; performed under fluoroscopy

   1. Preparation

      a. Obtain informed consent.

      b. Monitor coagulation studies (PT, aPTT, INR, platelet count).

      c. NPO 8 to 10 hr before procedure.

      d. Position on affected side to promote hemostasis.

      e. Monitor for bleeding complications.

H. **Paracentesis:** Needle inserted through abdominal wall into peritoneal cavity, withdrawing fluid accumulated due to ascites

   1. Have client void.

   2. Obtain baseline vital signs.

   3. Position upright.

   4. Administer mild sedation.

   5. Administer prescribed IV fluids or albumin to restore fluid balance (as much as 4 L of fluid is slowly drained from the abdomen).

   6. Monitor vital signs.

   7. Record weight before and after procedure.

   8. Measure abdominal girth before and after procedure.

   9. Monitor laboratory profile before and after procedure: albumin, amylase, protein, BUN, creatinine.

II Gastrointestinal Therapeutic Procedures

GASTROINTESTINAL TUBES

TUBE	PURPOSE	NURSING INTERVENTIONS
Nasogastric › **Levin:** single lumen › **Salem sump:** double lumen » Suction, aspiration » Vent	Decompress stomach (ileus, gastric atony, or intestinal obstruction) Obtain specimens for analysis (pH of gastric fluid and the presence of blood)	Elevate head of bed. Verify placement. Provide frequent mouth care. Maintain NPO.
Miller-Abbott: double lumen › Aspiration › Inflate balloon at tip	Small bowel suction	Reposition every 1 hr. Do NOT tape tube to nose. Monitor advancement of tube. Monitor color of gastric contents.
Sengstaken-Blakemore: triple lumen › Esophageal balloon › Gastric balloon › Suction, irrigation	For treatment of esophageal varices Can cause potential trauma and complications for the client, such as rebleeding, pneumonia, and respiratory obstruction	Monitor for respiratory distress (most clients have ETT). Keep scissors at bedside. Monitor signs of shock.

A. **Enteral Feeding Tubes:** delivery of a nutritionally complete feeding directly into the stomach, duodenum, or jejunum

KEY POINT: The auscultatory method of checking placement is NOT considered reliable. Initial placement of the nasogastric or nasointestinal tube should be checked by x-ray. Subsequent placement should be checked by aspirating stomach or intestinal contents and measuring pH. Gastric pH should be between 1.5 and 4; intestinal aspirate pH is around 6; respiratory aspirate pH is 7 or higher.

   1. Small-bore nasogastric feeding tubes

      a. Obtain x-ray to determine placement.

      b. Check gastric pH before each feeding; every 4 hr for continuous feeding.

      c. Maintain a semi-Fowler's position while feeding is infusing.

      d. Check residual in the stomach and refeed the residual, unless it exceeds the maximum.

      e. Provide nose and mouth care.

      f. Replace tube every 4 weeks.

KEY POINT: If residual exceeds 100 mL for intermittent feedings, or 2 hr worth of a continuous feeding, hold or stop the feeding. Do NOT refeed aspirate. Notify the provider.

2. Small-bore nasointestinal/jejunostomy tubes: inserted through the skin and occasionally sutured in place for long-term feeding

   a. Obtain x-ray to determine placement (prior to initial feeding).

   b. Check length of exposed tubing (tube migration).

   c. Check placement prior to feeding using intestinal pH.

   d. Maintain a semi-Fowler's position.

   e. Monitor residual (greater volume indicates upward migration).

3. Monitor for complications

   a. Refeeding syndrome can be life-threatening.

   b. Bleeding

   c. Infection

   d. Tube misplacement/dislodgement, aspiration: Immediately remove any tube suspected of being dislodged or misplaced.

   e. Abdominal distention, nausea, vomiting, diarrhea, constipation

   f. Fluid imbalance: hyperosmolar preparations can lead to dehydration

   g. Electrolyte imbalance: the most common are hyponatremia and hyperkalemia

4. Percutaneous endoscopic gastrostomy (PEG)

   a. Monitor skin integrity.

   b. Check residual volume.

   c. Allow feeding to infuse slowly (raise/lower syringe).

   d. Flush with 30 mL warm water before and after feeding.

   e. Maintain semi-Fowler's position 1 to 2 hr after feeding.

B. **Parenteral Nutrition:** IV administration of a hypertonic intravenous solution made up of glucose, insulin, minerals, lipids, electrolytes, and other essential nutrients. Used when the client cannot effectively use the GI tract for nutrition.

1. Partial or peripheral parenteral nutrition (PPN)

   a. Used when client can eat, but cannot take in enough nutrients to meet needs

   b. Administered through a large distal arm vein or PICC line

2. Total parenteral nutrition (TPN)

   a. Used when the client requires intensive nutritional support for an extended time period

   b. Delivered through a central vein

3. Contributing Factors

   a. Gastrointestinal mobility disorders

   b. Inability to achieve or maintain adequate nutrition for body requirements

   c. Short bowel syndrome

   d. Chronic pancreatitis

   e. Severe burns

   f. Malabsorption disorders

4. Collaborative Care

   a. **Nursing Interventions**

      1) Confirm placement by chest x-ray.

      2) Monitor central line insertion site for local infection.

      3) Maintain strict surgical asepsis for dressing change (every 72 hr).

      4) Change tubing and remaining TPN every 24 hr.

      5) Monitor for signs of systemic infection.

      6) Monitor glucose, electrolytes, and fluid balance.

      7) Prevent air embolism.

      8) Use infusion pump.

      9) Keep 10% dextrose/water available.

      10) For clients receiving fat emulsions, monitor for fat overload syndrome: fever, increased triglycerides, clotting problems and multi-system organ failure. Discontinue infusion and notify provider immediately.

III Oral and Esophageal Disorders

A. **Dental caries**

1. An erosive process of the tooth that occurs when acid is formed by the action of bacteria on fermentable carbohydrates

2. Contributing Factors

   a. Dental plaque

   b. Poor oral hygiene

   c. Lack of fluoridated water

   d. High intake of refined carbohydrates

   e. Decrease in saliva

3. Manifestations

   a. Halitosis

   b. Tooth pain

   c. Tooth erosion, discoloring

4. Collaborative Care

   a. Nursing Interventions

      1) Reinforce teaching about preventive measures

         a) Brush teeth after eating

         b) Floss

         c) Increase intake of fresh fruits and vegetables, nuts, cheese, plain yogurt

         d) If water is not fluoridated, obtain from other source

         e) Dental sealants

         f) Twice-yearly dental cleaning and screening

B. **Salivary Gland, Oral Mucosa, and Pharyngeal Disorders**

1. Salivary glands consist of the parotid, submandibular, sublingual, and buccal glands. Disorders can affect lubrication, protection from harmful bacteria, and digestion. Disorders include candidiasis (thrush), parotitis, sialoadenitis, salivary calculus, stomatitis, and cancer.

2. Contributing factors
   a. Tobacco use
   b. Alcohol use disorder
   c. Aging
   d. Dehydration
   e. Radiation
   f. Stress
   g. Malnutrition
   h. Poor oral hygiene
   i. Immunosuppression

3. Manifestations
   a. Pain
   b. Cheesy white plaque (candidiasis)
   c. Inflammation and redness
   d. Persistent, painless oral lesion that does not heal (cancer)
   e. Xerostomia

4. Collaborative Care
   a. **Nursing Interventions**
      1) Monitor nutritional status. Refer to dietitian PRN.
      2) Monitor swallowing ability.
      3) Implement alternatives to oral communication PRN.
      4) Ensure adequate food and fluid intake.
      5) Perform and reinforce teaching about regular and thorough oral hygiene.
      6) Minimize pain.
      7) Monitor for indications of infection.
      8) Promote a positive self-image.

C. **Gastroesophageal Reflux Disease**

1. A condition in which the lower esophageal sphincter (LES) does not close properly, allowing stomach contents to back up into the esophagus.

2. Contributing Factors
   a. Obesity
   b. Smoking
   c. Heavy alcohol use
   d. Ingestion of very large meals
   e. Obstructive sleep apnea

3. Manifestations
   a. Dyspepsia
   b. Regurgitation
   c. Eructation
   d. Flatulence
   e. Coughing, hoarseness, wheezing
   f. Water brash
   g. Dysphagia
   h. Odynophagia

4. Collaborative Care
   a. **Nursing Interventions**
      1) Reinforce education about dietary management.
         a) Limit or eliminate foods that decrease LES pressure: chocolate, caffeine, fried and fatty foods, alcohol, carbonated beverages, and spicy and acidic foods.
         b) Consume four to six small meals per day..
         c) Eat slowly and chew thoroughly
         d) Eat nothing for at least 3 hr before going to bed.
      2) Client should elevate the head of bed 6 to 12 inches.
      3) Client should sleep on right side.
      4) Encourage client to participate in smoking- and alcohol-cessation programs PRN.
      5) Encourage maintenance of proper weight.
      6) Client should wear loose clothing.
      7) Medications
         a) Histamine blockers: famotidine (Pepcid), ranitidine (Zantac), cimetidine (Tagamet)
         b) Antacids
         c) Proton pump inhibitors: omeprazole (Prilosec), esomeprazole (Nexium), or pantoprazole (Protonix) may be administered IV short term
      8) Endoscopic procedures

D. **Hiatal Hernia**

1. A portion of the stomach protrudes through the esophageal hiatus of the diaphragm into the chest.

HIATAL HERNIA

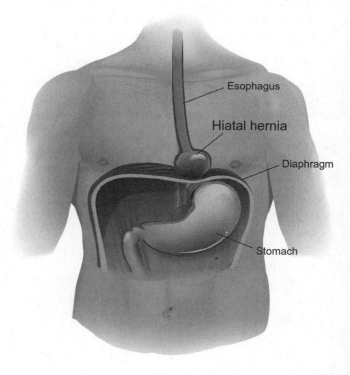

Esophagus

Hiatal hernia

Diaphragm

Stomach

ALLEN CROSWHITE
ASSESSMENT TECHNOLOGIES INSTITUTE

2. Contributing Factors

   a. High-fat diet

   b. Caffeinated beverages

   c. Tobacco products

   d. Medications: Ca⁺⁺ channel blockers, anticholinergics, nitrates

   e. Obesity

3. Manifestations

   a. Regurgitation

   b. Persistent heartburn and dysphagia

   c. Belching

   d. Epigastric pain

   e. Dysphagia

   f. Breathlessness or feeling of suffocation after eating

   g. Chest pain that mimics angina

   h. Symptoms that worsen after a meal or when supine

4. Collaborative Care

   a. **Nursing Interventions**

      1) Prepare for barium swallow with fluoroscopy.

      2) Collect data about diet history.

      3) Encourage small frequent meals.

      4) Avoid eating 3 hr prior to bedtime.

      5) Sit upright 1 to 2 hr after meals.

      6) Elevate head of bed.

      7) Encourage weight reduction for client's with BMI greater than 25.

      8) Avoid straining or vigorous exercise.

      9) Wear loose clothing around abdomen.

      10) Monitor for complications.

         a) Bleeding or esophageal ulcers

         b) Barrett's esophagus

         c) Aggravation of asthma, chronic cough, and pulmonary fibrosis

   b. Medications

      1) Antacids

      2) Histamine receptor antagonists

      3) Prokinetic agents

      4) Proton pump inhibitors

   c. Client Education

      1) Dietary medication regimen

      2) Precautions to prevent aspiration

   d. Therapeutic Measures

      1) Hiatal hernia—fundoplication if other measures ineffective

IV Gastrointestinal Disorders

A. **Peptic Ulcer Disease (PUD)**

   1. Ulcerations in the stomach or duodenum as a result of mucosal tissue destruction; high risk of perforation and bleeding. May be referred to as gastric, duodenal, or esophageal ulcer, depending on location.

   2. Contributing Factors

      a. NSAIDs

      b. Corticosteroids

      c. *H. pylori* infection

      d. Uncontrolled stress

      e. Smoking

      f. Caffeine

      g. Alcohol

      h. Type O blood

      i. Age 40 to 60 years

   3. Manifestations

      a. Dyspepsia

      b. Dull, gnawing, burning, mid-epigastric, and/or back pain with localized tenderness

      c. Symptoms worsen with empty stomach

      d. Relief noted with antacids

      e. Belching

      f. Bloating

      g. Vomiting of undigested food that may or may not be proceeded by nausea

      h. Melena

      i. Decreased hematocrit and hemoglobin

   4. Collaborative Care

      a. **Nursing Interventions**

         1) Refer to smoking- and alcohol-cessation programs PRN.

         2) Encourage stress-relieving techniques, such biofeedback, meditation, relaxation exercises.

         3) Reinforce teaching about dietary modifications.

            a) Avoid very cold and very hot foods.

            b) Eat three regular meals per day (small, frequent feedings are not necessary if an antacid or histamine blocker is taken).

            c) Avoid caffeine, alcohol, decaffeinated coffee, milk, and cream (diet is very individual—some may be able to tolerate these foods better than others).

         4) If other methods are not effective, prepare client for surgery (pyloroplasty, antrectomy).

b. Medications

   1) Triple therapy for 10 to 14 days: two antibiotics—metronidazole (Flagyl) or amoxicillin (Amoxil) and clarithromycin (Biaxin) plus a proton pump inhibitor (preferred treatment)

   2) Quadruple therapy that adds bismuth salts to the previous

   3) Mucosal healing agents

   4) Stool softeners

   5) Antacids

   6) Histamine receptor antagonists

   7) Prokinetic agents

   8) Proton pump inhibitors

c. Diagnostic Tests

   1) EGD

   2) Chest and abdominal x-ray

   3) Hematocrit and hemoglobin

   4) Stool specimen

d. Client Education

   1) Symptom management

   2) Medication therapy

   3) Nutrition therapy

   4) Stress reduction

B. **Irritable Bowel Syndrome (IBS)**

1. Chronic disorder with recurrent diarrhea, constipation, and/or abdominal pain and bloating (most common digestive disorder seen in clinical practice)

2. Contributing Factors

  a. Smoking

  b. Caffeine

  c. NSAIDs

  d. Stress

  e. Mental or behavioral illness

  f. High-fat diet

  g. Female gender

  h. Family history

  i. Dairy products

3. Manifestations

  a. Weight loss

  b. Fatigue and malaise

  c. Erratic bowel patterns

  d. Abdominal pain relieved by defecation

  e. Abdominal distention

  f. Mucus with passage of stool

  g. Colicky abdomen with diffuse tenderness

4. Collaborative Care

  a. **Nursing Interventions**

   1) Encourage a diet high in fiber.

   2) Encourage regular exercise such as walking and yoga.

   3) Reinforce teaching about stress-reduction techniques.

   4) Client should eat at regular times.

   5) Client should eat slowly and chew thoroughly.

   6) Reinforce teaching to consume adequate fluid intake but discourage fluids with meals.

   7) Encourage a food diary to identify triggers.

  b. Medications

   1) Bulk agents (e.g., psyllium [Metamucil])

   2) Antidiarrheals

   3) Antidepressants

   4) Anticholinergics

   5) Antispasmodics

   6) Probiotics

   7) Complementary agents

    a) Peppermint oil

    b) Artichoke leaf extract

    c) Caraway oil

  c. Diagnostic Tests

   1) Endoscopy

   2) Chest and abdominal x-ray

   3) Test for *H. pylori*

  d. Client Education

   1) Keeping diary to identify triggers

   2) Avoidance of causative agents

   3) Symptom management

   4) Medication therapy

   5) Nutrition therapy

   6) Stress reduction

C. **Inflammatory Bowel Disease**

> **KEY POINT:** Do not confuse inflammatory bowel disease with irritable bowel syndrome, which is much less severe. Inflammatory bowel disease is an autoimmune disorder that includes Crohn's disease and ulcerative colitis.

1. Crohn's Disease

  a. Inflammation of the GI tract that extends through all layers. It can occur anywhere in the intestinal tract, but most commonly occurs in the distal (terminal) ileum. It is characterized by the "cobblestone" appearance of ulcers that are separated by normal tissue.

CROHN'S DISEASE

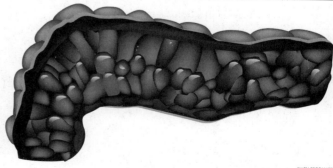

ALLEN CROSWHITE
ASSESSMENT TECHNOLOGIES INSTITUTE

b. Contributing Factors

1) Family history

2) Jewish ancestry

3) Bacterial infection

4) Smoking

5) Adolescents or young adults (ages 15 to 40)

6) Living in an urban area

c. Manifestations

1) Abdominal pain (right lower quadrant); does not resolve with defecation; pain is aggravated by eating

2) Low-grade fever

3) Diarrhea, steatorrhea

4) Weight loss (can become emaciated)

5) Formation of fistulas (abnormal tracts between bowel and skin/bladder or vagina)

6) Usually there is no bleeding (which helps differentiate from ulcerative colitis)

7) Low-grade fever, leukocytosis

8) Can be accompanied by arthritis, skin lesions, conjunctivitis, and/or oral ulcers

9) "String sign" on x-ray: indicates constriction in a segment of the terminal ileum

10) Decreased hematocrit and hemoglobin, elevated ESR

d. Collaborative Care

1) **Nursing Interventions**

a) Promote adequate rest periods.

b) Record color, volume, frequency, and consistency of stools.

c) Monitor and prevent fluid deficit.

d) Nutrition therapy includes high-calorie, high-protein, low-fiber, no dairy.

e) Provide supportive care.

f) Monitor for complications.

(1) Intestinal obstruction

(2) Perianal disease

(3) Fluid electrolyte imbalances

(4) Malnutrition

(5) Fistula, abscess

g) If the above measures are not effective, prepare for surgery: bowel resection with possible ileostomy or strictureplasty.

h) Encourage client to attend support group.

2) Medications

a) Steroids

b) Anti-infectives: metronidazole (Flagyl)

c) Aminosalicylates (5-ASAs)

d) Immune modulators: infliximab (Remicade), adalimumab (Humira), certolizumab (Cimzia), and natalizumab (Tysabri)

e) TPN

3) Therapeutic Measures

a) Bowel resection (possible ileostomy)

b) Strictureplasty

c) Laboratory profiles: Hct, hemoglobin, C-reactive protein, WBC, ESR

d) Abdominal x-ray

4) Client Education

a) Dietary

b) Health promotion and relaxation

2. Ulcerative Colitis

a. Recurrent ulcerative and inflammatory disease of the superficial mucosa of the colon. It usually begins in the rectum and spreads proximally through the entire colon. It is characterized by contiguous ulcers.

b. Contributing Factors

1) Family history

2) Jewish ancestry

3) Isotretinoin (Accutane) use

4) Young and middle-age adults (15 to 25 years; 55 to 65 years)

5) Caucasian ethnicity

c. Manifestations

1) Liquid, bloody stool (10 to 20 per day)

2) Low-grade fever

3) Abdominal distention along the colon

4) Rebound tenderness indicates perforation/peritonitis

5) Passage of mucous and pus from the bowel

6) Left, lower quadrant abdominal pain

7) Anorexia and weight loss

8) Vomiting and dehydration

9) Sensation of an urgent need to defecate

10) Hypocalcemia, anemia

11) Associated arthritis, conjunctivitis, skin lesions and/or liver problems

KEY POINT: Bleeding is common with ulcerative colitis. This helps differentiate it from Crohn's disease, in which bleeding is rare.

d. Collaborative Care

1) **Nursing Interventions**

a) Promote adequate rest periods.

b) Record color, volume, frequency, and consistency of stools.

c) Maintain NPO status during acute phase.

d) Monitor for dehydration. Maintain fluid balance.

e) Monitor electrolytes. IV fluids may be indicated for imbalances.

f) Provide dietary management and client education.

(1) Increase oral fluids.

(2) Low-residue, high-calorie, high-protein diet.

g) Administer multivitamin and supplemental iron.

h) Refer to support group.

i) If the above measures are not successful, prepare for surgery: proctocolectomy with ileostomy.

2) Medications

   a) Antidiarrheals (monitor for megacolon)

   b) Aminosalicylates (5-ASAs)

   c) Immune modulators: infliximab (Remicade), adalimumab (Humira), certolizumab (Cimzia), and natalizumab (Tysabri)

   d) TPN

   e) Corticosteroids (oral, parenteral, topical)

3) Therapeutic Measures

   a) Surgical management is indicated for bowel perforation, toxic megacolon, hemorrhage, and colon cancer.

     (1) Colectomy and ileostomy

     (2) Total proctocolectomy with permanent ileostomy

     (3) Laboratory profiles: Hct, hemoglobin, C-reactive protein, WBC, ESR

     (4) Abdominal x-ray

4) Client Education

   a) Support group

   b) Dietary

   c) Health promotion and relaxation

D. **Diverticular Disease**

1. Includes three conditions that involve numerous small sacs or pockets in the wall of the colon.

  a. Diverticulosis: the presence of pouchlike herniations (diverticula) along the wall of the intestines; most common in the Sigmoid colon

  b. Diverticular bleeding: results from injury of small vessels near the diverticula

  c. Diverticulitis: inflammation of one or more diverticula

2. Contributing Factors

  a. Aging

  b. Constipation

  c. Diet risk: low-fiber, high-fat, and red meat

  d. Connective tissue disorders causing weakness in the colon wall

3. Manifestations (Diverticulitis)

  a. Alternating diarrhea with constipation

  b. Painful cramps or tenderness in the lower abdomen (lower left quadrant)

  c. Chills or fever

4. Collaborative Care

  a. **Nursing Interventions**

   1) Dietary management

     a) Diverticulitis: Begin with clear liquids. Advance to a low-fiber diet.

     b) Diverticulosis: Provide a high-fiber diet.

     c) Review sources of dietary fiber.

     d) Avoid foods with nuts, seeds, or kernels (e.g., popcorn).

     e) Increase fluid intake to 3 L/day.

     f) Refer for nutritional counseling.

   2) Manage pain.

   3) Avoid laxatives.

   4) Monitor bowel elimination patterns.

   5) Monitor for complications (obstruction, hemorrhage, infection).

   6) In event of complications, prepare for surgery: colon resection.

  b. Medications

   1) Bulk laxatives (preventive)

   2) Metronidazole (Flagyl)

   3) Trimethoprim/sulfamethoxazole (Bactrim, Septra)

   4) Ciprofloxacin (Cipro)

   5) Antispasmodics (oxyphencyclimine [Daricon])

   6) Analgesics (meperidine [Demerol])

> **KEY POINT:** Morphine is contraindicated because it can increase pressure in the colon, exacerbating symptoms.

  c. Therapeutic Measures

   1) Emergency colon resection for peritonitis, bowel obstruction, or abscess

  d. Client Teaching

   1) High-fiber vs. low-fiber diet

   2) Collaborate with nutritionist

   3) Preventive measures

E. **Abdominal Hernia**

1. Protrusion of bowel through the muscle wall of abdominal cavity (umbilical, ventral, inguinal/femoral). Classified as reducible, irreducible, or strangulated.

> **KEY POINT:** Absent bowel sounds can indicate strangulation, which cuts off the blood supply to the bowel. This is a medical emergency that can result in ischemia and obstruction, leading to necrosis and perforation. Manifestations are abdominal distention, nausea, vomiting, pain, fever, and tachycardia.

FEMORAL HERNIA

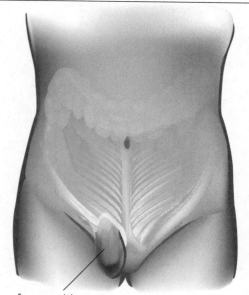

femoral hernia

ALLEN CROSWHITE
ASSESSMENT TECHNOLOGIES INSTITUTE

2. Contributing Factors

  a. Aging

  b. Male gender

  c. Obesity

  d. Heavy lifting or straining

  e. Abdominal surgery

  f. Pregnancy

  g. Congenital or acquired muscle weakness

  h. Ascites, distension

3. Manifestations

  a. Client reports "lump" felt at the involved site

  b. Pain in groin when bending, coughing, or lifting

  c. Absent bowel sounds (strangulated)

  d. Palpation of mass

4. Collaborative Care

  a. **Nursing Interventions**

    1) Wear abdominal binder for support of herniated tissue.

    2) Encourage increased fluid intake.

    3) Monitor for complications: strangulation, perforation.

    4) Prepare for surgery: minimally invasive inguinal hernia repair (MIIHR or herniorrhaphy) or laparoscopic repair, bowel resection for strangulation.

    5) Postsurgical care

      a) Allow to stand to void (males).

      b) For inguinal repair: elevate scrotum and apply ice.

      c) Client should avoid coughing during recovery period.

      d) Client should avoid lifting or straining for 4 to 6 weeks.

    6) Medications

      a) Analgesics

      b) Stool softeners

  b. Therapeutic Procedures

    1) Herniorrhaphy laparoscopic repair

  c. Client Education

    1) Avoid lifting for 4 to 6 weeks after surgery.

F. **Intestinal Obstruction**

1. Partial or complete blockage of intestinal contents that can be the result of mechanical obstruction (adhesions, tumors, volvulus), neurogenic (paralytic ileus), or vascular (mesenteric artery occlusion)

2. Etiologies: mechanical (adhesions, tumors, volvulus), neurogenic (paralytic ileus), or vascular (mesenteric artery occlusion)

3. Contributing Factors

  a. Crohn's disease

  b. Radiation therapy

  c. Fecal impaction

  d. Carcinomas

  e. Surgical procedures

  f. Narcotics

  g. Hypokalemia

  h. Diverticulitis

4. Manifestations

  a. Inability to pass flatus or stool for more than 8 hr

  b. Abdominal distention

  c. Hyperactive bowel sound above site of obstruction

  d. Hypoactive or active bowel sounds below site of obstruction

COMPARISON OF INTESTINAL OBSTRUCTION MANIFESTATIONS

Small Bowel	Large Intestine
Sporadic, colicky pain	Diffuse and constant pain
Visible peristaltic waves	Significant abdominal distention
Profuse, projectile vomitus with fecal odor (vomiting relieves pain)	Infrequent vomiting, leakage of fecal fluid around impaction

5. Collaborative Care

  a. **Nursing Interventions**

    1) NPO

    2) Monitor bowel sounds

    3) IV fluids

    4) Preoperative care

    5) NG tube for decompression

    6) Prevent fluid and electrolyte deficit

  b. Therapeutic Measures

    1) Abdominal x-rays

    2) Endoscopy

    3) CT scan

    4) Surgical intervention (remove obstruction, resection)

  c. Client Teaching

    1) Preventive measures based on etiology

    2) Diet

v Gastric Surgical Procedures

A. **Bariatric Surgery for Morbid Obesity**

1. Morbid obesity is more than 2 times ideal body weight, which places clients at high risk for multiple health problems. Bariatric surgery is performed when nonsurgical attempts at weight reduction fail. Methods include restrictive (gastric banding—reduces volume of the stomach) and malabsorptive (Roux-en-Y gastric bypass—interferes with food and nutrient absorption).

2. Indications for surgery

   a. BMI greater than 40

   b. BMI greater than 35 with other diseases

   c. Repeated failure of nonsurgical weight reduction

3. Collaborative Care

   a. **Nursing Interventions**

      1) Preoperative care

         a) Ensure thorough psychological preparation

         b) Reinforce teaching: diet of liquids and pureed foods for first 6 weeks

         c) Reinforce healthy lifestyle changes

         d) Ensure support systems are available

      2) Postoperative care

         a) Immediate priority is airway.

         b) Ensure abdominal binder is in place.

         c) Place in semi-Fowler's position.

         d) Assist client to ambulate as soon as able, the day of surgery.

         e) Measure and compare abdominal girth. Listen for bowel sounds.

         f) Collaborate with dietitian to introduce six small feedings per day. Begin with 1 oz servings of clear liquids. Increase amount as tolerated.

         g) Monitor for manifestations of dumping syndrome (tachycardia, nausea, diarrhea, abdominal cramping, diaphoresis) and anastomotic leak

> **KEY POINT:** Anastomotic leaks are the most common complication and can be life-threatening. Monitor for increasing back, shoulder, and abdominal pain; restlessness; tachycardia; oliguria. Report to provider immediately.

      3) Medications

         a) Analgesics

         b) Antispasmodics

         c) Multi-vitamin

      4) Long-term management

         a) To prevent dumping syndrome: eat slowly; avoid drinking liquids with meals, after beginning solid foods; avoid high-fat foods, refined carbohydrates, and sugar; lie flat with head slightly elevated for 1 hr after eating.

         b) Encourage increase in physical activity

         c) Provide ongoing psychological support

B. **Colostomy:** A surgical procedure that brings the end of the colon through the abdominal wall, creating an opening for the evacuation of fecal material. Can be temporary or permanent.

1. Indications

   a. Cancer or tumors

   b. Obstructive bowel disease

   c. Colectomy

   d. Severe diverticulitis or Crohn's disease

   e. Trauma

2. Collaborative Care

   a. **Nursing Interventions**

      1) Monitor ostomy site.

      2) Monitor output from stoma. (The higher an ostomy is placed in the small intestine, the more liquid and acidic the output will be.)

      3) Empty ostomy bag when ¼ to ½ full.

      4) Fit appliance to prevent leakage.

      5) Monitor for complications: fluid and electrolyte imbalances, ischemia of ostomy; bleeding, infection, peristomal skin irritation.

      6) Offer emotional support.

      7) Encourage attendance at a support group.

   b. Client Education

      1) Reinforce teaching how to fit, care for, and change appliance.

      2) Collaborate with ostomy nurse for additional teaching.

      3) A breath mint may be placed in bag to reduce odor.

      4) Dietary management

         a) Client should avoid hard-to-digest foods, such as nuts, popcorn, celery, seeds, and coconut.

         b) Client should maintain adequate fluid intake.

         c) Client should reintroduce foods one at a time.

         d) Identify foods that can contribute to odor and gas: cruciferous vegetables, asparagus.

vi Hepatic Disorders

A. **Cirrhosis:** A chronic disease characterized by extensive, irreversible scarring of the liver that disrupts structure and function. — liver failure

1. Contributing Factors

   a. Alcohol consumption (Laennec's)

   b. Postnecrotic (hepatitis, chemicals)

   c. Biliary disease

   d. Severe right-sided heart failure

2. Manifestations

   a. Early stage

      1) Enlarged liver

      2) Jaundice

      3) Gastrointestinal disturbances

      4) Weight loss

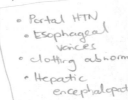

- Portal HTN
- Esophageal varices
- clotting abnorm.
- Hepatic encephalopathy
- Ascites / peritonitis
- Altered nutrient + vitamin metabolism

b. Late stage

  1) Liver becomes smaller and nodular

  2) Splenomegaly

  3) Ascites, distended abdominal veins; increased pressure in the portal system

  4) Bleeding tendencies; decreased vitamin K and prothrombin; anemia

  5) Esophageal varices; internal hemorrhoids; increased pressure in the portal area

  6) Dyspnea from ascites and anemia

  7) Pruritus from dry skin

  8) Clay-colored stools; no bile in stool

  9) Tea-colored urine; bile in urine

c. End stage

  1) Prodromal: slurred speech, vacant stare, restlessness, neurological deterioration

  2) Impending: asterixis (flapping tremors), apraxia, lethargy, confusion

  3) Stuporous: marked mental confusion, somnolence

  4) Coma: unarousable, fetor hepaticus, seizures, high mortality rate

3. Collaborative Care

a. **Nursing Interventions**

  1) Encourage rest.

  2) Weigh the client daily and measure abdominal girth.

  3) Monitor skin integrity frequently. — *paracentesis assist*

  4) Monitor I&O.

  5) Monitor for bleeding and hemorrhoids. — *Bleeding percautions*

  6) Avoid hepatotoxic medications.

  7) Maintain a high-calorie, low-protein (20 to 40 g/day), low-fat, low-sodium diet. (Maintain protein restriction during stages I and II of encephalopathy; no protein allowed during stages III and IV.)

  8) Limit sodium and fluid intake as prescribed.

  9) Monitor liver enzymes, bilirubin, hematologic testing: CBC, WBC, platelets, PT/INR, and ammonia levels.

b. Medications

  1) Diuretics: spironolactone (Aldactone), furosemide (Lasix)

  2) Neomycin and metronidazole (Flagyl): reduces intestinal bacteria

  3) Lactulose (Chronulac): decreases ammonia levels.

  4) Supplemental vitamins (B_1 and B complex; A, C, and K; folic acid; and thiamine) as prescribed

  5) Fat-soluble vitamin supplements and folic acid might need to be given IV

  6) Proton pump inhibitors and H_2 receptor antagonist

  7) Albumin IV to decrease ascites

c. Therapeutic Measures

  1) Liver biopsy

  2) EGD

  3) Paracentesis

  4) Transjugular intrahepatic portosystemic shunt (TIPS)

d. Client Education

  1) Alcohol abstinence

  2) Dietary guidelines

  3) Bleeding risk and precautions

4. Referral and Follow-up

a. Alcohol recovery program

b. Nutrition

c. Social services

B. **Hepatitis**

1. Inflammation of the liver caused by infectious organisms, chemicals, or toxins. Cases must be reported to the local health department.

CHARACTERISTICS OF HEPATITIS

Mode of transmission

TYPE A (HAV)	Fecal-oral route Person-to-person	Food contamination
TYPE B (HBV)	Unprotected sex Sharing needles Needlesticks	Blood products; organ transplant before 1992
TYPE C (HCV)	Blood-to-blood Illicit IV drug sharing	Blood products; organ transplant before 1992

Manifestations

TYPE A (HAV)	Mild course "Flu-like" Advanced age and chronic disease increase severity	
TYPE B (HBV)	May be asymptomatic RUQ pain Anorexia, N/V Fatigue	Febrile Dark urine Light-colored stool Jaundice
TYPE C (HCV)	Most are asymptomatic Diagnosis with blood testing Chronic inflammation progresses to cirrhosis	

Prevention

TYPE A (HAV)	Hand hygiene Vaccine for ages 2 and older Two doses 6 to 18 months apart
TYPE B (HBV)	Vaccine infants and high-risk populations Three doses during 6-month period
TYPE C (HCV)	Avoid high-risk behaviors

Treatment

TYPE A (HAV)	Symptom-specific May have change in medication regimen to "rest liver"
TYPE B (HBV)	Antiviral drugs
TYPE C (HCV)	Administer peginterferon-alpha 2B (PegIntron) Monitor kidney function

C. **Nonviral Hepatitis**

1. Definition: liver injury and inflammation caused by ingestion of drugs and chemicals (industrial toxins, alcohol, drugs)

2. Contributing Factors

   a. Inhalation of hepatotoxic agents

   b. Drug toxicity

   c. Alcohol

   d. Secondary infection can occur with Epstein-Barr, herpes simplex, varicella-zoster, and cytomegalovirus

3. Manifestations

   a. Jaundice

   b. Liver enlargement

   c. Liver necrosis

4. Collaborative Care

   a. Monitor signs of liver impairment.

   b. Monitor client for right upper quadrant pain.

   c. Monitor weight.

   d. Treatment is specific to symptoms and causative factors.

D. **Gallbladder Disease**

1. Types

   a. Cholecystitis: Inflammation of the gallbladder

   b. Cholelithiasis: Presence of stones in the gallbladder

2. Contributing Factors

   a. Female gender

   b. Age older than 40

   c. Overweight

   d. High consumption of cholesterol, fat

   e. Sedentary lifestyle

   f. Family history

   g. Diabetes mellitus

   h. American Indian ethnicity

3. Manifestations

   a. Right upper quadrant, epigastric, or shoulder pain

   b. Nausea and vomiting

   c. Dietary fat intolerance

   d. Murphy's sign

   e. Jaundice with pruritus; icterus

   f. Flatulence

   g. Dyspepsia

   h. Dark urine, clay-colored stool

4. Diagnostic Procedures

   a. Ultrasound

   b. Hepatobiliary scan

   c. Endoscopic retrograde cholangiopancreatography (ERCP)

   d. Cholangiography

5. Collaborative Care

   a. **Nursing Interventions**

      1) Administer analgesics as prescribed.

      2) Prevent F&E imbalances.

      3) Maintain low-fat diet.

      4) Provide postoperative care.

      5) Cholecystectomy client may have T-tube.

         a) Monitor drainage; keep below level of GB.

         b) Empty collection bag every 8 hr.

         c) Report drainage amounts greater than 1,000 mL/day.

         d) Never irrigate without physician order.

      6) Observe color of stool.

      7) Monitor for indications of postcholecystectomy syndrome (manifestations of cholecystitis after surgery) and report to physician.

   b. Medications

      1) Analgesics: morphine, hydromorphone (Dilaudid), ketorolac

> **KEY POINT:** Meperidine (Demerol) is contraindicated for acute biliary pain. It breaks down into a toxic metabolite that can cause seizures, especially in older adults.

      2) Antiemetics

      3) Anticholinergics

      4) Ursodeoxycholic acid (Urso, Actigall) and chenodiol (Chenix) can be used to nonsurgically dissolve stones

      5) Antibiotics

   c. Therapeutic Measures

      1) Sphincterotomy with stone removal may be done with ERCP

      2) Extracorporeal shock wave lithotripsy (ESWL) to break up stones (only for small cholesterol stones)

      3) Cholecystectomy

   d. Client Education

      1) Resume regular low-fat diet.

      2) Prevent dumping syndrome.

      3) Care of T-tube at home.

VII Pancreatic Disorders

A. **Acute Pancreatitis**

1. Inflammation of the pancreas caused by autodigestion by exocrine enzymes. It is life-threatening.

B. **Chronic Pancreatitis:** Progressive disease of the pancreas characterized by remissions and exacerbations resulting in diminished function

1. Contributing Factors

   a. Alcohol use disorder

   b. Gallstones

   c. Illegal drug use

   d. Infection

   e. Blunt abdominal trauma

   f. Operative manipulation and trauma

2. Manifestations
   a. Severe midepigastric or left upper quadrant pain
   b. Pain intensifies after meals and when lying down
   c. Nausea and vomiting
   d. Abdominal tenderness
   e. Elevated amylase and lipase
   f. Steatorrhea
   g. Turner's sign
   h. Cullen's sign
3. Diagnostic Procedures
   a. Laboratory profiles: liver enzymes, bilirubin, pancreatic enzymes
   b. CT scan with contrast
4. Collaborative Care

   a. **Nursing Interventions**
      1) Dietary management.
         a) NPO initially.
         b) After 24 to 48 hr, begin jejunal feedings.
         c) When food is tolerated, advance to small, frequent, moderate- to high-carbohydrate, high-protein, low-fat meals.
      2) Nasogastric tube for the severely ill, with intractable vomiting or biliary obstruction.
      3) Pain management.
      4) Position for comfort (fetal, sitting up, leaning forward).
      5) Monitor bowel sounds.
      6) I&O.
      7) Monitor for indications of hypocalcemia and hypomagnesemia.
      8) Monitor respirations.
      9) Reassure clients, and carefully explain procedures to reduce anxiety.
   b. Medications
      1) Antibiotics
      2) Opioid analgesics: morphine or hydromorphone (Dilaudid); **meperidine (Demerol) is contraindicated**
      3) Anticholinergics
      4) Pancreatic enzymes
      5) H_2 blockers or proton pump inhibitors
   c. Therapeutic Measures
      1) TPN
      2) ERCP to create an opening in sphincter of Oddi if cause is gallstones
      3) Cholecystectomy
      4) Pancreaticojejunostomy (Roux-en-Y) to "reroute" pancreatic secretions to the jejunum
   d. Client Education for Chronic Pancreatitis
      1) Take enzymes before meals and snacks.
      2) Follow up with all scheduled laboratory testing.
      3) Nutrition: high caloric needs.
      4) Abstain from alcohol.
      5) Limit fat intake.

5. Referral and Follow-up
   a. Alcohol recovery program.
   b. Home health for clients requiring long-term TPN.
   c. Collaborate with a dietitian.

C. **Pancreatic Cancer**
1. Carcinoma has vague symptoms and is usually diagnosed in late stages after liver or gallbladder involvement.
2. Contributing Factors
   a. Older adults
   b. Tobacco use
   c. Chronic pancreatitis
   d. Diabetes mellitus
   e. Cirrhosis
   f. High intake of red meat, processed meat
   g. Obesity
   h. Small number have an inherited risk
3. Manifestations
   a. Fatigue, anorexia, flatulence
   b. Pruritus
   c. Weight loss, palpable abdominal mass, abdominal pain that can radiate to the back
   d. Hepatomegaly, jaundice (late sign when cancer blocks the bile duct)
   e. Ascites
   f. Clay-colored stools; dark urine
   g. Glucose intolerance
4. Diagnostic Procedures
   a. Carcinoembryonic antigen (CEA) levels
      1) Expected findings: less than 2.5 ng/mL nonsmoker; less than 5 ng/mL smoker
      2) Critical findings: greater than 6 ng/mL
   b. Elevated serum amylase and lipase
   c. Elevated alkaline phosphatase and bilirubin
   d. ERCP
   e. Ultrasound, CT scan
5. Collaborative Care
   a. **Nursing Interventions**
      1) Palliative care measures.
      2) Pain management.
      3) Monitor blood glucose levels.
      4) Provide nutritional support (enteral supplements and TPN).
   b. Medications
      1) Opioid analgesics: morphine or hydromorphone (Dilaudid)
   c. Therapeutic Measures
      1) Chemotherapy may be used to shrink the tumor size. The nurse monitors for myelosuppression and pancytopenia.
      2) Radiation therapy
      3) Partial pancreatectomy for small tumors

4) Whipple procedure: Pancreatoduodenectomy is the most common operation to remove (resect) pancreatic cancers. Procedure done when cancer is located in the head of the pancreas. Involves removing the head of the pancreas, duodenum, parts of the jejunum and stomach, gallbladder, and possibly spleen. The pancreatic duct is reconnected to the common bile duct, and the stomach is connected to the jejunum. May be done laparoscopically.

   a) Nursing interventions

      (1) Provide routine postoperative care.

      (2) Monitor NG output. Observe for bloody or bile-tinged drainage, which can indicate anastomotic disruption.

      (3) Maintain a semi-Fowler's position to prevent stress on suture line.

      (4) Facilitate coughing and deep breathing and use of incentive spirometer.

      (5) Monitor blood glucose and administer insulin as needed.

      (6) Provide analgesia.

d. Client Education

   1) Encourage client to seek palliative care at home, cancer support group, and available community resources.

   2) Support measures for pain, anorexia and weight loss.

SECTION 5

Disorders of the Musculoskeletal System

I Diagnostic Tests for Musculoskeletal Disorders

A. **Bone Scan:** Radioactive medium is injected for viewing entire skeleton, primarily to detect tumors, arthritis, osteomyelitis, osteoporosis, vertebral compression fractures, and unexplained bone pain.

   1. Technician or physician administers the isotope 4 to 6 hr prior to testing.

   2. Client must lie still for 30 to 60 min as imaging is performed.

   3. Increase fluids post procedures.

B. **Dual-Energy X-ray Absorptiometry (DEXA) Scan:** Most common screening tool for measuring bone mineral density for diagnosis of osteopenia and osteoporosis

   1. Baseline for women in their 40s.

   2. Client should wear loose clothing without zippers or metal.

   3. Client must remove jewelry.

   4. Instruct client to stop vitamin D and calcium supplementation 48 hr prior to scan.

C. **Electromyography (EMG) and Nerve Conduction Studies:** Used to evaluate muscle weakness by emission of low-frequency electrical stimulation

   1. Client will be asked to perform activities for measurement of muscle activity.

   2. Observe needle insertion sites for hematoma.

   3. Support client with anxiety related to testing.

D. **Magnetic Resonance Imaging (MRI):** Imaging produced through interaction of magnetic fields, radio waves, and atomic nuclei to diagnose muscle, tissue, and bone disorders

   1. Client must remove all metal objects (inquire about surgical implanted devices, nonvisible piercings). Canes, crutches, and walkers generally must be left outside of the MRI room. Assist client as necessary to stretcher.

   2. Contraindicated for clients who have pacemakers, stents, and surgical clips.

   3. Clients who have titanium joint replacements may have MRI.

   4. Ask client about history of claustrophobia if closed scanner is used.

   5. Verify that client can lie still in supine position for 45 to 60 min.

E. **Laboratory**

   1. Serum calcium

   2. Serum phosphorus

   3. Alkaline phosphatase

   4. Creatine kinase

   5. Lactic dehydrogenase

   6. Aspartate aminotransferase

   7. Aldolase

II Arthritis

Inflammation of one or more joints, which results in pain, swelling, stiffness, and limited movement

A. **Osteoarthritis:** Progressive deterioration and loss of cartilage in one or more joints

   1. Contributing Factors

      a. Aging

      b. Female gender

      c. Metabolic disease

      d. Obesity

      e. Repetitive use or abuse of joints

      f. Smoking

   2. Manifestations

      a. Chronic joint pain and stiffness

      b. Pain diminished after rest and worsens after activity

      c. Crepitus

      d. Limited movement

      e. Heberden's nodes (closest to end of fingers and toes)

      f. Bouchard's nodes (middle joints of fingers or toes)

      g. Excess joint fluid (especially with knee involvement)

      h. Skeletal muscle atrophy from disuse

ARTHRITIS MANIFESTATIONS

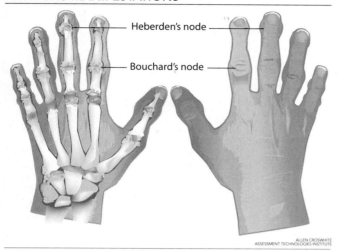

Heberden's node

Bouchard's node

ALLEN CROSWHITE
ASSESSMENT TECHNOLOGIES INSTITUTE

3. Diagnostic Procedures

a. X-rays

b. MRI

c. Erythrocyte sedimentation rate (ESR) and serum C-reactive protein (CRP) show slight elevation

4. Collaborative Care

a. **Nursing Interventions**

1) Monitor and manage pain.

2) Client may use ice or heat for comfort.

3) Encourage client to perform range of motion and isometric exercises.

4) Encourage adequate rest and sleep as needed to relieve pain.

5) Involve physical therapy as appropriate.

6) Use assistive devices to help increase independence and complete activities of daily living.

b. Medications

1) NSAIDs

2) Corticosteroids

3) Topical analgesics

c. Therapeutic Measures

1) Total joint arthroplasty

2) Total joint replacement

d. Client Education

1) Use of mobility devices and safety

2) Prevention of complications

3) Performing exercises per treatment plan

5. Referral and Follow-up

a. Physical therapy

b. Rehabilitation therapy

B. **Rheumatoid Arthritis:** Chronic, progressive autoimmune connective tissue disorder primarily affecting synovial joints

1. Contributing Factors

a. Physical and emotional stress

b. Female gender

c. Young to middle age

d. Family history

2. Manifestations

a. Morning stiffness and pain

b. Bilateral joint inflammation with decreased range of motion

c. Joint deformity in late stages

d. Warmth, redness, and edema of affected areas

e. Dry eyes and mouth (Sjögren's syndrome)

f. Numbness, tingling, or burning in the hands and feet

3. Diagnostic Procedures

a. X-ray

b. MRI

c. Positive rheumatoid factor

d. Synovial fluid analysis

e. Antinuclear antibody test

f. Erythrocyte sedimentation rate

g. C-reactive protein

4. Collaborative Care

a. **Nursing Interventions**

1) Client may use ice or heat for comfort.

2) Encourage physical activity to maintain joint mobility (within client's capacity).

3) Monitor client for indications of fatigue.

4) Monitor for complications related to therapy (secondary osteoporosis, vasculitis).

5) Complementary therapies

a) Hypnosis

b) Imagery

c) Acupuncture

d) Music therapy

e) Omega-3

f) Tai chi

b. Medications

1) NSAIDs

2) Corticosteroids

3) Disease-modifying antirheumatic drugs (DMARDs)

a) Methotrexate (Rheumatrex)

b) Leflunomide (Arava)

c) Hydroxychloroquine (Plaquenil)

4) Biologic-response modifiers (administered parenterally)

a) Etanercept (Enbrel)

b) Adalimumab (Humira)

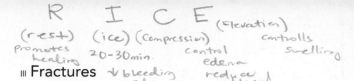

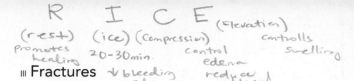

R I C E (elevation)
(rest) (ice) (compression) controlls
promotes 20-30min. control swelling
healing ↓bleeding edema reduce
edema bleed

c. Therapeutic Measures
   1) Plasmapheresis for severe, life-threatening exacerbation
   2) Synovectomy
   3) Total joint arthroplasty if unresponsive to medication
d. Client Education
   1) Use of mobility devices and safety
   2) Prevention of complications
   3) Perform exercises per treatment plan
5. Referral and Follow-up
   a. Occupational/physical therapy
   b. Rehabilitation therapy
   c. Arthritis support group

C. **Gouty Arthritis:** Systemic inflammatory disease caused by problems with purine metabolism (primary gout) or hyperuricemia (secondary gout)
   1. Contributing Factors
      a. Family history
      b. Excessive alcohol intake
      c. High intake of foods with purines (organ meats, yeast, sardines, spinach)
      d. Obesity
      e. Comorbid conditions of DM and/or kidney disease
   2. Manifestations
      a. Excruciating pain and inflammation in one or more small joints (great toe is most common joint; appears warm and red)
      b. Appearance of tophi (deposits of sodium urate crystals; generally appear after years of gouty arthritis)
      c. Progressive joint damage and deformity
      d. Increased incidence of uric acid renal stone
   3. Diagnostic Procedures
      a. Serum uric acid greater than 7 mg/dL
      b. ESR
      c. Synovial fluid analysis (will show uric acid crystals)
   4. Collaborative Care
      a. **Nursing Interventions**
         1) Maintain bed rest during acute attacks.
         2) Use bed cradle to keep linen elevated above affected joint.
         3) Promote fluid intake 3 L/day.
         4) Limit foods high in purine.
      b. Medications
         1) Acute phase: colchicine
         2) Chronic treatment: allopurinol
         3) NSAIDs
         4) Corticosteroids
         5) Injection of corticosteroid into affected joint by provider
      c. Client Education
         1) Foods to avoid (high in purine).
         2) Client should keep diary of triggering factors.
         3) Avoid alcohol.
         4) Lose weight slowly. (Rapid weight loss can precipitate a flare-up or increase the incidence of uric acid kidney stones.)

III **Fractures**
A break or disruption in the continuity of bone tissue

cold/heat applicats
*need order

A. **Types of Fractures**
   1. Closed
   2. Comminuted (fragmented)
   3. Compression
   4. Displaced
   5. Greenstick
   6. Impacted
   7. Oblique
   8. Open (compound)
   9. Pathologic (tumors, infection, bone disease)
   10. Spiral
   11. Stress (small crack in bone)

TYPES OF BONE FRACTURES

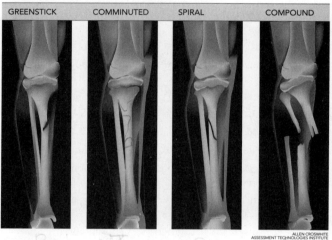

GREENSTICK COMMINUTED SPIRAL COMPOUND

ALLEN CROSWHITE
ASSESSMENT TECHNOLOGIES INSTITUTE

R I C E

B. **Collaborative Care**
   1. Monitor client's neurovascular status (6 P's), noting bilateral comparisons.
      a. Pain
      b. Pressure
      c. Paralysis
      d. Pallor
      e. Pulselessness
      f. Paresthesia

   Compartment Syndrome
   - pain w/ PROM

   2. Monitor for changes in skin temperature.
   3. Monitor for complications of fat embolism (most common with long bone fractures):
      a. Confusion, anxiety
      b. Tachycardia
      c. Tachypnea
      d. Hemoptysis
      e. Petechiae over neck, upper arms, chest, abdomen (late sign)

4. Monitor for complications of compartment syndrome (irreversible if compromise persists beyond 4 to 6 hr).

   a. Pain unrelieved by positioning or medication

   b. Cyanosis

   c. Tingling

   d. Paralysis

   − Monitor 6 P's
   − Position extremity @ ∅ level
   − Open / bivalve cast

5. Maintain correct body alignment.

6. Provide nursing care specific to therapeutic measures of fracture reduction.

C. **Therapeutic Measures**

   1. Cast: application of plaster or fiberglass to immobilize and maintain alignment of the bone

      a. Collaborative Care

         1) Monitor neurovascular status.

         2) Allow plaster cast to air dry. Handle cast with palms while drying.

         3) Elevate affected extremity.

         4) Monitor for complications.

         5) Client may "petal" plaster cast if irritation around edges develops.

         6) To help reduce risk of infection, remind client to not place objects down cast.

2. Traction

   a. Skin traction: provides a mechanical pulling force to overcome muscle spasms, to immobilize or relieve pain

      1) Buck's

      2) Bryant's

      3) Cervical halter

      4) Pelvic

   b. Skeletal traction: applied directly to a bone to reduce a fracture or maintain surgically manipulated bone alignment

      1) Pins or wires inserted through skin and soft tissue into the bone

      2) Balanced suspension using splints, slings, weights

D. **External Fixation Device:** Rigid metal frames with attached percutaneous pins or wires used to align and immobilize

   1. Collaborative Care

      a. Monitor pulses and vascular status.

      b. Maintain proper body alignment.

      c. Verify weights are free hanging.

      d. Monitor skin for pressure points or breakdown.

      e. Promote strengthening exercises for uninjured areas.

      f. Consult with physical therapy.

EXTERNAL FIXATION DEVICES

CERVICAL TRACTION

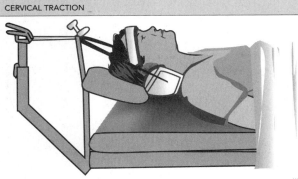

ALLEN CROSWHITE
ASSESSMENT TECHNOLOGIES INSTITUTE

BUCK'S TRACTION

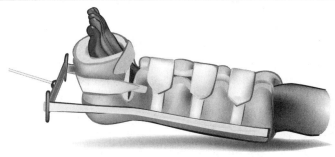

ALLEN CROSWHITE
ASSESSMENT TECHNOLOGIES INSTITUTE

BALANCED SUSPENSION SKELETAL TRACTION

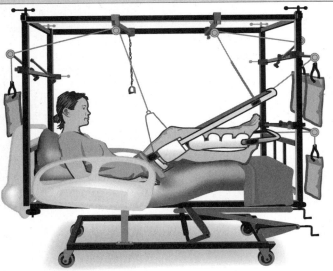

ALLEN CROSWHITE
ASSESSMENT TECHNOLOGIES INSTITUTE

HALO TRACTION

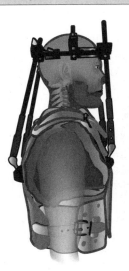
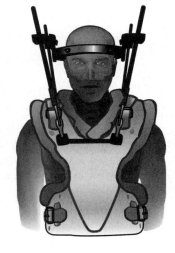

ALLEN CROSWHITE
ASSESSMENT TECHNOLOGIES INSTITUTE

IV Osteoporosis

Chronic disease in which bone loss causes decreased density and possible fracture. Osteopenia is the precursor of osteoporosis.

A. **Contributing Factors**

1. Primary Osteoporosis

   a. Women age 65 and older

   b. Men age 75 and older

   c. Asian and Caucasian ethnicity

   d. Family history

   e. Estrogen or androgen deficiency

   f. Protein deficiency

   g. Sedentary lifestyle

   h. Smoking and alcohol intake

2. Secondary Osteoporosis

   a. Bone cancer

   b. Cushing's syndrome

   c. Diabetes mellitus

   d. Medications: corticosteroids, phenytoin, cytotoxic agents, immunosuppressants, loop diuretics

   e. Paget's disease

   f. Prolonged immobilization

   g. Rheumatoid arthritis

B. **Manifestations**

1. Shortened height

2. History of fractures

3. Thoracic kyphosis

4. Decreased bone mass

C. **Collaborative Care**

1. **Nursing Interventions**

   a. Encourage safe weight-bearing exercises.

   b. Reinforce teaching about strengthening exercises; encourage walking.

   c. Client should increase foods rich in calcium and vitamin D.

   d. Client can benefit from smoking cessation program if applicable.

   e. Implement fall precautions.

2. Medications

   a. Bisphosphonates

   b. Calcium supplements

   c. Vitamin D supplements

   d. Estrogen agonists/antagonists

   e. Calcitonin

   f. Parathyroid hormone (prepared as teriparatide [Forteo]): teach to administer subcutaneously each day

3. Client Education

   a. Client should continue health screenings and diagnostic evaluations.

   b. Client should avoid activities with increased risk of falls (ice, slippery surfaces).

   c. Client should take medications as prescribed.

V Osteomyelitis

An acute or chronic bone infection

A. **Contributing Factors**

1. Diabetes

2. Hemodialysis

3. Injection drug use

4. Poor blood supply

5. Recent trauma

B. **Manifestations**

1. Bone pain

2. Fever

3. General discomfort, uneasiness, or ill feeling (malaise)

4. Local swelling, redness, and warmth

5. Other possible manifestations

   a. Chills

   b. Excessive sweating

   c. Low-back pain

   d. Swelling of the ankles, feet, and legs

C. **Diagnostic Procedures**

1. Bone biopsy (which is then cultured)

2. Bone scan

3. Bone x-ray

4. Complete blood count (CBC)

5. CRP

6. ESR

7. MRI of the bone

8. Needle aspiration of the area around affected bones

D. **Collaborative Care**

1. **Nursing Interventions**

   a. Initiate IV antibiotic therapy as soon as possible.

   b. In the presence of wound drainage, implement contact precautions.

   c. The full course of antibiotics must be completed, even if manifestations disappear.

   d. Implement wound irrigation.

   e. Refer to wound care nurse as needed.

2. Medications

   a. Antibiotics

   b. Analgesics

3. Therapeutic Measures

   a. Surgical excision of dead and infected bone can be needed.

   b. Bone grafting may be performed in large impacted areas.

VI Total Joint Arthroplasty (Replacement)

Surgical procedure performed to replace a joint with a prosthetic system. Arthroplasty may be performed for ankle, finger, elbow, shoulder, toe, and wrist. The hip and knee arthroplasties are the most commonly performed procedures.

KNEE REPLACEMENT

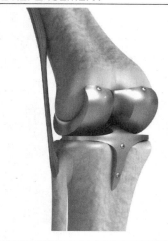

ALEXANDR MITIUC
GETTY IMAGES/ISTOCKPHOTO

A. **Contributing Factors**

1. Impaired mobility and uncontrolled pain related to osteoarthritis

2. Congenital anomalies

3. Trauma

4. Osteonecrosis

B. **Collaborative Care**

1. **Nursing Interventions**

a. Position client correctly, maintaining alignment.

1) Hip arthroplasty: keep abductor pillow in place while in bed; do not flex hip more than 90°

2) Knee arthroplasty: maintain continue passive motion (CPM) machine to promote joint mobility

b. Monitor for pain, rotation, and extremity shortening.

c. Monitor neurovascular status.

d. Use aseptic technique for wound care and emptying of drains.

e. Monitor for indications of infection.

f. Ambulate the day of surgery, after stabilization and discharge from PACU.

g. Use toilet seat extender.

h. Reinforce teaching about exercises to reduce risk of DVT: ankle dorsiflexion, circles with the feet, push feet into bed while tightening quads, and straight-leg raises.

2. Medications

a. Anticoagulants

b. NSAIDs

c. Opioid narcotics; extended-release epidural morphine or PCA

3. Client Education

a. Client should participate in exercise regimen.

b. Reinforce teaching about use of ambulatory devices.

C. **Referral and Follow-up**

1. Physical therapy for ambulation, transfer, and joint movement

2. Occupational therapy to meet goals of independence and self-care

VII Amputations

Removal of a part of the body; can be elective or traumatic

A. **Types of Amputations**

1. Above-the-knee

2. Below-the-knee

3. Mid-foot

4. Toe

B. **Contributing Factors**

1. Peripheral vascular disease

2. Severe crushing of tissues or significant vessels

3. Malignant tumors

4. Osteomyelitis

C. **Collaborative Care**

1. **Nursing Interventions**

a. Monitor neurovascular status.

b. Monitor psychosocial status.

c. Monitor client's willingness and motivation to withstand prolonged rehabilitation.

d. Manage phantom limb and residual limb pain.

e. Monitor for signs of wound healing.

f. Monitor for complications.

1) Hemorrhage

2) Infection

3) Phantom limb pain

4) Flexion contractures

g. Promote mobility and range of motion.

h. Promote independence.

i. Maintain aseptic technique with dressing changes.

j. Wrap stump with figure-8 elastic bandage after surgical dressing is removed.

FIGURE-8 BANDAGE

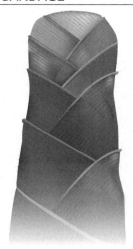

ALLEN CROSWHITE
ASSESSMENT TECHNOLOGIES INSTITUTE

2. Medications

   a. Opioids for residual limb pain

   b. Calcitonin to reduce phantom pain

   c. Antispasmodics for muscle spasms

   d. Beta blockers for constant, dull, burning pain

   e. Antiepileptic drugs for knifelike or sharp burning pain

3. Client Education

   a. Types of pain and management regimen

   b. Measures to prevent contractures

   c. Use of ambulatory devices or prosthetics

D. **Referral and Follow-up**

1. Rehabilitation therapy

2. Support group

SECTION 6

Endocrine System Functions and Disorders

Overview of the endocrine system: The endocrine system is made up of glands, organs, and hormones. The endocrine system works with the nervous system to regulate body function and maintain homeostasis through feedback loops. Endocrine glands include the hypothalamus, pituitary gland, adrenal glands, thyroid gland, parathyroid glands, islet cells of the pancreas, and gonads.

I Pituitary Gland

A. **Anterior pituitary gland**: secretion of these hormones is controlled by the hypothalamus.

1. Adrenocorticotropic hormone (ACTH)

2. Follicle-stimulating hormone (FSH)

3. Luteinizing hormone (LH)

4. Gonadotropic hormones

5. Prolactin

6. Growth hormone (GH)

7. Thyroid-stimulating hormone (TSH)

B. **Posterior pituitary gland**

1. Vasopressin (antidiuretic hormone [ADH])

2. Oxytocin

II Disorders of the Anterior Pituitary Gland

A. **Acromegaly:** Hypersecretion of growth hormone (GH) that occurs after puberty

1. Manifestations

   a. Enlargement of skeletal extremities; increase in adult height; change in ring or shoe size

   b. Protrusion of the jaw and orbital ridges

   c. Headache, visual problems, and blindness

   d. Muscle weakness

   e. Organ enlargement

   f. Decalcification of the skeleton

   g. Endocrine disturbances similar hyperthyroidism

2. Diagnostic Procedures

   a. Serum studies, showing elevated GH levels

   b. CT and MRI of pituitary may show pituitary tumor

   c. X-rays show abnormal bone growth

3. Collaborative Care

   a. **Nursing Interventions**

     1) Provide emotional support.

     2) Provide symptomatic care.

     3) Prepare client for surgery or radiation if indicated for tumor treatment.

   b. Medications

     1) Octreotide (Sandostatin): synthetic GH analogue

     2) Bromocriptine mesylate (Parlodel) or pergolide (Permax): dopamine agonists

   c. Therapeutic Measures

     1) Surgical removal of pituitary gland (transsphenoidal hypophysectomy); surgery is generally the first treatment option.

     2) Replacement therapy will be needed following surgical removal of the pituitary gland and can be needed following radiation therapy.

       a) Corticosteroids

       b) Thyroid hormones

     3) Radiation therapy.

4. Client Education and Referral

   a. Medication adherence

   b. Continued compliance with follow-up appointments with all providers

B. **Gigantism:** Hypersecretion of GH that occurs in childhood prior to closure of the growth plates

1. Manifestations

   a. Proportional overgrowth in all body tissue

2. Diagnostic Procedures/Collaborative Care: same as acromegaly

C. **Dwarfism:** Hyposecretion of GH during fetal development or childhood that results in limited growth congenital or result from damage to the pituitary gland.

1. Manifestations

   a. Head and extremities are disproportionate to torso

     1) Face can appear younger than peers'

   b. Short stature; slow or flat growth rate

   c. Progressive bowed legs and lordosis

   d. Delayed adolescence or puberty

2. Diagnostic Procedures

   a. Comparison of height/weight against growth charts; slowed growth rate will be noted

   b. Serum growth hormone level; most providers will also evaluate other hormonal levels to ensure that no secondary deficiencies exist

   c. MRI of the head (to assess pituitary gland)

3. Collaborative Care

   a. **Nursing Interventions**
      1) Reinforce education with child and family about adaptive measures available for ADLs.
      2) Reinforce teaching with child and family how to administer supplemental GH.
         a) The earlier the therapy is initiated, the better the prognosis.
         b) GH therapy does not work in all children.
      3) Provide positive feedback to child to promote positive self-esteem.
   b. Medications
      1) Human growth hormone injections

III Disorders of the Posterior Pituitary Gland

A. **Diabetes Insipidus (DI):** A deficiency of antidiuretic hormone (ADH or vasopressin) due to a disorder of the posterior pituitary gland that results in the inability of the kidneys to conserve water appropriately. DI is caused by head trauma, tumor, surgery, radiation, CNS infections, malignant tumors, or failure of renal tubules. The underlying cause of DI should be identified and treated.

   1. Manifestations
      a. Urine chemistry (dilute)
         1) Decreased urine specific gravity
         2) Decreased urine osmolality
      b. Serum chemistry (concentrated)
         1) Hypernatremia
         2) Increased serum osmolality
         3) Hypokalemia
      c. Polyuria and polydipsia
         1) Increased urinary output
         2) Clients may crave ice water in excessive amounts
      d. Dehydration, weight loss, and dry skin
      e. Hemoconcentration
   2. Diagnostic Procedures
      a. Water (fluid) deprivation test
         1) Monitor body weight, hourly urine output
         2) Assess serum and urine osmolality
      b. Vasopressin test
         1) Performed only if fluid deprivation test is inconclusive
         2) IV vasopressin is administered
         3) Client urine and serum chemistries will improve
      c. MRI of hypothalamus and pituitary
      d. 24-hr urine
   3. Collaborative Care

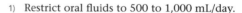

      a. **Nursing Interventions**
         1) Weigh client daily.
         2) Monitor urine output and urine specific gravity.
         3) Monitor the client's blood pressure and heart rate.
         4) Maintain fluid and electrolyte balance.

   b. Medications
      1) Desmopressin acetate (DDAVP)
      2) Vasopressin
      3) If DI is nephrogenic in origin, thiazide diuretics will be prescribed
   c. Client Education and Referral
      1) Lifetime vasopressin replacement therapy.
      2) Report weight gain or loss, polyuria, or polydipsia to the provider.
      3) Monitor fluid intake and urine output.
      4) Avoid foods with diuretic action.

B. **Syndrome of Inappropriate Secretion of Antidiuretic Hormone (SIADH):** The excessive release of ADH resulting in the inability to excrete an appropriate amount of urine, thus developing fluid retention and dilutional hyponatremia. Caused by neoplastic tumors, head injury, meningitis, respiratory disorders, and some medications (vincristine, phenothiazines, tricyclic antidepressants, thiazide diuretics) and nicotine.

   1. Manifestations
      a. Urine chemistry (concentrated)
         1) Increased urine specific gravity and osmolality
      b. Serum chemistry (dilute)
         1) Hyponatremia
         2) Decreased serum osmolality
         3) Hyperkalemia
      c. Mental confusion, irritability, lethargy, and seizures (due to hyponatremia)
      d. Weakness, anorexia, nausea, and vomiting (due to hyponatremia)
      e. Increased ADH (vasopressin) levels
      f. Weight gain
   2. Collaborative Care
      a. **Nursing Interventions**
         1) Restrict oral fluids to 500 to 1,000 mL/day.
         2) Monitor I&O.
         3) Weigh client daily.
         4) Monitor mental status frequently; initiate seizure precautions.
      b. Medications
         1) Hypertonic saline infusion (3% to 5% sodium chloride)
         2) Loop diuretics; used to treat hypervolemic hyponatremia
         3) Declomycin (Demeclocycline)
         4) Vasopressin receptor antagonists
            a) Conivaptan (Vaprisol)
      c. Therapeutic Measures
         1) Underlying cause is treated with surgery, chemotherapy, and/or radiation.

IV Adrenal Gland

The adrenal cortex produces glucocorticoids (cortisol), mineralocorticoids (aldosterone), and sex hormones. The adrenal medulla produces the catecholamines epinephrine and norepinephrine.

V Disorders of the Adrenal Cortex

A. **Addison's Disease (adrenal insufficiency):** The hyposecretion of adrenal cortex hormones caused by autoimmune disease, TB, histoplasmosis, adrenalectomy, tumors, HIV; can be induced by abrupt cessation of steroid medications

> **MEMORY HINT:** With Addison's you need to **add** cortisol.

1. Manifestations
   a. Weakness and fatigue
   b. Nausea and vomiting
   c. Hyperpigmentation
   d. Hypotension; increased heart rate
   e. Hypoglycemia, hyponatremia, hyperkalemia, hypercalcemia
   f. Craving salty foods
   g. Emotional lability and depression
   h. Diminished libido

2. Diagnostic Procedures
   a. Serum adrenocortical hormone levels
   b. ACTH stimulation test
   c. Electrolyte panels
   d. Abdominal/renal CT scan

3. Collaborative Care
   a. **Nursing Interventions**
      1) Monitor blood pressure and heart rhythm.
      2) Monitor fluid and electrolyte balance.
      3) Monitor and treat hypoglycemia.
      4) Monitor for Addisonian crisis (also known as adrenal crisis): characterized by signs of shock (hypotension, tachycardia, tachypnea, pallor). It occurs secondary to stressors such as infection, trauma, surgery, pregnancy, or emotional stress. The client will require IV fluid replacement and IV steroids and can require respiratory support.
      5) Monitor for adverse effects of hormone replacement therapy, which are the same manifestations as hypersecretion of the adrenal cortex.
   b. Medications—adrenocorticoid replacement
      1) Hydrocortisone (Cortef)
      2) Prednisone
      3) Cortisone (Cortisone Acetate)
   c. Client Education and Referral
      1) Provide emotional support to the client and provide instruction on lifelong disease management (medications, prompt treatment of infection and illness, and stress management).
      2) Reinforce education about lifelong medication replacement, including the potential need for increased steroid therapy during times of stress or illness.
         a) Reinforce teaching about manifestations of excessive or insufficient hormone replacement
         b) Client should promptly notify the provider in cases of infection, injury, and stress. Doses of hormones will need to be individually adjusted during these times.
      3) Client should recognize indications of Addisonian crisis.
      4) Client should avoid using caffeine and alcohol.
      5) Client should wear appropriate medical identification at all times in case of emergency.
      6) Client should eat a high-protein, high-carbohydrate diet.

B. **Cushing's Disease and Cushing's Syndrome:** The hypersecretion of the glucocorticoids caused by hyperplasia of the adrenal cortex or pituitary gland tumor. Cushing's syndrome is caused by exogenous use of steroid medications.

1. Manifestations
   a. Upper body obesity and thin extremities; moon face, buffalo hump, and neck fat
   b. Skin fragility with purple striae
   c. Osteoporosis
   d. Hyperglycemia, hypernatremia, hypokalemia, and hypocalcemia
   e. Hirsutism
   f. Amenorrhea
   g. Elevated triglycerides and hypertension
   h. Sexual dysfunction; decreased libido, erectile dysfunction in men
   i. Immunosuppression
   j. Peptic ulcer disease
   k. In children: slower growth rate
   l. Backache, bone pain, or tenderness
   m. Increased thirst and urination

2. Diagnostic Procedures
   a. Dexamethasone suppression test (dexamethasone administered at 2300; plasma cortisol levels obtained at 0800. Suppression of cortisol indicates the hypothalamic-pituitary-adrenal axis is functioning properly.
   b. Nighttime salivary cortisol levels

3. Collaborative Care

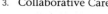

  a. **Nursing Interventions**

    1) Monitor the client for infection.

    2) Protect the client from accidents and falls.

    3) Monitor and treat hyperglycemia.

    4) Monitor blood pressure and heart rhythm.

  b. Medications

    1) Adrenal enzyme inhibitors (metyrapone [Metopirone], aminoglutethimide [Cytadren], mitotane [Lysodren], and ketoconazole)

  c. Therapeutic Measures

    1) For a pituitary adenoma, the client can need a transsphenoidal adenomectomy.

    2) For an adrenal carcinoma, the client can need a unilateral or bilateral adrenalectomy.

    3) Monitor for adrenal insufficiency following postsurgery.

    4) Slowly taper corticosteroid therapy.

  d. Client Education and Referral

    1) For clients prescribed exogenous steroid therapy, educate concerning long-term self-administration of hormone suppression therapy in Cushing's disease and the need for tapering steroid doses in Cushing's syndrome.

    2) Advise the client to eat foods high in protein and calcium, low in carbohydrates and sodium, with potassium supplementation.

    3) Reinforce client education about infection prevention, fall precautions, and skin care.

4 S's OF CUSHING'S AND ADDISON'S DISEASE

	CUSHINGS DISEASE (BIG S's) ↑	ADDISONS DISEASE (SMALL S's) ↓
Steroid	↑	↓ (need to "add")
Sugar	↑	↓
Sodium	↑	↓
Skin	Thin, fragile, striae	Hyperpigmented

C. **Hyperaldosteronism (Conn's syndrome):** The hypersecretion of aldosterone from the adrenal cortex (usually due to a tumor).

  1. Manifestations

    a. Hypokalemia and hypernatremia

    b. Hypertension

    c. Muscle weakness, numbness, and cardiac problems

    d. Fatigue

    e. Headache

    f. Polyuria and polydipsia

    g. Alkalosis

  2. Diagnostic Procedures

    a. Abdominal CT

    b. ECG

    c. Serum aldosterone/renin and potassium

    d. Urine aldosterone

3. Collaborative Care

  a. **Nursing Interventions**

    1) Provide a quiet environment.

    2) Monitor blood pressure and cardiac activity.

    3) Monitor potassium level and be prepared to replace potassium.

    4) Closely monitor I&O.

  b. Medications

    1) Antihypertensive medications: spironolactone (Aldactone)

    2) Eplerenone (Inspra): blocks action of aldosterone

  c. Therapeutic Measures

    1) Surgical removal of tumor/adrenal gland if primary cause

VI Disorders of the Adrenal Medulla

A. **Pheochromocytoma:** A usually benign tumor of the adrenal medulla that causes hypersecretion of epinephrine and norepinephrine

  1. Manifestations

    a. Most common signs are the 5 H's

      1) Hypertension

      2) Headache

      3) Hyperhidrosis (excessive sweating)

      4) Hypermetabolism

      5) Hyperglycemia

  2. Diagnostic Procedures

    a. Plasma levels of catecholamines and metanephrine (catecholamine metabolite)

    b. 24-hr urine level of catecholamines and their metabolites

    c. CT, MRI, or PET scan

    d. Adrenal biopsy

    e. Clonidine (Catapres) suppression test (in clients who have pheochromocytoma, catecholamines are not suppressed)

  3. Collaborative Care

    a. **Nursing Interventions**

      1) Monitor vital signs.

      2) Provide a high-calorie, nutritious diet, and avoid caffeine.

      3) Encourage frequent rest periods.

      4) Provide a quiet environment.

      5) Prevent stroke secondary to hypertensive crisis.

      6) Do not palpate or assess for CVA tenderness, as this can cause rupture of the tumor.

    b. Medications

      1) Alpha- (phentolamine [Regitine]) and beta-blocker (propranolol [Inderal]) to diminish the effect of norepinephrine prior to surgery

      2) Sodium nitroprusside (Nipride)

      3) Calcium channel blockers (nifedipine [Procardia])

    c. Therapeutic Measures

      1) Surgical removal of tumor

VII Thyroid Gland

The thyroid gland has a rich blood supply and produces thyroxine (T_4), triiodothyronine (T_3), and calcitonin. T_4 and T_3 regulate metabolism, and calcitonin helps regulate serum calcium levels.

VIII Disorders of the Thyroid Gland

A. **Hypothyroidism:** Suboptimal levels of thyroid hormone resulting in decreased metabolism. Occurs most frequently in older women.

1. Manifestations
   a. Fatigue and weakness
   b. Increased sensitivity to cold
   c. Constipation
   d. Dry skin, brittle hair and nails
   e. Weight gain
   f. Deepened, hoarse voice
   g. Joint pain
   h. Hyperlipidemia and anemia
   i. Depression
   j. Menstrual disturbances

2. Diagnostic Procedures/Findings
   a. Low serum T_4 and T_3
   b. Elevated TSH (seen in primary hypothyroidism)

3. Myxedema coma is a rare, life-threatening condition seen in untreated or uncontrolled hypothyroidism. The client is hypothermic with changes in mental functioning ranging from depression to unconsciousness. The severely decreased metabolism causes respiratory depression and cardiovascular collapse. Management is to provide intensive supportive measures along with hemodynamic therapy. High mortality rate.

4. Collaborative Care
   a. **Nursing Interventions**
      1) Provide a warm environment.
      2) Provide a diet low in calories, cholesterol, and fat.
      3) Increase roughage and fluids.
      4) Avoid sedatives.
      5) Plan rest periods for the client.
      6) Weigh the client daily.
      7) Observe for manifestations of overdose of thyroid preparations (palpitations, insomnia, increased appetite, and tremors).
   b. Medications
      1) Levothyroxine (Synthroid)
   c. Client Education and Referral
      1) Client will require lifelong medication therapy.
      2) Continue follow-up with provider.
      3) Take medication on an empty stomach each morning.
      4) Know manifestations of medication toxicity.
      5) Eat a diet high in fiber.
      6) Monitor need for sleep.

B. **Hyperthyroidism:** The excessive secretion of thyroid hormones. Graves' disease is the most common type of hyperthyroid disease and causes overstimulation of the thyroid by circulating immunoglobulins.

1. Manifestations
   a. Anxiety and irritability
   b. Insomnia and fatigue
   c. Tachycardia
   d. Tremors
   e. Diaphoresis
   f. Intolerance of heat
   g. Weight loss (despite food intake)
   h. Exophthalmos
   i. Diarrhea
   j. Light or absent menstrual cycle

2. Diagnostic Procedures/Findings
   a. Elevated T_4 and T_3
   b. Decreased TSH

3. Thyroid storm is a life-threatening condition seen in untreated or uncontrolled hyperthyroidisms. Manifestations include hyperpyrexia, tachycardia, hypertension, and other exaggerated symptoms of hyperthyroidism.

4. Collaborative Care
   a. **Nursing Interventions**
      1) Monitor vital signs.
      2) Promote comfort.
      3) Encourage the client to get adequate rest in a cool, quiet environment.
      4) Provide a high-calorie diet without extra stimulants.
      5) Weigh the client daily.
      6) Provide the client emotional support.
      7) Provide eye protection for the client who has exophthalmos by giving ophthalmic medicine, taping the client's eyes at night, and decreasing sodium and water.
      8) Elevate head of the bed.
   b. Medications
      1) Beta-blocker medications to manage tachycardia, anxiety, and tremors.
      2) Propylthiouracil (Propyl-Thyracil or PTU): blocks thyroid hormone production.
      3) Methimazole (Tapazole): short-term use to block production of thyroxine; usually used no more than 8 weeks. Monitor CBC frequently for occurrence of agranulocytosis.
      4) Iodides decrease vascularity and inhibit the release of thyroid hormones. Give through a straw to prevent staining of teeth.
         a) Lugol's solution
         b) Saturated solution of potassium iodide (SSKI); used prior to thyroidectomy
      5) A radioactive iodine treatment shrinks the thyroid gland; may be used alone or prior to surgery. Teach client appropriate radiation precautions.

c. Therapeutic Measures

1) Thyroidectomy: the removal of all or part of the thyroid gland. Requires a lifelong intake of levothyroxine (Synthroid) and possible calcium supplementation.

a) Preoperative goal: decrease thyroid function toward normal range (euthyroid) using saturated solution of potassium iodide (SSKI) and antithyroid medication.

b) Postoperative interventions

(1) Place the client in the semi-Fowler's position.

(2) Monitor dressings, especially the back of the neck.

(3) Observe for respiratory distress. Keep a tracheostomy tray, oxygen, and suction apparatus at the client's bedside.

(4) Monitor for signs of hemorrhage.

(5) Note any hoarseness, which is indicative of laryngeal nerve injury; limit talking.

(6) Observe for signs of tetany (Chvostek's and Trousseau's sign), which can indicate damage or accidental removal of parathyroid glands and subsequent hypocalcemia.

(7) Keep calcium gluconate IV at the bedside.

(8) Observe for thyroid storm caused by an increased release of the thyroid hormone due to manipulation of the thyroid gland.

(9) Gradually increase the range of motion to the neck and support the client when sitting up.

(10) Recognize and report change in client's condition.

IX Parathyroid Gland

Parathormone (parathyroid hormone) maintains calcium and phosphate balance

X Disorders of the Parathyroid Gland

A. **Hypoparathyroidism:** The hyposecretion of parathyroid hormone (PTH), resulting in hypocalcemia and hyperphosphatemia usually caused by surgical removal of parathyroid gland tissue during parathyroidectomy, thyroidectomy, or radical neck dissection.

1. Manifestations of Hypocalcemia

a. Paresthesia

b. Muscle cramps and tetany

c. Chvostek's sign: tapping the side of the cheek causes muscle spasms and twitching around the mouth, throat, and cheeks

d. Trousseau's sign: pressure from the blood pressure cuff induces muscle spasms in the distal extremity

e. Circumoral paraesthesia with numbness and tingling of the fingers

f. Severe tetany can lead to bronchospasm, laryngeal spasm, carpopedal spasm, dysphagia, cardiac dysrhythmias, and seizures

2. Collaborative Care

a. **Nursing Interventions**

1) Monitor ECG.

2) Monitor the client for signs of neuromuscular irritability.

3) Provide a high-calcium, low-phosphorous diet.

4) Institute seizure precautions.

b. Medications

1) Acute: IV calcium gluconate

2) Chronic

a) Oral calcium salts (generally calcium carbonate) and phosphate binders

b) Vitamin D

B. **Hyperparathyroidism:** A hypersecretion of PTH (caused by tumor or renal disease) that leads to the loss of calcium from the bones into the serum, resulting in hypercalcemia and hypophosphatemia

1. Manifestations: might not have symptoms

a. Kidney stones (containing calcium)

b. Osteoporosis

c. Hypercalcemia and hypophosphatemia

d. Abdominal pain, constipation, nausea, and vomiting

e. Muscle weakness and fatigue; skeletal and joint pain

f. Polyuria and polydipsia

g. Hypertension

h. Cardiac dysrhythmias

2. Collaborative Care

a. **Nursing Interventions**

1) Encourage a minimum of 2,000 mL of fluids daily.

2) Provide a diet low in calcium and vitamin D.

3) Prevent constipation and fecal impaction.

4) Strain all urine.

5) Reinforce teaching about safety measures to prevent fractures.

6) Encourage cranberry juice to lower urinary pH.

7) Monitor for hypercalcemic crisis, which is life-threatening. It usually occurs with serum calcium levels greater than 15 mg/dL).

a) IV rehydration

b) Phosphate therapy

c) Calcitonin

d) Dialysis

b. Medications

1) Calcimimetics, such as cinacalcet (Sensipar), mimic calcium in the blood and can cause the parathyroid to decrease the release of parathormone.

2) Calcitonin decreases the release of skeletal calcium and increases the kidney excretion of calcium; enhanced if given along with glucocorticoids.

3) Hydration and diuretics: furosemide (Lasix) promotes excretion of excess calcium (avoid thiazide diuretics).

4) Biphospates

c. Therapeutic Measures

1) Surgical removal of the parathyroid gland

XI Pancreas

The pancreas has exocrine (secretion of the pancreatic enzymes amylase, trypsin, and lipase, which aid in digestion) and endocrine (secretion of insulin, glucagon, and somatostatin) functions. Insulin lowers blood glucose by facilitating glucose entry into the cell. Somatostatin also lowers blood glucose levels. Glucagon raises blood glucose by converting glycogen to glucose in the liver.

XII Disorders of the Pancreas

A. **Diabetes mellitus:** A group of metabolic disorders characterized by hyperglycemia caused by altered insulin production, action, or a combination of both.

1. Type 1 is usually characterized by an acute onset before 30 years of age. In Type 1 diabetes, the pancreatic beta cells are destroyed by either genetic predisposition (not inherited), immunologic, environmental, or a combination of these factors. *Pancreas don't make enough insulin*

2. Type 2 usually occurs after 30 years of age and is comprised of inadequate insulin production and insulin resistance.

   a. Contributing Factors *Pancreas makes insulin but body is resistant*

      1) Family history of diabetes

      2) Obesity

      3) Race/ethnicity (more common in African Americans, Hispanic Americans, Native Americans, Asian Americans, and Pacific Islanders)

      4) Hypertension

      5) History of gestational diabetes

      6) Sedentary lifestyle

3. Metabolic Syndrome

   a. Insulin resistance leads to increase insulin production in attempt to maintain glucose at a normal level.

   b. Characterized by hypertension, hypercholesterolemia, and abdominal obesity.

   c. If the beta cells cannot produce enough insulin to meet the demands, type 2 diabetes develops.

4. Diagnostic Criteria

   a. Symptoms of diabetes plus casual plasma glucose of 200 mg/dL or greater, or

   b. Fasting plasma glucose of 126 mg/dL or greater, or

   c. 2-hr postload glucose of 200 mg/dL or greater during an oral glucose tolerance test

5. Glycemic Control

   a. Glucose control is monitored on a day-to-day basis by capillary blood glucose levels.

   b. Glucose control is monitored on a long-term basis by HbA1c (glycosylated hemoglobin).

6. Manifestations

   a. "3 Polys"

      1) Polyuria

      2) Polydipsia

      3) Polyphagia

   b. Fatigue and weakness

   c. Sudden vision changes

   d. Recurrent infections

   e. Slow wound healing

   f. Type 1 diabetes

      1) Sudden weight loss

      2) Nausea, vomiting, or abdominal pain

7. Long-Term Complications

   a. Neuropathy

   b. Nephropathy

   c. Retinopathy

   d. Cardiovascular disease

   e. Infection and slow wound healing

8. Collaborative Care

   a. **Nursing Interventions**

      1) Monitor blood glucose.

      2) Administer medication as prescribed.

      3) Reinforce education. (See Client Education.)

      4) Monitor vital signs and I&O.

      5) Collaborate with a diabetic educator.

      6) Monitor for complications.

   b. Possible Complications

      1) Hypoglycemia occurs when the blood glucose level falls below 60 mg/dL.

         a) Causes: decreased dietary intake, excess insulin, and increased exercise

         b) Manifestations

            (1) Tachycardia *Palpitations*

            (2) Diaphoresis *Hunger*

            (3) Weakness, fatigue *blurred vision*

            (4) Irritability, anxiety *cool/clammy skin*

            (5) Confusion

      2) Transient Hyperglycemia: Elevated blood glucose; generally treated with sliding scale insulin to return serum blood glucose to normal range

         a) Prompt treatment is necessary to avoid hyperglycemic emergencies.

            (1) Treat with regular insulin.

            (2) Do not hold insulin when blood glucose is in the normal range.

            (3) Provide education on importance and strategies to maintain blood glucose in the normal range.

Hyperglycemic *Polyuria* *Polydipsia* *Polyphagia* *Fruity breath Kussmaul Resp.*

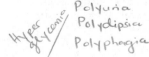

b) **Nursing Interventions**

(1) Administer 15 g of fast-acting simple carbohydrates.

　(a) Three or four glucose tablets for the equivalent to 15 g of carbohydrates

　(b) 4 oz fruit juice or regular soda

　(c) 6 to 10 hard candies

　(d) 2 to 3 teaspoons sugar or honey

(2) If the client is unconscious or unable to swallow, administer glucagon IM or subcutaneous. Repeat in 10 min if client is still unconscious and notify provider.

(3) Follow the 15/15/15 rule.

　(a) Administer 15 g simple carbohydrates.

　(b) Wait 15 min and recheck blood glucose.

　(c) Administer another 15 g carbohydrates if blood glucose remains less than 70 mg/dL.

　(d) Give 7 g protein when blood glucose is within normal limits.

　　i) 2 tablespoons peanut butter

　　ii) 1 oz cheese

　　iii) 8 oz milk

c. Medications (see Unit Four: Pharmacology in Nursing)

1) Insulin pump: An external device that provides a basal dose of rapid-acting or regular insulin with a bolus dose for meals, which is calculated by the client using a predetermined insulin-to-carbohydrate ratio. Does not read blood glucose.

　a) Needles are inserted into subcutaneous abdominal tissue (change site at least every 3 days).

　b) Complications are secondary to continuous administration of insulin or from disruption of insulin infusion.

　c) Allows for flexibility of diet.

d. Client Education

1) Nutritional therapy as prescribed (exchange, carbohydrate counting, calories, healthy food choices)

2) Importance of consistent exercise

3) Self-monitoring of glucose and interpretation of results

4) Medication administration

　a) Medication importance and schedule

　b) Medication route (PO, subcutaneous, insulin pump)

　c) Rotation of injection within an anatomic area

5) Manifestations and management of hypo and hyperglycemia

6) Wear medic alert bracelet

7) Foot care

　a) Cleanse feet daily in warm, soapy water. Rinse and dry carefully.

　b) Trim nails straight across.

　c) Wear supportive, protective shoes.

　d) Inspect feet daily, including between the toes.

8) Guidelines during illness ("Sick Day Rules")

　a) Take usual doses of insulin or antidiabetic agents.

　b) Test blood glucose and urine for ketones every 3 to 4 hr.

　c) Report elevated blood glucose or urine ketones to provider.

　d) Encourage to consume 4 oz sugar-free, noncaffeinated fluids every 30 min to prevent dehydration.

　e) Eat small, frequent meals of soft foods or liquids to meet carbohydrate needs.

B. **Diabetic Ketoacidosis:** An acute, life-threatening complication of diabetes mellitus due to insufficient insulin. Main clinical manifestations are hyperglycemia (blood glucose levels vary between 300 to 800 mg/dL) , acidosis, dehydration and fluid loss; most common in type 1 diabetes mellitus.

1. Contributing Factors

　a. Decreased or missed dose of insulin

　b. Illness or infection

　c. Undiagnosed or untreated diabetes

2. Manifestations

　a. Exacerbated polyuria, polydipsia, polyphagia

　b. Anorexia, nausea, vomiting, abdominal pain

　c. Metabolic acidosis with ketonuria

　d. Kussmaul's respirations

　e. Acetone breath (fruity odor)

　f. Altered mental status, blurred vision, headache

　g. Weak, rapid pulse

　h. Orthostatic hypotension

3. Collaborative Care

　a. **Nursing Interventions**

　　1) Monitor blood glucose, LOC, vital signs, and strict I&O.

　　2) Administer prescribed IV fluids to promote perfusion.

　　　a) Normal saline infusion to maintain perfusion.

　　　b) Follow with 45% saline infusion to replace total body fluid losses

　　　c) Add fluids containing dextrose when blood glucose is approximately 250 mg/dL

　　3) Administer insulin.

　　　a) Insulin infusion usually at 0.1 mg/kg/hr. Regular insulin is the only insulin that may be given IV.

　　　b) Usually blood glucose checks hourly while on an insulin infusion.

　　　c) Resume subcutaneous when possible.

　　4) Monitor potassium levels and replace as prescribed.

　　5) Monitor acid-base balance.

　　6) Reinforce education about strategies to prevent DKA and hyperglycemic hyperosmolar state.

C. **Hyperglycemic Hyperosmolar State (HHS):** An acute, life-threatening complication of diabetes (more commonly in type 2). It is characterized by elevated blood glucose levels of greater than 600 mg/dL, a hyperosmolar state, which leads to fluid and electrolyte losses.

1. Contributing Factors

   a. Acute illness (e.g., surgery, infection, CVA)

   b. Medications that exacerbate hyperglycemia (thiazides)

   c. Treatments (e.g., dialysis)

2. Manifestations

   a. Clinical signs of dehydration

      1) Hypotension and tachycardia

      2) Elevated BUN

   b. Generally not seen with ketosis

   c. Altered mental status

3. Collaborative Care

   a. **Nursing Interventions**

      1) Replace fluids as prescribed (monitor for fluid overload).

      2) Administer insulin and electrolytes as prescribed.

      3) Monitor blood glucose, LOC, vital signs, electrolyte levels and acid-base balance.

      4) Teach strategies to prevent HHS.

ENDOCRINE END-OF-SECTION REVIEW

1. A client who is taking levothyroxine (Synthroid) for hypothyroidism is experiencing palpations and tremors. The most likely cause of these manifestations is _____ thyroid medication.

2. It is important for a client on long-term steroid therapy not to suddenly _____ taking the medication without provider instructions.

3. A client who is on long-term steroid therapy is at risk for fractures due to _____, which is a potential adverse effect of long-term steroid therapy.

4. A medication that may be used to manage Addison's disease is _____.

5. A PN should monitor _____ for a client who has pheochromocytoma.

6. A client who has returned to the room following a thyroidectomy is at risk to develop thyroid storm. It is important for the PN to monitor for _____, _____, and/or _____.

7. A PN is administering Lugol's solution to a client who has hyperthyroidism. To prevent staining of the client's teeth, the medication needs to be given with a _____.

8. Appropriate foot care for a client who has diabetes includes wearing cotton socks and protective _____, daily _____, and _____ feet thoroughly after washing.

9. A PN checks the capillary blood glucose level for a client who has diabetes and finds that it is 55 mg/dL. The client is awake and alert. An appropriate intervention would be to give the client _____ and recheck the blood glucose in _____ minutes.

10. When the blood glucose for the client above is rechecked, it is 90 mg/dL. An appropriate intervention would be to give the client _____.

WORD BANK	
15	Insufficient
30	Osteoporosis
4 oz orange juice	Prednisone
8 oz milk	Restriction
Blood pressure	Shoes
Excessive	Straw
Drying	Synthroid
Hyperpyrexia	Stop
Hypotension	Tachycardia
Hypertension	Thyroid storm
Inspection	Weighed

Answer Key: 1. Excessive; 2. Stop; 3. Osteoporosis; 4. Prednisone; 5. Blood pressure; 6. Hyperpyrexia, Tachycardia, Hypertension; 7. Straw; 8. Shoes, Inspection, Drying; 9. 4 oz juice, 15; 10. 8 oz milk

SECTION 7

Hematologic Disorders

A. **Anemia:** A deficiency of RBCs characterized by a decreased RBC count, Hgb/Hct, or both. Anemia is a clinical sign that results in decreased oxygen delivery to the cells.

1. Contributing Factors

   a. Acute or chronic blood loss (gastrointestinal bleeding)

   b. Greater than normal destruction of RBCs (spleen diseases)

   c. Abnormal bone marrow function (chemotherapy)

   d. Decreased erythropoietin (renal failure)

   e. Inadequate maturation of RBCs (cancer)

   f. Nutritional deficiencies (iron, B_{12}, folic acid, intrinsic factor)

2. Manifestations

   a. Fatigue and weakness

   b. Dizziness and headaches

   c. Pallor: first seen in conjunctival area (Caucasian) and oral area (dark-skinned population), as well as the nail beds, the palmar creases, and around the mouth

   d. Tachycardia, murmurs and gallops, and orthostatic hypotension

   e. Decreased activity tolerance

   f. Decreased Hgb, Hct, and RBC levels

   g. Shortness of breath and dyspnea; decreased oxygen saturation levels

3. Collaborative Care

   a. **Nursing Interventions**

   1) Monitor labs (RBC, Hgb, and Hct).

   2) Encourage activity as tolerated by the client with frequent rest periods.

   3) Monitor skin integrity and implement measures to prevent breakdown.

   4) Provide oxygen therapy to the client as needed.

   5) Administer medications as prescribed. (See individual anemias.)

   6) Monitor client receiving blood products.

   7) Encourage foods high in iron (meats, poultry, fish).

B. **Types of Anemia**

1. Anemia secondary to renal disease: Anemia due to lack of erythropoietin

   a. Medications

   1) Erythropoietin (Procrit, Epogen)

2. Iron deficiency anemia: Anemia resulting from low iron levels; the iron stores are depleted first, followed by hemoglobin stores

   a. Contributing Factors

   1) Chronic blood loss (bleeding ulcer)

   2) Nutritional deficiency

   3) Common in infants, older adults, and young adult women (due to pregnancy or menses)

   b. Manifestations

   1) Microcytic red blood cells

   2) Weakness and pallor

   3) Low serum ferritin levels

   c. Collaborative Care

   1) **Nursing Interventions**

   a) Monitor for symptoms of bleeding.

   b) Monitor labs.

   2) Medications

   a) Administer iron preparations.

   3) Therapeutic Measures

   a) Follow prescriptions for ulcer treatment.

3. Aplastic anemia: Bone marrow suppression of new stem cell production resulting in a deficiency of circulating WBCs, platelets, or RBCs. Can be due to medications, viruses, toxins, or radiation exposure.

   a. Manifestations

   1) Hypoxia, fatigue, and pallor (related to anemia)

   2) Increased susceptibility to infection (related to leukopenia)

   3) Hemorrhage, ecchymosis/petechiae (related to thrombocytopenia)

   4) Pancytopenia (decrease in RBCs, WBCs, and platelets)

   b. Collaborative Care

   1) **Nursing Interventions**

   a) Monitor labs.

   b) Provide protective isolation.

   c) Monitor for manifestations of infection.

   d) Provide emotional and psychological support.

   e) Implement protective barrier precautions.

   2) Medications

   a) Immunosuppressive therapy (prednisone, cyclosporine)

   b) Chemotherapy medications (Cytoxan, Procytox)

   3) Therapeutic Measures

   a) Hematopoietic stem cell transplantation

   b) Splenectomy

   c) Cautious use of blood transfusions

4. B$_{12}$ deficiency anemias (megaloblastic and pernicious anemia): Anemia due to a lack of dietary intake or absorption of vitamin B$_{12}$

   a. Contributing Factors

      1) Atrophy of the gastric mucosa/hypochlorhydria (underproduction of hydrochloric acid by the stomach)

      2) Total gastrectomy (lack of intrinsic factor decreases intestinal vitamin B$_{12}$ absorption)

      3) Malnutrition

   b. Manifestations

      1) Numbness and tingling of extremities (paresthesia)

      2) Hypoxemia

      3) Pallor

      4) Jaundice

      5) Glossitis

      6) Poor balance

   c. Diagnostic Procedures

      1) Shilling test measures the presence of vitamin B$_{12}$ in the urine after the client receives an oral dose of radioactive vitamin B$_{12}$.

      2) CBC: megaloblastic RBCs (macrocytic)

   d. Collaborative Care

      1) **Nursing Interventions**

         a) Monitor labs.

         b) Promote rest and encourage a balanced dietary intake.

      2) Medications

         a) Cobalamin (vitamin B$_{12}$): standard dose is 1,000 mcg IM daily for 2 weeks, then weekly until Hct level is therapeutic, then monthly for life. Cyanocobalamin (Nascobal) intranasally maintains vitamin B$_{12}$ levels.

5. Folic acid deficiency anemia: Anemia due to folic acid deficiency. Symptoms similar to vitamin B$_{12}$ deficiency, but nervous system functions remain normal.

   a. Contributing Factors

      1) Poor nutrition

      2) Malabsorption (secondary to Crohn's disease)

      3) Drugs (chronic alcohol abuse, anticonvulsants, and oral contraceptives)

   b. Collaborative Care

      1) **Nursing Interventions**

         a) Identify high-risk clients: alcohol use disorder, elderly, debilitated clients

      2) Medications

         a) Folic acid replacement

6. Hemolytic anemia: A group of anemias that occur when the bone marrow is unable to increase production to make up for the premature destruction of red blood cells. Sickle cell and thalassemia are hemolytic anemias.

   a. Contributing Factors

      1) Trauma, crushing injuries

      2) Lead poisoning

      3) Tuberculosis

      4) Infections

      5) Transfusion reactions

      6) Toxic agents

   b. Manifestations

      1) Chills

      2) Dark urine

      3) Enlarged spleen

      4) Pallor

      5) Rapid heart rate

      6) Shortness of breath

      7) Jaundice

   c. Collaborative Care

      1) **Nursing Interventions**

         a) Treat the underlying cause.

         b) Hydrate the client.

         c) Blood transfusion when kidney function is normal.

      2) Medications

         a) In severe immune-related hemolytic anemia, steroid therapy is sometimes necessary.

7. Sickle cell anemia: A genetic defect found in clients of African American or Mediterranean origin, in which the Hgb molecule assumes a sickle shape and delivers less oxygen to tissues. The sickle cells become lodged in the blood vessels, especially the brain and the kidneys.

   a. Contributing Factors (precipitate crisis by enhancing sickling)

      1) Stress

      2) Dehydration

      3) Hypoxia

      4) High altitudes

      5) Infections

   b. Manifestations

      1) Severe pain and swelling

      2) Fever

      3) Jaundice

      4) Susceptibility to infection

      5) Hypoxic damage to organs: spleen, liver, heart, kidney, brain

c. Diagnostic Procedures

   1) Percentage of hemoglobin S (Hb S) seen on electrophoresis. Sickle cell trait has less than 40% Hb S and sickle cell disease can have 80% to 100% Hb S.

d. Collaborative Care

   1) **Nursing Interventions**

      a) Maintain adequate hydration.

      b) Provide oxygen therapy to the client.

      c) Encourage the client to rest and avoid high altitudes, alcohol, and temperature extremes.

      d) Reinforce teaching to identify triggers, get immunizations in a timely manner, and refer for genetic counseling.

   2) Medications

      a) Morphine sulfate or hydromorphone (Dilaudid) to manage pain

      b) Hydroxyurea (Droxia) to reduce the amount of sickling and number of painful episodes

8. Thalassemia: Inherited blood disorder in which the body makes an abnormal form of hemoglobin, resulting in excessive destruction of red blood cells, which leads to anemia.

   a. Contributing Factors

      1) Must inherit the defective gene from both parents to develop thalassemia major

      2) Asian, Mediterranean, or African American ethnicity

      3) Family history of the disorder

   b. Manifestations

      1) Develops during the first year of life

      2) Bone deformities in the face

      3) Fatigue

      4) Growth failure

      5) Shortness of breath

      6) Yellow skin (jaundice)

   c. Diagnostic Procedures

      1) Red blood cells appear small and abnormally shaped.

      2) CBC reveals anemia.

      3) Hemoglobin electrophoresis shows the presence of an abnormal form of hemoglobin.

      4) Mutational analysis detects alpha thalassemia that cannot be seen with hemoglobin electrophoresis.

d. Collaborative Care

   1) **Nursing Interventions**

      a) Encourage increase of folate in the diet by including dark green leafy vegetables, dried beans and peas (legumes), and citrus fruits and juices.

      b) Monitor administration of blood transfusions.

      c) Encourage rest.

      d) Provide genetic counseling.

   2) Therapeutic Measures

      a) Treatment often involves regular blood transfusions.

      b) Clients receiving blood transfusions should not take iron supplements because this can cause high iron levels in the blood.

      c) Chelation therapy can be necessary to remove excess iron from the body.

      d) Bone marrow transplant can help treat the disease in some clients, especially children.

   3) Medications

      a) Folic acid

Cardiovascular System Disorders

I Cardiovascular Overview

A. Efficiently pumps blood to all parts of the body, indicating healthy working cardiac muscles and system.

B. Circulates adequate blood volume to meet the body's needs.

C. Adequate blood pressure is maintained by peripheral vasculature.

D. Normal heart rate is 60 to 100/min.

II Diagnostic Procedures

A. **Laboratory tests**

   1. Serum electrolytes

   2. Erythrocyte sedimentation rate (ESR)

   3. C-reactive protein

   4. Blood coagulation tests

      a. PTT: most significant if the client is receiving heparin therapy

      b. PT: most significant if the client is receiving warfarin (Coumadin) therapy

      c. INR

5. BUN and creatinine: reflect renal function and perfusion; levels may increase in MI, CHF, and cardiomyopathy

6. Total serum cholesterol

   a. Low-density lipids (LDL)

   b. High-density lipids (HDL)

   c. Triglycerides

7. B-type natriuretic peptide (BNP): indicator for diagnosing heart failure

8. Enzymes: test indicates death of myocardial muscles, heart attack

   a. Creatinine phosphokinase MB (CK-MB) isoenzyme increases within 4 to 6 hr following a MI and remains elevated from 24 to 72 hr.

   b. Troponin is a protein that is considered the gold standard in diagnosing MI. It remains elevated for 2 to 3 weeks following an event. Normal level is less than 0.2 ng/dL.

DIAGNOSTIC TESTING: CARDIAC ENZYMES

Important Lab Findings

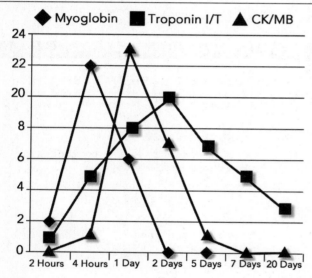

B. **Electrocardiogram (ECG):** A recording of electrical activity in the heart. A 12-lead ECG should be obtained within 10 min of onset of chest pain to identify areas of myocardial damage.

   1. T wave inversion: ischemia

   2. ST-segment elevation: injury

   3. Q-wave enlargement: infarction

ECG WAVE ELEMENTS

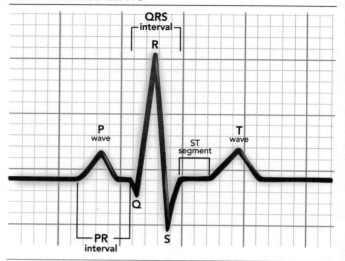

P wave represents atrial depolarization (contraction).

QRS complex (interval) represents ventricular depolarization (contraction) and should be less than 0.12 seconds.

T wave represents ventricular repolarization (relaxation)/reset. T wave depression (inversion) indicates myocardial ischemia.

PR interval represents time between SA node and AV node. Should be between 0.12 and 0.20 seconds.

ST segments represents elevation. Indicates myocardial injury.

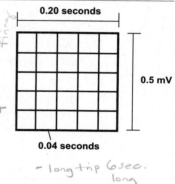

(handwritten notes)
5 large squares = second
300 lg sq = 1 min.
15 blocks = 3 sec. strip
30 blocks = 6 sec. strip
- measure R tips for pattern

C. **Cardiac catheterization:** A procedure involving the advancement of a catheter, usually through the femoral artery, into the coronary arteries. Dye may be injected to visualize blockages, which can then be treated with percutaneous coronary intervention (PCI). The femoral vein can also be accessed to perform other assessments of cardiac function.

   1. Types of PCI

      a. **Coronary Angioplasty:** A balloon-tipped catheter is used to press the coronary blockage open to improve blood flow.

      b. **Coronary Stent:** A procedure performed during angioplasty that leaves a metal mesh in place as a structural support to prevent the blockage from reoccurring.

2. Purpose
   a. Perform angiography.
   b. Perform PCI.
   c. Obtain information about cardiac structure and blood flow.
   d. Obtain blood samples.
   e. Determine cardiac output.

3. **Nursing Interventions**
   a. Prior to catheterization
      1) Verify that procedural consent has been obtained.
      2) Know approach for shave prep: right (venous) side, or left (arterial) side.
      3) NPO for 6 hr prior to the procedure.
      4) Mark distal (baseline) pulses.
      5) Explain to the client that the procedure can leave a metallic taste, and the client might feel flushed when the dye is injected.
      6) Verify that the client does not have any history of allergy to dye or shellfish.

D. **After catheterization**
   1. Monitor blood pressure and apical pulse every 15 min for 2 to 4 hr.
   2. Perform a neurovascular assessment every 15 min for the first 2 hr, then every 30 min until the client is able to sit up.
   3. Monitor for bleeding or hematoma at catheter insertion site.
   4. Apply pressure for a minimum of 15 min to prevent bleeding or hematoma formation.
   5. Monitor for vasospasm, dysrhythmia, or rupture of the coronary vessel.
   6. Monitor for chest pain.
   7. Keep the extremity extended for 4 to 6 hr.
   8. Maintain bed rest; no hip flexion and no sitting up in bed.
   9. Increase fluid intake to enhance flushing of dye.

III Cardiovascular Disorders

A. **Angina (stable, unstable, and variant)**: A manifestation of myocardial ischemia caused by arterial stenosis or blockage, uncontrolled blood pressure, or cardiomyopathy.
   1. **Stable angina.** Usually triggered by physical exertion. Factors such as emotional stress, cold temperatures, heavy meals, and smoking also can trigger angina. *predictable. Relieved by rest / nitroglycerin*
   2. **Unstable angina.** If fatty deposits in a blood vessel rupture or a blood clot forms, it can quickly block or reduce flow through a narrowed artery, suddenly and severely decreasing blood flow to the heart muscle. Unstable angina also can be caused by conditions such as severe anemia when narrowed coronary arteries are present. It is not relieved by rest or medications. *→ 911 Preinfarction; no relief*
   3. **Variant angina.** Also called Prinzmetal's angina, it is caused by a spasm in a coronary artery in which the artery temporarily narrows. Accounts for about 2% of angina cases.
   - no fatty deposits
   - cal channel blockers for relief

B. **Contributing Factors** *✳ modifi modifiable factors*
   1. Coronary artery disease (CAD)
      a. Family history *- uncontrolled stress*
      b. Advanced age
      c. Hyperlipidemia *- African American*
      d. Tobacco use
      e. Hypertension
      f. Diabetes mellitus
      g. Obesity
      h. Physical inactivity

C. **Manifestations** *- any location*
   1. Chest pain or discomfort *- Pallor*
   2. Pain in arms, neck, jaw, shoulder, or back *- Palpitations*
   3. Nausea
   4. Fatigue
   5. Shortness of breath
   6. Anxiety
   7. Diaphoresis
   8. Dizziness

D. **Diagnostic Procedures**
   1. 12-lead ECG
   2. Stress test
   3. Cardiac catheterization
   4. Echocardiogram
   5. Cardiac enzymes and biomarkers

E. **Collaborative Care**
   1. **Nursing Interventions**
      a. Collect data about the client's pain.
         1) Location: jaw and/or arm, as well as chest
         2) Character
         3) Duration: relieved with rest and/or nitroglycerine
         4) Precipitating factors (once identified, eliminate or minimize to avoid attacks)
      b. Administer oxygen as needed.
      c. Provide environment conducive to rest; avoid activities
      d. Administer medications.
         1) Aspirin
         2) Nitrates
         3) Beta blockers
         4) Statins
         5) Calcium channel blockers
         6) Angiotensin-converting enzyme (ACE)

e. Client Education

   1) Lifestyle changes

      a) Avoid constipation.

      b) Avoid excessive activity in cold weather.

      c) Decrease stress.

      d) Exercise.

      e) Consume low-sodium, low-fat diet.

      f) Maintain healthy weight.

      g) Rest after meals.

      h) Promote tobacco cessation.

   2) Reinforce client education about the correct use of nitroglycerin.

      a) Take as needed at onset of chest pain or tightness or in preparation of exertional activity.

      b) Take nitroglycerin as prescribed, at onset of attack, and every 5 min up to three doses. If pain is not relieved after first sublingual tablet, call 911.

      c) Store nitroglycerin in a dark, dry spot, and replace every 6 months.

      d) Side effects of nitroglycerin include headache and hypotension.

      e) Types of nitroglycerin are tablets, ointment, patch, and spray.

      f) If the client receives nitroglycerin for prevention, the client must be nitroglycerine-free daily for 12 hr to prevent developing a tolerance.

      g) If the client uses a nitro patch, remind to apply it in the morning and remove it at bedtime.

      h) Client should take nitroglycerine (Nitrostat) while sitting down and stopping all activity.

      i) Erectile dysfunction medication is contraindicated with the use of nitrates.

F. **Myocardial infarction (MI)**: The process by which myocardial tissue is destroyed due to reduced coronary blood flow and lack of oxygen. Actual necrosis of the heart muscle (myocardium) occurs.

   1. Contributing Factors

      a. Atherosclerotic heart disease

      b. Coronary artery embolism

   2. Manifestations

      a. Severe chest pain, unrelieved with nitroglycerin or rest.

      b. Crushing quality, radiates to jawline, left arm, neck, and/or back.

      c. Women, older adults, and clients who have diabetes mellitus often report no pain.

      d. Diaphoresis, nausea, vomiting, anxiety, fear.

      e. Vital sign changes: tachycardia, hypotension, dyspnea, dysrhythmias.

3. Diagnostic Procedures

   a. Laboratory results: elevated troponin and CK-MB enzymes, elevated LDH

   b. 12-lead ECG: Should be obtained ASAP to identify ST changes. Can be ST elevation MI (STEMI) or non-ST elevation MI (NSTEMI)

4. Collaborative Care

   a. **Nursing Interventions** (aimed at resting the myocardium and preserving the heart muscle)

      1) Early

         a) Administer oxygen.

         b) Administer medications.

            (1) Aspirin

            (2) Antidysrhythmics: amiodarone (Cordarone), lidocaine (Xylocaine)

            (3) Analgesics: morphine sulfate

            (4) Anticoagulants: heparin IV

            (5) Thrombolytics within 6 hr of a cardiac event: alteplase recombinant (Activase)

            (6) Vasodilators: nitroglycerine

            (7) Beta blockers: metoprolol (Lopressor)

            (8) Calcium channel blockers: verapamil (Calan), nifedipine (Procardia)

         c) Frequently monitor vital signs, O_2 saturation, and ECG.

         d) Provide emotional support to the client.

      2) Later

         a) Administer stool softeners to prevent straining with bowel movements or Valsalva maneuver.

         b) Provide a soft diet low in fat, cholesterol, and sodium.

         c) Use a bedside commode, which requires less energy than using a bedpan.

         d) Promote self-care, but remind the client to stop at the onset of pain.

         e) Plan for cardiac rehabilitation.

         f) Encourage an exercise program, but to stop if fatigue or chest pain occurs.

         g) Reinforce teaching and encourage the use of stress management techniques.

         h) Reinforce client education to modify risk factors.

            (1) Obesity

            (2) Stress

            (3) Diet

            (4) Hypertension

            (5) Tobacco use

            (6) Physical inactivity

i) Recognize risk factors that cannot be modified.

  (1) Heredity

  (2) Race

  (3) Age

  (4) Gender

j) Ensure bleeding precautions with anticoagulant and antiplatelet therapy.

k) Initiate long-term medication therapy.

  (1) Anticoagulants/antiplatelets: heparin, aspirin, warfarin (Coumadin), enoxaparin (Lovenox), clopidogrel (Plavix)

  (2) Antihypertensives

    (a) Beta-blockers: metoprolol (Lopressor)

    (b) Calcium channel blockers: diltiazem (Cardizem)

  (3) Vasodilators: nitroglycerin

  (4) Antilipidemics: simvastatin (Zocor), atorvastatin (Lipitor)

G. **Heart failure:** The inability of the heart to meet the tissue requirements for oxygen. Characterized by manifestations of fluid overload or inadequate tissue perfusion. Has been called congestive heart failure due to the frequent occurrence of pulmonary and peripheral congestion. Most often a chronic condition with a goal of preventing acute exacerbations.

1. Left-sided heart failure: Manifestation primarily related to pulmonary congestion

  a. Dyspnea

  b. Cough

  c. Crackles

  d. Orthopnea

  e. Paroxysmal nocturnal dyspnea

  f. Low oxygen saturation levels

  g. Elevated PAWP

2. Right-sided heart failure: Manifestations primarily related to systemic congestion

  a. Dependent edema

  b. Hepatomegaly

  c. Ascites

  d. Anorexia and vomiting

  e. Weakness

  f. Weight gain

  g. Jugular vein distention

  h. Elevated CVP

3. Collaborative Care

  a. **Nursing Interventions**

    1) Respiratory status

      a) Auscultate lung sounds to detect crackles or wheezes

      b) Oxygen therapy as needed

      c) Fowler's position to help work of breathing

    2) Fluid volume

      a) Fluid restriction depending on severity

      b) Low-sodium diet: 2,000 to 3,000 mg day

      c) Report 2- to 3-lb weight increase in 1 day

    3) Pharmacological therapy

      a) ACE inhibitors

      b) ARBs

      c) Hydralazine and nitrates

      d) Beta-blockers

      e) Calcium channel blockers

      f) Diuretics

      g) Digitalis

      h) IV nesiritide (Natrecor)

      i) IV milrinone (Primacor)

      j) IV dobutamine (Dobutrex)

H. **Valvular disorders:** Result in narrowing of valve that prevents or impedes blood flow (stenosis) or impaired closure that allows backward leakage of blood (regurgitation); can affect mitral, aortic, or tricuspid valve.

1. Contributing Factors

  a. History of endocarditis and rheumatic fever is frequently the cause.

2. Manifestations

  a. Right-sided heart failure (caused by mitral stenosis, mitral regurgitation, tricuspid stenosis)

  b. Left-sided heart failure (caused by aortic stenosis, aortic regurgitation)

  c. Murmurs

  d. Decreased cardiac output

3. Collaborative Care

  a. **Nursing Interventions**

    1) Management: similar as for heart failure.

    2) Valvuloplasty: postprocedure care is similar to that of PCI. Watch for signs of systemic emboli, which might have dislodged from the valve.

    3) Valve replacement

      a) Mechanical: will require lifelong anticoagulants using warfarin (Coumadin). Maintain INR 2.0 to 3.0.

      b) Biologic: will only require prophylactic anticoagulants for 3 months.

      c) All clients who have undergone valve surgery will require prophylactic antibiotics prior to any future invasive procedures or tests, including dental procedures to prevent infective endocarditis.

I. **Aortic aneurysm**: Local distention of the aortic artery wall, usually thoracic or abdominal. Monitored until greater than 5 cm, when the rate of rupture increases and surgery is usually required.

1. Contributing factors

    a. Atherosclerosis (most common cause)

    b. Infections/inflammatory disorders

    c. Connective tissue disorders

2. Manifestations (frequently asymptomatic)

    a. Thoracic: pain, dyspnea, hoarseness, cough, dysphagia

    b. Abdominal: abdominal pain; persistent or intermittent low-back or flank pain; pulsating abdominal mass

3. Diagnostic Procedures

    a. CT scan, MRI

    b. X-ray, ultrasound

4. Collaborative Care

    a. **Nursing Interventions**

        1) Treatment often includes surgery.

            a) Preoperative: Maintain systolic pressure at 100 to 120 mm Hg with beta-blockers and/or antihypertensives such as hydralazine (Apresoline). Continuous IV nipride can be required. Monitor closely for manifestations of rupture (e.g., intense pain, decreasing blood pressure).

            b) Postoperative: careful monitoring of peripheral circulation below the level of the aneurysm. Continue close monitoring of blood pressure. Low BP can indicate hemorrhage. High BP places stress on the arterial suture line.

            c) Postoperative complications

                (1) Arterial occlusion

                (2) Hemorrhage

                (3) Infection

                (4) Kidney failure

J. **Hypertension**: Persistent blood pressure above 140/90 mm Hg; often called the "silent killer."

1. Primary hypertension

    a. Most common type (90% of cases)

    b. Hereditary disease; cause unknown

    c. More common among African Americans

    d. Late manifestations: headaches, fatigue, dyspnea, edema, nocturia, blackouts

    e. Usually no manifestations until end-organ involvement occurs

2. Secondary hypertension

    a. Due to identifiable cause

    b. Pheochromocytoma

    c. Renal pathology

3. Collaborative Care

    a. **Nursing Interventions**

        1) Reinforce weight-control methods.

        2) Encourage tobacco cessation.

        3) Decrease alcohol and caffeine intake.

        4) Promote a program of regular physical exercise.

        5) Promote a lifestyle with reduced stress.

        6) Encourage a sodium-restricted diet.

        7) Encourage the DASH diet—increased fruits, vegetables, low-fat dairy, limited saturated fats.

    b. Medications: Initial medications include diuretics and beta-blockers.

        1) Loop diuretic: furosemide (Lasix), bumetanide (Bumex)

        2) Thiazide-hydrochlorothiazide (HCTZ), chlorothiazide (Diuril)

            a) Interventions for loop and HCTZ diuretics

                (1) Administer potassium supplements as prescribed.

                (2) Encourage intake of potassium-rich foods.

                (3) Hypokalemia increases the risk of digitalis toxicity.

        3) Potassium-sparing diuretics

            a) Spironolactone (Aldactone)

            b) Triamterene (Dyrenium)

            c) Monitor for increased potassium level.

        4) Beta-blockers

            a) Propranolol HCl (Inderal)

            b) Atenolol (Tenormin)

            c) Metoprolol (Lopressor)

                (1) **Nursing Interventions** for beta blockers

                    (a) Monitor for major side effects of bradycardia.

                    (b) Monitor pulse daily.

                    (c) Monitor for manifestations of heart failure.

                    (d) Noncardioselective beta-blockers can be contraindicated in clients who have asthma.

                    (e) Monitor for hypoglycemia in clients who have diabetes mellitus; can mask manifestations.

        5) Central-acting alpha-blockers (sympatholytics)

            a) Clonidine HCl (Catapres)

            b) Guanfacine HCl (Tenex)

            c) Methyldopa (Aldomet)

        6) Angiotensin-converting enzyme (ACE) inhibitors

            a) Captopril (Capoten)

            b) Enalapril (Vasotec)

            c) Lisinopril (Zestril)

        7) Calcium-channel blockers

            a) Nifedipine (Procardia)

            b) Verapamil (Calan), diltiazem (Cardizem)

GERONTOLOGIC CONSIDERATIONS

1. Medications start at half the dose used in younger clients.
2. Monotherapy desirable due to simplicity and decreased expense.
3. At increased risk for postural hypotension secondary to medications.

K. **Venous Thromboembolism (VTE):** The collective condition of deep-vein thrombosis (DVT) and pulmonary embolism (PE).

1. Contributing Factors
   a. Immobility
   b. Surgery
   c. Trauma
   d. Obesity
   e. Age greater than 65
   f. Spinal cord injury
   g. Disorders of coagulation
   h. Pregnancy
   i. Oral contraceptives
2. Manifestations of DVT
   a. Edema of affected limb
   b. Local swelling, bumpy, knotty
   c. Red, tender, local induration
   d. Venous ulcers usually around the ankle; reddened and bluish; edema often present
3. Diagnostic Procedures
   a. MRI, CT scan, ultrasound
4. Collaborative Care

   a. **Nursing Interventions**
      1) Heparin: Monitor PTT.
      2) Warfarin (Coumadin): Monitor INR or PT.
      3) Thrombolytic therapy: alteplase (Activase)
      4) Monitor for bleeding and thrombocytopenia.
      5) Elevate affected extremity and apply warm, moist compresses.
      6) Monitor for manifestations of PE: dyspnea, chest pain, tachycardia, anxiety.

KEY NURSING INTERVENTIONS: Prevention of VTE: Early mobilization, leg exercises, compression stockings or intermittent pneumatic compression devices, prophylactic antithrombotic therapy.

L. **Varicose veins**

1. Contributing Factors
   a. Prolonged standing
   b. Pregnancy
   c. Obesity
   d. Heredity
2. Manifestations
   a. Enlarged, tortuous veins in lower extremities
   b. Pain
   c. Edema (after upright)
3. Collaborative Care
   a. **Nursing Interventions**
      1) Client should avoid prolonged sitting or standing.
      2) Client should wear supportive antiembolism stockings, especially during air flights and pregnancy.
      3) Client should avoid crossing legs, engage in daily exercise, and maintain an ideal body weight.
      4) Elevate lower extremities to reduce edema and promote venous return.
      5) Promote circulation with thigh-high antiembolism stockings, ambulation, and elevation.
4. Medical Management
   a. **Sclerotherapy:** chemical injection
   b. **Ligation and stripping:** surgery
   c. **Thermal ablation:** nonsurgical use of energy or lasers

M. **Peripheral Arterial Occlusive Disease**

1. Manifestations
   a. Intermittent claudication: pain/cramping when walking; resolves with rest
   b. Calf muscle atrophy
   c. Shiny skin with hair loss and thickened toenails
   d. Poor neurovascular integrity
   e. Necrotic ulcers (looks punched-out; no edema present)
   f. Tingling and numbness of the toes
   g. Cool extremities with poor pulses
2. Collaborative Care
   a. **Nursing Interventions**
      1) Exercise therapy: walk to the point of pain three times per week.
      2) Encourage tobacco cessation.
      3) Promote weight reduction.
      4) Dependent position relieves pain.
3. Administer Medications
   a. Administer pentoxifylline (Trental) and cilostazol (Pletal).
4. Therapeutic Measures
   a. Surgical treatment
      1) Femoral popliteal bypass surgery
      2) Angioplasty or stenting

N. **Buerger's disease (thromboangiitis obliterans):** Recurring inflammation of the arteries and veins of the lower and upper extremities, resulting in thrombus with occlusion (cause unknown).

1. Contributing Factors

    a. Thought to have a genetic predisposition.

    b. Cigarette smoking and chewing tobacco use.

    c. Occurs most often in men ages 20 to 35.

2. Manifestations

    a. Intermittent pain in the legs, feet, arms and hands. Pain eases when activity is stopped (claudication).

    b. Inflammation along a vein below the skin's surface (due to a blood clot in the vein).

    c. Cold sensitivity of the Raynaud type frequently occurs in the hands.

    d. Painful open sores on fingers and toes.

    e. Ulcerations and gangrene with amputation are common.

3. Collaborative Care

    a. Interventions

        1) Promote smoking cessation.

        2) Avoid exposure to cold temperatures.

        3) Do not wear constrictive clothing.

O. **Raynaud's syndrome:** Vasospastic or obstructive condition of the arteries/arterioles of upper and lower extremities resulting from exposure to cold/stress; more common in women.

1. Contributing Factors

    a. Factors that cause Raynaud's attacks are not clearly understood.

    b. Blood vessels in hands and feet appear to overreact to cold or stress.

2. Manifestations

    a. Coldness, pallor, and pain in extremities secondary to vasospasm

    b. Occasional ulceration of the fingertips

    c. Color changes from white to blue to red (can be bilateral or symmetrical)

3. Diagnostic Procedures

    a. Cold-stimulation test: placing the hands in cool water or exposing to cold air to trigger an episode of Raynaud's

4. Collaborative Care

    a. **Nursing Interventions**

        1) Client should avoid exposure to cold temperatures and keep extremities warm. Wear warm, nonconstrictive gloves.

        2) Encourage the client to stop smoking and to limit caffeine intake.

    b. Medications

        1) Administer nifedipine (Procardia).

IV Shock

Inadequate delivery of oxygen and nutrients to support vital organs and cellular function. Results in impaired tissue perfusion.

A. **Types**

1. Cardiogenic: failure of the heart to pump adequately

2. Hypovolemic: decreased circulating blood volume

3. Distributive (circulatory): vasodilation that causes blood to pool in the peripheral vessels

    a. Neurogenic: Caused by spinal cord injury, certain medications, or hypoglycemia. Characterized by warm, dry skin and bradycardia.

    b. Anaphylactic: Hypersensitivity reaction that causes a sudden onset of hypotension and is life-threatening. Can also experience respiratory distress and cardiac arrest.

    c. Septic: Most common type of circulatory shock. It results from a systemic infection and is characterized by warm, dry skin, bounding pulses, and tachypnea.

B. **Manifestations (related to decreased tissue perfusion)**

1. Tachycardia with hypotension

2. Tachypnea

3. Oliguria

4. Cold, moist skin (except neuro and septic)

5. Color ashen, pallor

6. Metabolic acidosis

7. Decreased level of consciousness

C. **Collaborative Care**

1. **Nursing Interventions**

    a. Position the client in modified Trendelenburg.

    b. Secure a large-bore IV line (16- or 18-gauge).

    c. Administer oxygen.

    d. Record vital signs every 5 min.

    e. Promote rest and decrease movement.

    f. Monitor urine output.

2. Treatment

    a. Hypovolemic: volume replacement

    b. Cardiogenic: increase contractility and reduce afterload (BP)

    c. Septic: IV fluids and vasopressors

    d. Anaphylactic: epinephrine and diphenhydramine

    e. Neurogenic: treat cause (e.g., stabilize spinal cord)

ᵥ Cardiopulmonary Resuscitation (CPR)

A. **Indications**

1. Absence of palpable carotid pulse

2. Absence of breath sounds

B. **Purpose**

1. Establish effective circulation and respiration.

2. Prevent irreversible cerebral anoxic damage.

C. **Procedure**

1. Follow American Heart Association recommendations.

   a. Call 911.

   b. Send someone for the automated external defibrillator.

   c. Immediately begin CPR if an adult victim is unresponsive and not breathing normally.

   d. Early, uninterrupted chest compressions are important. Follow the acronym CAB (Compressions, Airway, Breathing).

   e. Untrained rescuers should perform hands-only compressions. Push hard and fast on the center of the victim's chest or follow the directions of EMS dispatchers.

   f. Trained rescuers should provide 30 compressions and two rescue breaths to improve outcomes.

   g. Depth: Compress the chest at least 2 inches (5 cm) in adults and ⅓ the depth of chest in children and infants.

   h. Rate: Provide compressions 100/min, to the beat of the Bee Gees song "Stayin' Alive."

   i. Recoil: Allow the chest to recoil fully between compressions.

   j. Minimize interruptions: Do not delay or interrupt chest compressions to check pulse or rhythm.

   k. When necessary to check for a pulse, do not exceed 10 seconds.

2. Complications

   a. Fractured ribs

   b. Punctured lungs

   c. Lacerated liver

   d. Abdominal distension

3. Stop CPR when

   a. A provider pronounces the client dead.

   b. The rescuer is exhausted.

   c. Help arrives.

   d. The client's heartbeat returns.

4. Automated external defibrillator: A computerized defibrillator that analyzes cardiac rhythm once pads are placed on the client's chest

   a. A mechanical voice tells the rescuer when to deliver shock to the client.

   b. AED is frequently found in public locations because it is easy for nontrained individuals to use.

5. Obstructed airway

   a. Conscious

      1) Establish that the client is choking.

      2) Perform the Heimlich maneuver until it is successful or the client becomes unconscious.

   b. Unconscious

      1) If a conscious choking adult becomes unresponsive, look for the foreign object in the pharynx. If object is seen, perform a finger sweep.

      2) If not breathing, begin CPR. Every time you open the airway to give breaths, look for the object.

      3) Continue CPR.

HEART

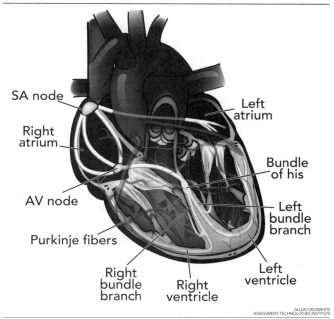

SA node
Right atrium
AV node
Purkinje fibers
Right bundle branch
Right ventricle
Left atrium
Bundle of his
Left bundle branch
Left ventricle

ALLEN CROSWHITE
ASSESSMENT TECHNOLOGIES INSTITUTE

VI Adjunctive Management

If medications are ineffective in eliminating dysrhythmias, electrical cardioversion and defibrillation may be used for tachydysrhythmias and pacemaker therapy for bradycardias.

A. **Cardioversion**: Treats tachydysrhythmias by delivering an electrical current to the heart in an effort to convert the client to a normal rhythm

   1. Synchronized (timed to coincide with the client's own electrical cardiac cycle).

   2. Used when the client has a pulse.

   3. May be scheduled.

   4. Sedation is commonly used.

B. **Defibrillation**: Also delivers an electrical current to the heart, but used only for life-threatening dysrhythmias in an effort to convert the client to a more stable rhythm

   1. Used for VF or pulseless VT.

   2. Unsynchronized (not timed as with cardioversion).

   3. Delivery is required immediately (not scheduled).

   4. Used ONLY when client is pulseless.

   5. Not effective for treatment of asystole.

C. **Pacemaker Therapy**: An electronic device that provides repetitive electrical stimuli to the heart muscle, in order to control the heart rate

   1. Types

      a. Permanent pacemakers

         1) Surgically placed in the subcutaneous tissue of the chest.

         2) Client should avoid raising arm above head until wound heals.

         3) Observe for hiccups (sign of accidental dislodgement).

         4) Reinforce client education.

            a) Avoid large magnets (MRIs).

            b) Know set rate and check pulse daily.

            c) Recognize and report signs of battery failure.

            d) Wear loose-fitting clothing.

            e) Avoid contact sports.

      b. Temporary pacemakers (transvenous)

         1) Monitor ECG.

         2) Check heart rate.

         3) Monitor site for hematoma and infection.

         4) Administer analgesics as needed.

         5) Maintain electrically safe environment.

      c. Transcutaneous (skin)

         1) Externally placed for use in emergency situations only.

         2) Causes significant discomfort.

         3) Prepare for alternate interventions (temporary pacemaker).

   2. Settings

      a. Ventricular demand: Fires at a preset rate when heart rate drops below a predetermined/preprogrammed rate.

      b. Ventricular fixed: Fires constantly at a preset/preprogrammed rate, regardless of heart rate.

      c. Dual chamber: Stimulates both the atria and the ventricles.

      d. Atrial demand: Fires as needed when the atria do not originate a rhythm.

      e. Variable rate: Senses oxygen demands and increases the firing rate to meet the client's needs.

IDENTIFY THE FOLLOWING ECG RHYTHMS

Calculating Heart Rate: To estimate the client's heart rate, count the number of R waves in 6 seconds and multiply by 10. In the ECG rhythm below, there are seven R waves. The estimated heart rate is 70/min (7 x 10 = 70).

1. Name the Rhythm: NORMAL SINUS

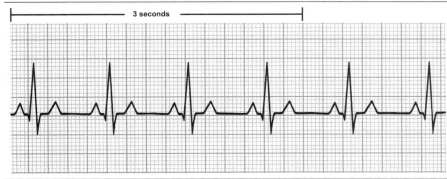

Characteristics

› Rate: Atrial (P wave) and ventricular (QRS complex) rates are 60 to 100/min.
› Rhythm: Atrial (P wave) and ventricular (QRS complex) rhythms are regular.
› P waves: Consistent and one before each QRS complex.

2. Name the Rhythm: SINUS TACHYCARDIA

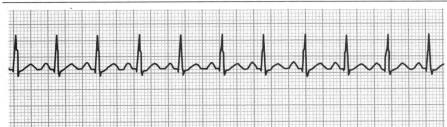

- Bronchodilator
- Stable vs. unstable?
- transiet vs. sustained?

Characteristics

› Rate: Atrial (P wave) and ventricular (QRS complex) rates greater than 100/min.
› Rhythm: Atrial (P wave) and ventricular (QRS complex) rhythms are regular.
› P waves: Consistent and one before each QRS complex.

Causes: Shock, fever, stress, exercise, anxiety, pain, stimulants.

Treatment: Usually none other than treating the cause.

3. Name the Rhythm: SINUS BRADYCARDIA

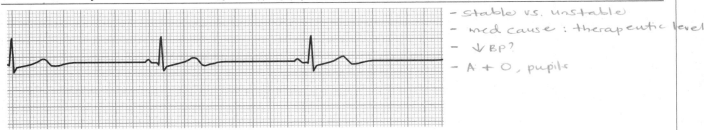

- Stable vs. unstable
- med cause: therapeutic level
- ↓ BP?
- A + O, pupils

Characteristics

› Rate: Atrial (P wave) and ventricular (QRS complex) rates less than 60/min.
› Rhythm: Atrial (P wave) and ventricular (QRS complex) rhythms are regular.
› P waves: Consistent and one before each QRS complex.

Causes: Lower metabolic needs (e.g., sleep, hypothyroidism, athletic individuals), vagal stimulation (e.g., vomiting, straining during a bowel movement), medications (e.g., beta-blockers, calcium channel blockers).

Treatment: Directed at the cause if possible (e.g., discontinuing medication, preventing vagal stimulation) or signs of hemodynamic instability (e.g., hypotensive, dyspneic, altered mental status, angina). If the client is unstable, IV atropine 0.5 mg is the medication of choice.

4. Name the Rhythm: _ATRIAL FIBRILLATION_ *(handwritten)*

(handwritten, top right) HX, rate, symptoms, new?
↓ BP ← less time for blood to fill
CONCERN: BLOOD CLOTS TO BRAIN
ATRIA QUIVERING CAUSE CLOTS
Ⓛ → BRAIN
Ⓡ → LUNGS
→ STROKE!

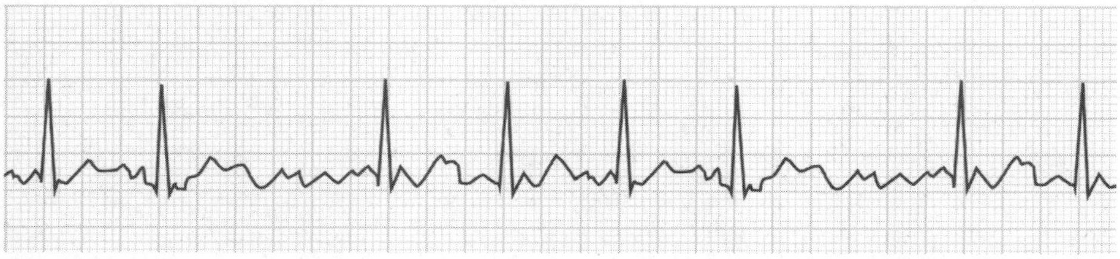

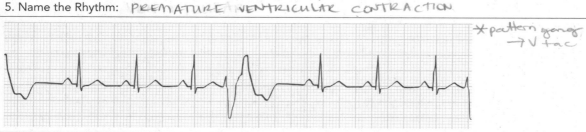

Characteristics
(handwritten: arrhythmic / synchronized a-fib.)

› Rate
  » Atrial: Multiple rapid impulses from many areas of the atria result in a fibrillatory line.
  » Ventricular: Usually responds at a rate of 120 to 200/min.
› Rhythm: Ventricular rhythm is irregular.
› P waves: No clear P wave.
› PR interval: No clear P wave so unable to determine.

Causes: Usually occurs in older adults who have heart disease.

Treatment: Depends on the cause and the duration of the dysrhythmia. Many clients convert to a NSR spontaneously within 24 hr. If a client is unstable (e.g., hypotensive, dyspneic, altered mental status, angina), electrical cardioversion may be indicated. If a client has been in this rhythm for more than 48 hr, treatment with anticoagulants should occur first with warfarin (Coumadin) for 3 to 4 weeks to avoid the formation of emboli, which can cause a cerebrovascular accident (CVA). Heart failure can occur due to loss of atrial kick. Medications can also be effective in converting the client back to a NSR. If atrial fibrillation is chronic, treatment with daily anticoagulant is common to prevent CVA.

5. Name the Rhythm: _SINUS RHYTHM w/ PREMATURE VENTRICULAR CONTRACTION_ *(handwritten)*

(handwritten, right) *pattern gang → V tac*

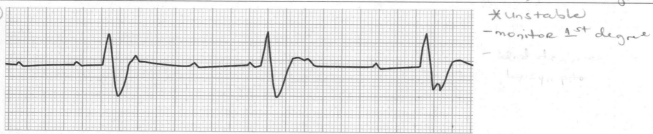

Characteristics: Not a rhythm, but are isolated abnormal beats that arise from an irritable area within a ventricle that causes the ventricle to contract prematurely. Can cause palpitations.

Causes: May occur in healthy individuals. Often associated with nicotine, caffeine, and alcohol intake. Can be caused by myocardial ischemia or infarction, heart failure, acidosis, hypoxia, and electrolyte imbalances, especially hypokalemia.

Treatment: If they occur in the absence of heart disease and are not causing a problem for the client, there might not be any treatment indicated. Treating the cause if possible and administering amiodarone or sotalol can be indicated depending on the severity and symptoms of the client. Manifestations can include slowing of the heart rate, decreased BP, and signs of impaired tissue perfusion.

6. Name the Rhythm: _ATRIAL VENTRICULAR DISOCIATION (HEART BLOCK) - 3rd degree_ *(handwritten)* *Complete*

(handwritten, right) *unstable
- monitor 1st degree
- [illegible]
- [illegible] symptoms*

(handwritten, left margin, vertical) Divorce

Characteristics
› Rate: Atrial rate is faster than the ventricular rate.
› Rhythm: Atrial and ventricular rhythms are usually regular.
› P waves: Consistently present, but not consistently followed by a QRS complex.
› PR interval: Inconsistent and no identifiable relationship between the P-wave and QRS complex.
› QRS complex: Usually consistent and can be wider than normal.

› Atrioventricular (AV) heart block: Cardiac electrical conduction transmission is blocked, not allowing any impulses to be conducted through the AV node. The atria and ventricles are beating independently from each other. Ventricular pacing is slow and unreliable.

Causes: Can be caused by medication (e.g., digitalis, beta-blockers, calcium channel blockers), myocardial ischemia and infarction, cardiomyopathy, inflammatory heart disease, or valvular disorders.

Treatment: Depends on the cause but often requires the placement of a pacemaker. Atropine is not effective.

(handwritten, bottom left) Defibrillator
- synch
- paco

IDENTIFY THE FOLLOWING ECG RHYTHMS (CONTINUED)

7. Name the Rhythm: VENTRICULAR TACHYCARDIA

"brushing teeth" ex.

2 forms:
w/ pulse or no pulse CPR wait for
↳ synchronized cardiovert defib
unstable reading → check pt!

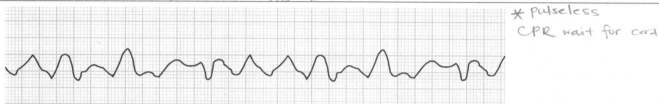

Characteristics
› Rate: Ventricular rate usually 140 to 180/min. → 200-300
› Rhythm: Irregular.
› P waves: Not usually seen.
› PR interval: Not identifiable.
› QRS complex: Wide.

Causes: Similar to those for PVCs and more lethal if associated with myocardial infarction or low ejection fraction (percent of blood ejected from the heart with each contraction).

Treatment: The client with this rhythm might not have a pulse. If the client has a pulse, cardioversion and the administration of antidysrhythmic IV medications are indicated. If the client does not have a pulse, the treatment is immediate defibrillation and CPR.

8. Name the Rhythm: VENTRICULAR FIBRILLATION

* pulseless CPR wait for cart

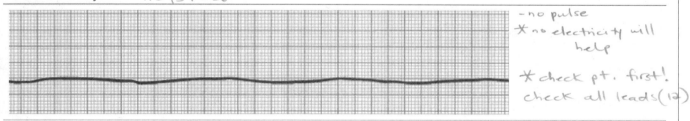

Characteristics: The electrical chaos in the heart causes the ventricles to fibrillate resulting in a fibrillatory wave pattern. There are no recognizable waves or patterns. They do not contract and there is no pulse. There is no cerebral or systemic perfusion occurring. This rhythm is usually fatal if not reversed in 3 to 5 min.

Causes: Most commonly caused by myocardial infarction and is the most common dysrhythmia resulting in cardiac arrest.

Treatment: There is never a pulse with this rhythm. In addition to CPR, immediate defibrillation is critical to survival. The chance for survival decreases by 7% to 10% for every 1 min delay in defibrillation.

9. Name the Rhythm: ASYSTOLE

- no pulse
* no electricity will help
* check pt. first!
check all leads (12)

Characteristics: There is no electrical activity in the heart. This results in a flat line with no identifiable waves or pattern. Because there is no electrical activity, there is no contraction, pulse, or perfusion occurring. The prognosis for these clients is usually poor.

Causes: Hypoxia, acidosis, severe electrolyte imbalances, drug overdose, hypovolemia, cardiac tamponade, tension pneumothorax, myocardial infarction, hypothermia, or trauma.

Treatment: High-quality CPR. Identify and treat cause. Medications such as epinephrine and vasopressin can be beneficial. If this does not correct the rhythm, resuscitation efforts are usually ceased.

Answer Key: 1. Normal sinus rhythm; 2. Sinus tachycardia; 3. Sinus bradycardia; 4. Atrial fibrillation; 5. Premature ventricular contractions; 6. Third-degree heart block; 7. Ventricular tachycardia; 8. Ventricular fibrillation; 9. Asystole

Genitourinary System Disorders

A. **Assessment of the Kidney and Urinary System**

1. Functions of the kidney

    a. Regulates acid-base balance.

    b. Regulates fluid and electrolyte balance.

    c. Excretes metabolic wastes (creatinine, urea).

    d. Regulates blood pressure: Renin (stimulated by decreased blood pressure or blood volume) stimulates the production of angiotensin I, which is converted to angiotensin II in the lungs; angiotensin II is a strong vasoconstrictor and stimulates aldosterone secretion; vasoconstriction and sodium reabsorption result in increased blood volume and increased blood pressure.

    e. Secretes erythropoietin.

    f. Converts vitamin D to its active form for absorption of calcium.

    g. Excretes water-soluble medications and medication metabolites.

    h. Minimum urine output 0.5 ml/kg/hr.

2. Contributing Factors

    a. History of genitourinary disorder

    b. History of hypertension

    c. History of diabetes

    d. Family history of kidney disease, such as PKD

    e. Incontinence, BPH, cancer, or kidney stones

    f. Nephrotoxic medications

3. Manifestations

    a. Flank pain radiating to upper thigh, testis, or labium

    b. Changes in voiding: hematuria, proteinuria, dysuria, frequency, urgency, burning, nocturia, incontinence, polyuria, oliguria, anuria

    c. Thirst, fatigue, generalized edema

B. **Diagnostic Tests**

1. Urinalysis

    a. Specific gravity

    b. Color: yellow, amber, or clear

    c. Negative glucose, protein, nitrites, RBCs, and WBCs

    d. pH

    e. First voided morning sample preferred: 15 mL

    f. Sent to laboratory immediately or refrigerated

    g. If clean catch, get urine for culture prior to starting antibiotics.

        1) Cleanse labia, glans penis.

        2) Obtain midstream sample.

2. Renal function tests (several tests over a period of time are necessary)

    a. BUN

    b. An increased BUN can indicate

        1) Hepatic or renal disease

        2) Dehydration or decreased kidney perfusion

        3) A high-protein diet

        4) Infection

        5) Stress

        6) Steroid use

        7) GI bleeding

    c. Creatinine

        1) Creatinine is the best measure of renal function.

    d. 24-hr creatinine clearance: 75 to 120 mL/min

        1) Have the client void and discard the first specimen.

        2) Obtain serum creatinine.

        3) Collect all urine from the client for the next 24 hr (refrigerate or keep container on ice).

        4) At the completion of the 24 hr, the test is stopped following the client's last void.

    e. Uric acid (serum)

    f. Prostate-specific antigen: greater than 10 indicates risk of prostate cancer

3. Radiologic tests

    a. Kidneys, ureters, bladder (x-ray): shows the size, shape, and position of kidneys, ureters, and bladder. No preparation necessary (verify that the client is not pregnant).

    b. IV pyelography (contrast dye): to help in visualization of the urinary tract

        1) Collaborative Care

            a) **Nursing Interventions**

                (1) Verify that informed consent has been signed.

                (2) Verify the client's last creatinine level.

                (3) The client should remain NPO for 8 hr; fluids may be permitted.

                (4) Administer laxatives as prescribed.

                (5) Administer an enema or suppository on the morning of the test (as necessary).

                (6) Check for allergies to iodine or shellfish.

                (7) Reinforce teaching about potential sensations during the exam (flushing, warmth, nausea, metallic or salty taste, incontinence).

                (8) Emergency equipment should be readily available during the test.

                (9) Encourage fluids to help flush out the dye.

4. Renal angiography: Visualization of renal arterial supply; contrast material injected through a catheter

   a. **Nursing Interventions** (preprocedure)
      1) Approach is through the femoral or brachial artery.
      2) Locate and mark peripheral pulses.
      3) Have the client void before the procedure.
      4) Explain that the procedure can create a feeling of warmth along the vessel.

   b. **Nursing Interventions** (postprocedure)
      1) Maintain bed rest for 6 to 8 hr.
      2) Monitor vital signs until stable.
      3) Observe for swelling and hematoma.
      4) Palpate peripheral pulses/vascular checks.
      5) Monitor I&O, including urinary status.

5. Cystoscopy: An invasive procedure in which a scope is passed to view the interior of the bladder, urethra, or the position of urethral orifices to remove calculi from the urethra, bladder, and ureter; to treat lesions of the bladder, urethra, and prostate.

   a. **Nursing Interventions** (preoperative)
      1) Maintain NPO if the client is given general anesthesia.
      2) Administer preoperative cathartics/enemas as prescribed.
      3) Encourage deep breathing and relaxation exercises to relieve bladder spasms.
      4) Monitor for postural hypotension.
      5) Inform the client that pink-tinged or tea-colored urine is common following the procedure, but bright, red urine or clots should be reported.
      6) Provide nonpharmacological pain management techniques following the procedure.

   b. **Nursing Interventions** (postoperative)
      1) Monitor for leg cramps due to lithotomy position.
      2) Monitor for back pain or abdominal pain.
      3) Offer warm sitz baths for comfort.
      4) Push fluids and provide analgesics.
      5) Monitor I&O.

6. Renal biopsy

   a. **Nursing Interventions** (preprocedure)
      1) Obtain bleeding, clotting, and prothrombin times.
      2) Obtain results of prebiopsy x-rays of kidney.
      3) Administer IV fluids.
      4) Maintain NPO status for 6 to 8 hr.
      5) Position the client with a pillow under the abdomen and shoulders on the bed.
      6) Verify that the informed consent is signed.
      7) Client should remain still during the procedure.

   b. **Nursing Interventions** (postprocedure)
      1) Maintain the client in the supine position. The client should remain in bed for 24 hr.
      2) Monitor vital signs every 5 to 15 min for 4 hr.
      3) Maintain pressure to the puncture site for 20 min.
      4) Observe for any pain, nausea, vomiting, and blood pressure changes.
      5) Encourage fluid intake.
      6) Check Hct and Hgb 8 hr after procedure.
      7) Monitor urine output.
      8) Make sure the client avoids strenuous activity, sports, and heavy lifting for at least 2 weeks.

7. Indwelling urinary catheterization: A sterile procedure to empty the contents of the bladder, obtain a sterile specimen, determine residual urine, initiate irrigation of the bladder, or bypass an obstruction.

   a. Collaborative Care
      1) **Nursing Interventions**
         a) Maintain a closed system.
         b) Measure output every shift.
         c) Provide meticulous perineal care.
         d) Keep a drainage bag below the level of the bladder.
         e) Increase daily fluid intake.
         f) Prevent dependent loops in the catheter tubing.
         g) Discontinue as soon as possible due to increased risk for urinary tract infection.

C. **Specific Disorders**

   1. Cystitis: Inflammation of the urinary bladder

      a. Contributing Factors
         1) Wiping back to front after toileting, secondary to ascending infection from *Escherichia coli*
         2) Prolonged baths with excessive soap (common in females)
         3) Benign prostatic hyperplasia (males)

      b. Manifestations
         1) Frequency and urgency, and only voiding small amounts of urine each time
         2) Dysuria with hematuria
         3) Suprapubic tenderness; pain in the bladder region or flank pain
         4) Fever, malaise, chills
         5) Cloudy, foul-smelling urine

c. Collaborative Care

 1) **Nursing Interventions**

  a) Obtain clean catch urine sample for culture and sensitivity before initiating antibiotic therapy.

  b) Maintain acidic urine pH.

  c) Push fluids (greater than 3,000 mL/day).

  d) Encourage the client to drink cranberry juice.

  e) Apply heat to the perineum for comfort.

 2) Medications

  a) Antimicrobial medications: Sulfonamides are the medications of choice unless the client is allergic (sulfamethoxazole-trimethoprim [Bactrim] and nitrofurantoin macrocrystal [Macrodantin]).

  b) Urinary analgesics (phenazopyridine [Pyridium]): Inform the client that the medication will temporarily turn urine orange.

  c) Antispasmodics: Hyoscyamine (Anaspaz, Cystospaz).

 3) Client Education and Referral

  a) Follow appropriate perineal care (wiping front to back).

  b) Wear cotton underwear.

  c) Avoid bubble baths (can irritate urethra).

  d) Maintain an increased fluid intake.

  e) Void after sexual intercourse.

  f) Drink cranberry juice daily.

2. Acute Glomerulonephritis: An acute renal disease involving the renal glomeruli of both kidneys. Thought to be an antigen-antibody reaction that damages the glomeruli of the kidney. Can be a secondary response to infection in other areas of the body that usually occurs in children. Prognosis is good if treatment is implemented.

 a. Contributing Factors

  1) Beta-hemolytic streptococci

  2) Can follow tonsillitis or pharyngitis

 b. Manifestations

  1) Hematuria (cola- or tea-colored urine) with proteinuria

  2) Edema (especially facial and periorbital; ascites)

  3) Oliguria or anuria

  4) Hypertension with headache

  5) Azotemia

  6) Flank or abdominal pain

  7) Anemia

 c. Collaborative Care

 1) **Nursing Interventions**

  a) Maintain bed rest to protect the kidney.

  b) Restrict fluids.

  c) Increase calories and reduce protein and sodium in the diet.

  d) Monitor daily weight.

 2) Medications

  a) Penicillin for streptococcal infection (substitute other antibiotics for clients allergic to penicillin)

  b) Corticosteroids for inflammatory disease

  c) Antihypertensives for increased blood pressure

3. Nephrosis: A clinical disorder associated with protein wasting; secondary to diffuse glomerular damage

 a. Contributing Factors

  1) Can be autoimmune; the glomerular membrane is more permeable, especially to proteins.

 b. Manifestations

  1) Insidious onset of pitting edema (generalized edema is anasarca)

  2) Proteinuria

  3) Anemia

  4) Hypoalbuminemia

  5) Anorexia, malaise, and nausea

  6) Oliguria

  7) Ascites

 c. Collaborative Care

 1) **Nursing Interventions**

  a) Maintain bed rest (during severe edema only) to preserve renal function.

  b) Maintain a low-sodium, low-potassium, moderate-protein, high-calorie diet.

  c) Protect the client from infection.

  d) Monitor I&O.

  e) Weigh the client and measure abdominal girth daily.

 2) Medication therapy

  a) Loop diuretics: furosemide (Lasix)

  b) Steroids: prednisone

  c) Immunosuppressive agents: cyclophosphamide (Cytoxan)

4. Urolithiasis (urinary calculi): Stones in the urinary system

 a. Contributing Factors

  1) Obstruction and urinary stasis

  2) Uric acid stones (excessive purine intake)

  3) Immobilization

  4) More common in men ages 20 to 40 and tends to reoccur

 b. Manifestations (based on location and size of the stone)

  1) Pain: severe renal colic (ureter); dull, aching (kidney); radiates to the groin

  2) Nausea, vomiting, diarrhea, or constipation

  3) Hematuria

  4) Manifestations of a urinary tract infection

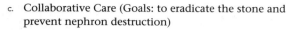

c. Collaborative Care (Goals: to eradicate the stone and prevent nephron destruction)

   1) **Nursing Interventions**

      a) Increase fluids—at least 3,000 mL/day (IV or by mouth)

      b) Strain all urine

      c) Provide pain control

      d) Maintain proper urine pH (depends on type of stone)

   2) Medications

      a) Opioids (morphine IV for rapid pain relief). NSAID ketorolac in acute phase.

      b) Administer allopurinol (Zyloprim) for uric acid stones.

   3) Therapeutic Measures

      a) Lithotripsy to crush the stone via sound waves

   4) Client Education

      a) Avoid foods high in oxalates (spinach, black tea, rhubarb, chocolate) for calcium oxalate stones.

      b) Maintain fluid intake to maintain hydration.

5. Acute renal failure: An abrupt decrease in renal function; can be the result of trauma, allergic reactions, drug overdose, kidney stones, or shock

   a. Contributing Factors

      1) Prerenal: disrupted blood flow to the kidneys; hypovolemic shock, dehydration, heart failure, burn injury, and anaphylaxis

      2) Renal: renal tissue damage; trauma, hypokalemia, acute glomerulonephritis, hemolytic uremic syndrome (infection caused by *Escherichia coli*; common in children), substance abuse

      3) Postrenal: urine flow from the kidney is compromised; kidney stones, prostate hyperplasia, tumors, and strictures

   b. Manifestations (four phases)

      1) Onset: begins with the onset of the event and lasts for hours to days.

      2) Oliguric (1 to 3 weeks): sudden onset, less than 400 mL in 24 hr, edema, elevated BUN, creatinine and potassium; increased specific gravity; acidosis; heart failure; dysrhythmias

      3) Diuretic: urine output increases followed by diuresis of up to 5,000 mL/day, indicating recovery of damaged nephrons; decreased specific gravity; hypotension and fluid and electrolyte imbalances are a concern

      4) Recovery: can take up to 1 year until renal function returns to normal (baseline); older adults are at increased risk for residual impairment

c. Collaborative Care

   1) **Nursing Interventions**

      a) Eliminate or prevent cause.

      b) Correct metabolic acidosis, hyperkalemia, hyperphosphatemia, and hypocalcemia.

         (1) Kayexalate (an ion exchange resin given orally or by enema to treat hyperkalemia)

         (2) IV glucose and insulin (causes potassium to enter cells)

         (3) Calcium IV or sodium bicarbonate to stabilize cell membrane

      c) Implement diet.

         (1) For oliguric phase, low-protein, high-carbohydrate diet and restricted potassium intake

         (2) For diuresis phase, low-protein, high-calorie diet and restricted fluids as indicated

            (a) Encourage bed rest in the oliguric phase.

            (b) Monitor daily weights.

            (c) Monitor I&O.

            (d) Implement dialysis as prescribed until renal function returns.

            (e) Monitor for pericarditis (friction rubs).

   2) Medications

      a) Phosphate binders to lower phosphorus while replacing calcium (PhosLo, calcium acetate)

      b) Epogen (Procrit) to treat anemia

6. Chronic Kidney Disease: Progressive failure of kidney function that results in death unless hemodialysis or transplant is performed; is irreversible

   a. Contributing Factors

      1) Diabetes mellitus (leading cause)

      2) Uncontrolled hypertension (second-leading cause)

      3) Chronic glomerulonephritis

      4) Pyelonephritis

      5) Congenital kidney disease, such as PKD

      6) Ethnicity—African American, Native American, and Asian

   b. Manifestations (progressively worsen)

      1) Fatigue secondary to anemia

      2) Headache and hypertension

      3) Nausea, vomiting, diarrhea

      4) Irritability

      5) Edema

      6) Hypocalcemia, hyperkalemia

      7) Pruritus, uremic frost

      8) Pallid, gray-yellow complexion

      9) Metabolic acidosis; elevated BUN and creatinine; decreased glomerular filtration rate

      10) Convulsions, coma

c. Collaborative Care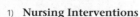

1) **Nursing Interventions**

a) Maintain bed rest.

b) Implement a renal diet—low-protein, low-potassium, high-carbohydrate, low-sodium, and low-phosphate with vitamins and calcium supplements.

c) Monitor for and treat hypertension as prescribed.

d) Strict I&O; fluid replacement—500 to 600 mL more than previous 24-hr urine output.

e) Monitor electrolytes, especially potassium.

f) Do not administer antacids with magnesium or enemas with phosphorous.

g) Maintain dialysis.

h) Administer diuretics in early stages.

i) Provide meticulous skin care.

j) Provide emotional support to the client and family.

k) Monitor for bleeding tendencies.

2) Medications

a) Phosphate binders (aluminum hydroxide gel [Amphojel], calcium acetate [PhosLo], sevelamer hydrochloride [Renagel])

b) Epoetin alfa/erythropoietin (Epogen, Procrit) for anemia to stimulate RBC formation and transfuse as necessary

7. Dialysis

a. Goals

1) Remove end products of metabolism (urea and creatinine) from the blood.

2) Maintain safe concentration of serum electrolytes.

3) Correct acidosis.

4) Remove excess fluid from the blood.

b. Hemodialysis: The process of cleansing blood of accumulated waste products and fluids; used for ESRD or clients who are acutely ill and require short-term treatment

1) Collaborative Care

a) **Nursing Interventions**

(1) Weigh the client before and after the procedure.

(2) Monitor blood pressure continuously during the procedure.

(3) Provide care to the access site to prevent clotting and infection.

(4) Monitor for presence of thrill and bruit.

(5) Provide adequate nutrition as prescribed.

(6) Post a sign above the bed that warns of no blood pressure readings or blood work on the side of the fistula.

(7) Maintain fluid restrictions.

(8) Withhold regular morning medications prior to dialysis.

(9) Instruct the client to notify the nurse of muscle cramps, headache, nausea, or dizziness during the procedure.

(10) Provide emotional support. Offer activities, such as books, magazines, music, cards, or television, to occupy the client.

c. Peritoneal dialysis: An alternative method using the peritoneum to remove fluids, electrolytes, and waste products from the blood. Dialysis is accomplished via a catheter surgically placed into the peritoneal cavity.

1) Collaborative Care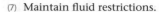

a) **Nursing Interventions**

(1) Assist the client to void prior to the procedure.

(2) Weigh the client daily.

(3) Monitor vital signs and baseline electrolytes.

(4) Maintain asepsis.

(5) Perform sterile dressing changes per facility policy.

(6) Keep an accurate record of fluid balance.

(7) Procedure

(a) Warm dialysate (1 to 2 L of 1.5%, 2.5%, or 4.25% glucose solution).

(b) Allow to flow in by gravity.

(c) 5 to 10 min inflow time; close clamp immediately.

(d) 30 min of equilibration (dwell time).

(e) 10 to 30 min of drainage (should be clear and pale yellow).

(f) Monitor for complications (peritonitis, bleeding, respiratory difficulty, abdominal pain, and bowel or bladder perforation).

d. Continuous ambulatory peritoneal dialysis (CAPD): Peritoneal dialysis performed by the client without the use of a machine (cycler)

1) Procedure (differs from acute peritoneal dialysis)

a) Permanent indwelling catheter inserted into peritoneum

b) Fluid infused by gravity (1.5 to 3 L)

c) Dwell time: 4 to 8 hr

d) Dialysate drains by gravity: 20 to 40 min

e) Four to five exchanges daily, 7 days/week (some clients may elect to do at night with automatic cycling machines; 10 to 14 hr, 3 times/week); continuous cycling peritoneal dialysis (CCPD)

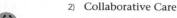

2) Collaborative Care

  a) **Nursing Interventions**

    (1) Monitor for complications.

    (2) Monitor for peritonitis (rebound tenderness, fever, cloudy outflow).

    (3) Monitor for bladder perforation (yellow outflow).

    (4) Monitor for hypotension.

    (5) Monitor for bowel perforation (brown outflow).

  b) Advantages to CAPD

    (1) More independence.

    (2) Clients may continue normal activities during CAPD.

    (3) Free dietary intake and better nutrition.

    (4) Satisfactory control of uremia.

    (5) Least expensive dialysis.

    (6) Decreased likelihood of future transplant rejection.

    (7) More closely approximates normal renal function.

8. Renal and urinary tract surgery

  a. Kidney transplantation

    1) For clients who have ESRD

    2) Requires a well-matched donor

      a) Living donors (most desirable)

      b) Cadaver donors

    3) Preoperative management

      a) Interventions are prescribed to correct metabolic status.

      b) Administer immunosuppressive therapy.

      c) Perform hemodialysis within 24 hr.

      d) Provide emotional support.

    4) **Nursing Interventions** (postoperative management)

      a) Monitor labs (CBC, electrolytes, BUN/creatinine).

      b) Administer immunosuppressive medications, such as azathioprine (Imuran), cyclosporine (Sandimmune), or steroids.

      c) Monitor for rejection. This can include oliguria, edema, fever, tenderness over graft site, fluid and electrolyte imbalance, hypertension, elevated BUN, creatinine, and elevated WBCs.

      d) Monitor for infection and maintain protective isolation.

      e) Provide emotional support and monitor for depression.

9. Urinary diversion: Removal of the bladder and surrounding structures to reroute urinary flow through a pouch and abdominal stoma

  a. Collaborative Care

    1) **Nursing Interventions**

      a) Monitor vital signs. (Hemorrhage and shock are frequent complications.)

      b) Monitor stoma.

      c) Provide pain control.

      d) Observe for manifestations of paralytic ileus, which are very common.

      e) Provide adequate fluid replacement.

      f) Weigh the client daily.

      g) Maintain function and patency of the drainage tubes.

        (1) Indwelling urinary catheter (dependent position, tape tubing to the thigh)

        (2) Nephrostomy tube

          (a) Never clamp.

          (b) Irrigate only with prescription for 10 mL of 0.9% sodium chloride.

          (c) Monitor for leakage of urine.

        (3) Ureteral catheters

          (a) Each catheter drains half of the urinary system.

          (b) Bloody drainage is expected after surgery, but should clear within 24 to 48 hr.

          (c) Never irrigate the surgical implant.

          (d) Aseptic technique is required.

10. Benign prostatic hyperplasia: Enlargement of the prostate that can accompany the aging process in males; exact cause is unknown.

  a. Manifestations

    1) Difficulty starting stream/dribbling

    2) Decrease in force of the urinary stream

    3) Frequent urinary tract infections

    4) Nocturia

    5) Hematuria

  b. Diagnosis

    1) Digital rectal exam or cystoscopy

    2) Prostate-specific antigen (PSA) for diagnosis

  c. Treatments

    1) Urinary antibiotics

    2) Alpha-blocker medications to promote urinary flow: terazosin, tamsulosin (Flomax), alfuzosin (Uroxatral), silodosin (Rapaflo), and doxazosin (Cardura)

    3) Enzyme inhibitors to decrease the size of the prostate gland: dutasteride (Avodart) and finasteride (Proscar)

4) Transurethral resection of prostate (TURP): Enlarged portion of the prostate is removed through an endoscopic instrument

   a) **Nursing Interventions** (preoperative)

      (1) Insert indwelling urinary catheter.

      (2) Administer antibiotics as prescribed.

   b) **Nursing Interventions** (postoperative)

      (1) Monitor for shock and hemorrhage.

      (2) Client should avoid heavy lifting, prolonged sitting, constipation, or straining (which could cause a rebleed).

      (3) Monitor for continuous bladder irrigation (expect bloody drainage; monitor I&O carefully).

      (4) Encourage fluid intake (at least 3,000 mL/day).

      (5) Monitor for TURP syndrome: a cluster of manifestations resulting from absorption of irrigating fluids through prostate tissue (hyponatremia, confusion, bradycardia, hypo/hypertension, nausea, vomiting, and visual changes).

      (6) Medicate for pain control: the client might need medication and narcotics to decrease bladder spasm.

      (7) Keep the catheter taped tightly to the client's leg (for hemostasis at the surgical site by catheter balloon).

      (8) Reinforce teaching about Kegel exercises (there can be temporary or permanent loss of sexual function or urinary control).

11. Prostate cancer: A slow-growing cancer of the prostate gland

   a. Contributing Factors

      1) Men age 50 and older

      2) African American

      3) Family history

      4) Elevated testosterone levels

      5) High-fat diet

   b. Manifestations

      1) Asymptomatic in early stages

      2) Hematuria

      3) Prostate-specific antigen (PSA) greater than 10

      4) Rectal exam: hard, pea-sized nodule

      5) Frequent UTIs

   c. Treatment

      1) Radical prostatectomy

      2) External radiation therapy

      3) Internal radioactive seeds

      4) Hormone therapy

12. Testicular Cancer: Rare cancer affecting one or both testes. Testicular self-examination (TSE) should begin during adolescence.

   a. Contributing Factors

      1) Men 20 to 54 years of age

      2) Higher risk in males who have an undescended testis

      3) Family history

   b. Manifestations

      1) Swelling or painless lump in one or both testes

      2) Possible heaviness or aching in lower abdomen or scrotum

   c. Treatment

      1) Offer sperm banking prior to surgery.

      2) Orchiectomy to remove affected testicle.

      3) Chemotherapy.

      4) Provide emotional support.

13. Incontinence

   a. Types

      1) Urge: Cannot hold urine when stimulus to void occurs

      2) Functional: Cannot physically get to the bathroom or is not aware of the stimulus to void

      3) Stress: Pressure such as coughing, straining, lifting, bearing down, or laughing causes incontinence; very common in middle-age women

   b. Collaborative Care

      1) **Nursing Interventions**

         a) Use adult incontinence devices.

         b) Decrease fluid intake after 6 p.m.

         c) Maintain a regular toilet schedule.

         d) Perform Credé maneuver as needed.

         e) Monitor for signs of cystitis.

         f) Reinforce importance of Kegel exercises to strengthen the sphincter.

         g) Ensure that the physical environment enhances the ability to get to the bathroom.

14. Urine retention: Caused by a physical obstruction of the urethra from acute or chronic causes (edema, BPH, tumor, inflammation or inability of the bladder to work; postanesthesia, stroke); at risk for hydronephrosis

   a. Collaborative Care

      1) **Nursing Interventions**

         a) Stimulate relaxation of the urethral sphincter by providing privacy, placing the client's hands in warm water (or just turning on the water), and encouraging guided imagery.

         b) Administer bethanechol chloride (Urecholine).

         c) Position the client upright.

         d) Ensure adequate fluid intake.

      2) Medications

         a) Urge incontinence

            (1) Anticholinergics: tolterodine (Detrol) and oxybutynin (Ditropan)

         b) Stress incontinence

            (1) Tricyclic antidepressant: imipramine (Tofranil)

GENITOURINARY SYSTEM END-OF-SECTION REVIEW

1. The important function of the kidneys includes regulation of _____ and _____.

2. Renal function tests are monitored over time. Two selective ones for the kidneys include _____ and _____.

3. A client who has cystitis should be advised to maintain _____. Nursing interventions include _____ and voiding frequently.

4. Urolithiasis (urinary calculi) can be extremely painful to the client. Priority interventions include _____ and _____.

5. Acute kidney failure can be the result of trauma, allergic reactions, kidney stones, or shock. The client is experiencing _____ when output is less than 400 mL/24 hr.

6. A significant component of any type of dialysis includes weighing the client _____ dialysis. The PN also needs to _____ when providing care.

7. A client undergoing continuous ambulatory peritoneal dialysis (CAPD) is at risk for _____. One advantage of this type of dialysis is _____ for the client.

8. When caring for a client who has an indwelling urinary catheter, the tubing should be taped to the client's _____, and the collection bag should not be lifted above the _____.

9. Monitoring for transurethral resection of prostate (TURP) syndrome is important postoperative care for clients having this procedure. Manifestations include _____ and _____.

10. A client who has incontinence needs specific instructions to decrease her symptoms. Females should be encouraged to perform _____ and limit _____ after 6:00 p.m.

WORD BANK

Acid-base balance

Acidic urine pH

Before and after

Bladder

Blood pressure

BUN

Confusion

Creatinine

Drinking more than 3,000 mL fluids

Fluids

Hyponatremia

Kegel exercises

Monitor the fistula

More independence

Oliguria

Peritonitis

Provide pain control

Straining urine

Thigh

Answer Key: 1. Acid-base balance, blood pressure; 2. BUN, creatinine; 3. Acidic urine pH, drinking more than 3,000 mL fluids; 4. Straining urine, provide pain control; 5. Oliguria; 6. Monitor the fistula, before and after; 7. Peritonitis, more independence; 8. Thigh, bladder; 9. Hyponatremia, confusion; 10. Kegel exercises, fluids.

SECTION 10

Neurosensory Disorders

A. **Neurological Assessment**

1. History of present illness

2. Mental status

   a. Level of consciousness (alert, lethargic, obtunded, stuporous, comatose)

   b. Orientation (person, place, time)

   c. Affect

   d. Mood

   e. Speech (clarity, consistency, word-finding ability)

   f. Cognition (judgment and abstraction ability)

3. Cranial nerves (I through XII)

   a. CN I, olfactory: sensory, smell

   b. CN II, optic: sensory, vision

   c. CN III, oculomotor: motor, eye

   d. CN IV, trochlear: motor, eye

   e. CN V, trigeminal: sensory, face; motor, chewing

   f. CN VI, abducens: motor, eye

   g. CN VII, facial: sensory, face and hands

   h. CN VIII, acoustic: sensory, hearing and balance

   i. CN IX, glossopharyngeal: sensory, posterior taste

   j. CN X, vagus: sensory, throat; motor, swallow, speech; cardiac innervation (slows down)

   k. CN XI, accessory: motor, throat, neck muscles, upper back

   l. CN XII, hypoglossal: motor, tongue

4. Motor function

   a. Muscles

      1) Size

      2) Symmetry

      3) Tone

      4) Strength

   b. Coordination

   c. Movement

      1) Voluntary control/involuntary movements

      2) Tremors

      3) Twitches

      4) Balance and gait

d. Posturing

1) Decorticate: An abnormal posturing indicated by rigidity, flexion of the arms to the chest, clenched fists, and extended legs. Indicative of damage to the corticospinal tract (the pathway between the brain and the spinal cord).

DECORTICATE POSTURING

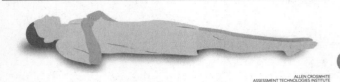

ALLEN CROSWHITE
ASSESSMENT TECHNOLOGIES INSTITUTE

2) Decerebrate: An abnormal body posturing indicated by rigid extension of the arms and legs, downward pointing of the toes, and backward arching of the head. Indicative of deterioration of structures of the nervous system, particularly the upper brain stem.

DECEREBRATE POSTURING

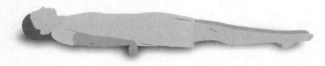

ALLEN CROSWHITE
ASSESSMENT TECHNOLOGIES INSTITUTE

5. Reflexes

a. Deep-tendon reflexes (DTRs)

1) Biceps, triceps, brachioradial, quadriceps

b. Superficial reflex

1) Plantar, abdominal, Babinski

c. Reflex activity

1) Absent, no response = 0

2) Weaker than normal = 1+

3) Normal = 2+

4) Stronger/more brisk = 3+

5) Hyperactive = 4+

6. Glasgow coma scale: neurologic assessment tool

a. Rating: 3 (least responsive) to 15 (most responsive)

GLASGOW COMA SCALE

EYE OPENING RESPONSE (E)	VERBAL RESPONSE (V)	MOTOR RESPONSE (M)
4 = Spontaneous	5 = Normal conversation	6 = Normal
3 = To voice	4 = Disoriented conversation	5 = Localizes to pain
2 = To pain	3 = Words, but not coherent	4 = Withdraws to pain
1 = None	2 = No words, only sounds	3 = Decorticate posture
	1 = None	2 = Decerebrate
		1 = None
E Score	V Score	M Score

E + V + M = Total score

7. Pupil check: PERRLA

a. **Pupils Equal in size, Round and regular in shape, Reactive to Light and Accommodation**

8. Vital signs

a. Blood pressure or heart rate changes can indicate increased intracranial pressure.

B. **Diagnostic Procedures**

1. Lumbar puncture: Procedure that inserts a needle into the subarachnoid space to measure pressure, obtain CSF for analysis, and inject contrast, anesthetics, and certain medications.

a. **Nursing Interventions**

1) Verify that informed consent has been signed.

2) Have the client empty his bladder and bowel.

3) Position the client on his side with knees pulled toward his chest and chin tucked downward.

4) Assist providers with measuring pressure and collecting fluid.

5) Postprocedure

a) Encourage fluid intake.

b) Check puncture site for redness, swelling, and clear drainage.

c) Evaluate movement of extremities.

d) Monitor for complications.

2. Computed tomography (CT) scan

a. **Nursing Interventions**

1) Preprocedure

a) Verify that informed consent has been signed.

b) Check for any allergies to iodine, contrast dyes, or shellfish.

c) Verify BUN and creatinine.

d) Instruct the client to lie still and flat.

2) Postprocedure

a) Increase fluids to clear dye from the client's system.

b) Monitor dye injection site.

c) Monitor for allergic reaction to dye.

d) Recognize and report change in client's condition.

3. Cerebral arteriography: Injection of dye usually via the femoral artery to allow visualization of the cerebral arteries

a. **Nursing Interventions**

1) Preprocedure

a) Verify that informed consent has been signed.

b) Check for allergies to iodine, contrast dyes, or shellfish.

c) Verify BUN and creatinine.

d) Keep client NPO 4 to 6 hr before the procedure.

e) Mark distal peripheral pulses.

f) Reinforce teaching that the client's face can feel warm during the procedure.

2) Postprocedure

   a) Monitor for an altered level of consciousness and sensory or motor deficits.

   b) Monitor for bleeding or hematoma at the insertion site. Movement is restricted for 8 to 12 hr.

   c) Monitor peripheral pulses, color, and temperature of extremities.

4. Electroencephalogram (EEG): Noninvasive assessment of the electrical activity of the brain. Test may be performed awake, asleep, or sleep-deprived. Electrodes are placed over multiple areas of the scalp to detect and record patterns of electrical activity, and they also check for abnormalities such as seizure disorders, evaluation of head injuries, tumors, infections, degenerative diseases, metabolic disturbances, or to confirm brain death.

  a. **Nursing Interventions**

   1) Verify which medications should be administered before the EEG. Depressive, stimulant, and antiseizure medications are usually not given.

   2) Client should avoid caffeine 8 hr before the test.

   3) Client should wash hair before the test because it must be free of oils, sprays, and conditioners.

5. Magnetic resonance imaging (MRI): A noninvasive procedure that uses a magnetic field to construct clear, detailed, cross-sectional images of the body.

  a. **Nursing Interventions**

   1) Verify that informed consent has been signed.

   2) Verify client history of claustrophobia.

   3) Remove all metal objects such as body piercings, jewelry, credit cards, and watches.

   4) No special test, diet, or medications are required.

C. **Disorders**

1. **Head injury:** Any trauma that leads to injury of the scalp, skull, or brain, ranging from concussion to skull fracture; classified as either closed or open (scalp, skull, and dura open).

  a. Closed-head injury

   1) Head sustains blunt force trauma

   2) Concussion (temporary loss of neurological function with no apparent structural damage)

   3) Contusion (brain is damaged; characterized by loss of consciousness and confusion)

   4) Diffuse axonal injury (shearing and rotational forces produce brain damage)

  b. Basilar skull fracture

   1) Manifestations

    a) Bleeding from the nose and ears

    b) Otorrhea, rhinorrhea: CSF from the ears or nose; differentiate between CSF and mucus by checking glucose content of the drainage

    c) Raccoon eyes (periorbital edema and ecchymosis)

    d) Battle's sign (postauricular ecchymosis) noted on mastoid bone

c. Hematomas

  1) Epidural hematoma: bleeding into the space between the skull and the dura

   a) Commonly involves the middle meningeal artery

   b) Typical presentation: Client sustains the injury, followed by a brief loss of consciousness. This is followed by a lucid interval, then rapid deterioration

   c) Emergency management: burr holes and placement of drain to relieve increasing intracranial pressure

  2) Subdural hematoma: bleeding below the dura

   a) Usually venous

   b) Can be acute, subacute, or chronic

   c) Manifestations

    (1) Acute: symptoms develop over 24 to 48 hr and include change in LOC, pupillary changes, and hemiparesis

    (2) Subacute: symptoms develop from 48 hr to 2 weeks after injury

    (3) Chronic: seen frequently in the elderly; symptoms can mimic CVA

    (4) Management: surgical evacuation of hematoma and/or burr holes and drain placement

  3) **Nursing Interventions**

   a) Monitor frequently for signs of increased intracranial pressure (ICP).

   b) Prevent or minimize increased ICP.

   c) Recognize and report change in client condition.

2. **Increased ICP:** A rise in pressure within the skull that can result from or cause a brain injury

  a. Contributing Factors

   1) Head injury with subdural or epidural hematoma

   2) Cerebrovascular accident or cerebral edema

   3) Brain tumor

   4) Hydrocephalus

   5) Ruptured aneurysm and subarachnoid hemorrhage

   6) Meningitis, encephalitis

  b. Manifestations (vary depending on cause and location; will affect level of consciousness)

   1) Changes in LOC such as restlessness, confusion, drowsiness, lethargy, or stupor; motor and sensory changes

   2) Headache, irritability

   3) Nausea and vomiting, often projectile

   4) Pupil changes: dilated, unequal, nonreactive

   5) Diplopia

   6) Changes in vital signs

    a) Cushing's triad: hypertension with widening pulse pressure, bradycardia, and irregular breathing

    b) Irregular respirations (Cheyne-Stokes respirations)

    c) Elevated temperature

STROKE:
- hemorrhagic
- ischemic

↑ICP
- change in LOC (early)
- cushing triad fixed (late)
  dilated pupils
  Posturing

c. Collaborative Care

   1) **Nursing Interventions**

     a) Monitor vital signs and neurological function.

     b) Keep head of bed elevated 30° to 45°.

     c) Keep the client's head in a neutral position to enhance drainage.

     d) Avoid coughing, sneezing, straining, and suctioning.

     e) Maintain maximum respiratory exchange. (Hypercapnia causes vasodilation, thus increasing ICP.)

     f) Administer oxygen to increase the supply to the brain.

     g) Monitor fluid I&O. May restrict fluids to prevent increased cerebral edema.

     h) Administer medications as prescribed.

     i) Use hypothermia as prescribed to decrease ICP.

     j) Decrease environmental stimuli.

     k) Intensive care is required when monitoring ICP (ventriculostomy).

   2) Medications

     a) Avoid opiates and sedatives unless ventilated. Will restrict neurological assessment.

     b) Barbiturates to place the client into a therapeutic coma with ventilator support and close monitoring of cardiac status.

     c) Acetaminophen (Tylenol) may be used for fever.

     d) Osmotic diuretics (mannitol [Osmitrol]) and steroids (dexamethasone) may be used to decrease cerebral edema.

3. **Hyperthermia:** Elevated temperature can be caused by infection or damage to the hypothalamic temperature regulating center. This increases cerebral oxygen demand.

  a. Contributing Factors

   1) Infections

   2) Cerebral edema

   3) Environmental heat

  b. Manifestations

   1) Temperature elevation, shivering

   2) Hypoxia

  c. Collaborative Care

   1) **Nursing Interventions**

     a) Monitor neurologic status and vital signs.

     b) Use a hypothermia blanket or cool sponge bath.

     c) Monitor ECG for tachycardia and dysrhythmias.

     d) Monitor for manifestations of dehydration by checking I&O and weighing the client daily.

     e) Initiate seizure precautions. Benzodiazepines may be prescribed to suppress seizure activity.

     f) Prevent shivering, which can occur if temperature is reduced quickly, to decrease risk of increased ICP and oxygen consumption

       (1) Chlorpromazine (Thorazine)

       (2) Benzodiazepines: diazepam (Valium)

4. **Seizure disorders:** Abnormal, sudden, uncontrolled, excessive discharge of electrical activity within the brain

  a. Contributing Factors

   1) Drug or alcohol withdrawal

   2) Trauma

   3) Brain tumors

   4) Toxicity or infection

   5) Fever

  b. Classifications

   1) Generalized seizures

     a) Tonic-clonic (formerly grand mal)

     b) Absence (formerly petit mal)

     c) Myoclonic

     d) Atonic or akinetic (drop attacks)

   2) Partial seizures

     a) Complex (usually with impairment of consciousness)

     b) Simple (usually without alteration of consciousness)

  c. Collaborative Care

   1) **Nursing Interventions**

     a) Maintain patent airway (position side-lying).

     b) Monitor respiratory status and loosen constrictive clothing.

     c) Protect the client from injury.

     d) Do not restrain the client.

     e) Do not put anything in the client's mouth.

     f) Turn client's head to the side to prevent aspiration.

     g) Document observations before, during, and after seizure.

     h) Observe for prodromal signs of an aura (a sensory warning that the seizure is about to occur).

     i) Document how long the client remains unconscious.

     j) Determine if there is any incontinence.

     k) Identify precipitating factors.

     l) Monitor and document behavior during the postictal phase (period following seizure).

     m) Initiate seizure precautions.

       (1) Bed rest should include padded side rails.

       (2) Ensure that immediate access is available for oxygen administration and suction.

   2) Medications

     a) Phenytoin (Dilantin)

     b) Carbamazepine (Tegretol)

     c) Valproic acid (Depakene, Depakote)

     d) Phenobarbital (Luminal)

     e) Levetiracetam (Keppra)

     f) Topiramate (Topamax)

(handwritten margin notes: "- nutritional support", "- glasgow coma scale")

3) Client Education

   a) Take medications consistently. Never stop abruptly.

   b) Teach manifestations of medication toxicity.

   c) Get adequate rest to minimize fatigue.

   d) Avoid alcohol.

   e) Wear medical alert bracelet.

   f) Follow state laws regarding operating vehicles and machinery.

   g) Keep all follow-up appointments.

   h) Identify seizure triggers.

5. **Status epilepticus**: A life-threatening condition characterized by a series of generalized seizures without full recovery of consciousness between. Can be caused by a sudden withdrawal of anticonvulsant medications. Can lead to brain damage or death.

  a. Collaborative Care

   1) **Nursing Interventions**

    a) Initiate seizure precautions.

    b) Collaborate with health care team.

    c) Recognize and report changes in client condition.

   2) Medications

    a) Lorazepam (Ativan): medication of choice

    b) Diazepam (Valium)

    c) Phenytoin (Dilantin)

    d) Fosphenytoin (Cerebyx)

6. **Transient ischemic attack (TIA)**: Sudden temporary episode of neurological dysfunction lasting usually less than 1 hr secondary to decreased blood flow to the brain. Can be a warning sign of an impending stroke.

  a. Contributing Factors

   1) Nonmodifiable

    a) Older adults

    b) Gender (male)

    c) Genetics

   2) Modifiable

    a) Hypertension

    b) Hyperlipidemia

    c) Diabetes mellitus

    d) Smoking

    e) Atrial fibrillation

  b. Manifestations

   1) Sudden change in visual function

   2) Sudden loss of sensory or motor functions

  c. Diagnostic Procedures

   1) Carotid ultrasound

   2) CT scan, MRI

   3) Arteriography

   4) 12-lead ECG

  d. Collaborative Care

   1) **Nursing Interventions**

    a) Encourage client to stop smoking and limit alcohol intake.

    b) DASH diet (high in fruits and vegetables, moderate in low-fat dairy products, and low in animal protein)

    c) Stress the importance of maintaining ideal body weight with regular exercise.

   2) Medications

    a) Antiplatelet medications

     (1) Clopidogrel (Plavix): may add low-dose aspirin

     (2) Dipyridamole (Persantine) plus aspirin

     (3) Ticlopidine (Ticlid)

    b) Anticoagulant medications

     (1) Warfarin (Coumadin)

    c) Lipid-lowering agents

   3) Therapeutic Measures

    a) Angioplasty

    b) Carotid endarterectomy (removal of plaque from one or both carotid arteries)

7. **Cerebrovascular accident (CVA)**: Commonly referred to as a stroke or "brain attack." The sudden loss of brain function resulting from a disruption of blood supply to the involved part of the brain. Causes temporary or permanent neurological deficits.

  a. Contributing Factors

   1) Hypertension and obesity

   2) Smoking or cocaine use

   3) Hyperlipidemia

   4) Diabetes mellitus

   5) Peripheral vascular disease

   6) Aneurysm or cranial hemorrhage

  b. Manifestations: The severity of the neurological deficit is determined by location and the extent of tissue ischemia; physical manifestations occur on the side opposite of damage to the brain.

   1) Change in mental status

   2) Slurred speech, aphasia, and dysphagia

   3) Numbness or weakness of the face or extremities, especially on one side of the body

   4) Visual disturbance

   5) Cranial nerve disturbance

   6) Loss of balance or coordination

   7) Sudden severe headache

  c. Collaborative Care

   1) **Nursing Interventions**

    a) Maintain airway.

    b) Monitor neurological function and vital signs.

    c) Establish baseline level of function and Glasgow coma scale.

    d) Maintain fluid and electrolyte balance.

e) Monitor for aspiration due to risk of dysphagia. Feed the client slowly, placing food in the back of the mouth and to the unaffected side.

f) Provide psychological support to the client and family.

g) Establish means of communication with a client who is experiencing aphasia (expressive, receptive, global).

h) Encourage slow, deliberate speech.

i) Range of motion: To prevent flexion contractures, keep extremities in a position of extension or neutrality.

j) Maintain skin integrity.

k) Hemiparesis, hemiplegia: Will cause safety issues in the client.

l) Help the client to achieve bowel and bladder control.

m) Hemianopsia: Place articles within visual range.

2) Therapeutic measures

a) Thrombolytic therapy (ischemic CVA)

b) Surgical management (usually hemorrhagic CVA)

3) Client Education and Referral

a) Occupational and physical therapy

b) Speech therapy

8. **Spinal cord injury**: Partial or complete disruption of nerve tracts and neurons; resulting in paralysis, sensory loss, altered activity, and autonomic nervous system dysfunction.

a. Contributing Factors

- location of injury determines deficit in neurosystem
⤷ higher affects breathing
⤷ lower paralysis

1) Males age 16 to 30 years

2) Motor vehicle crashes

3) Falls

4) Violence

5) Sporting activities

b. Types

1) Contusion

2) Laceration

3) Compression of the cord

4) Complete transection (paralyzed below the level of injury)

c. Manifestations (determined by the level of injury)

-spinal / neurogenic shock
-orthostatic hypotension
-immobility complications

1) Cervical: Partial or complete quadriplegia/tetraplegia

a) Respiratory dysfunction (the client can be ventilator-dependent)

b) Partial or complete paralysis of all four extremities

c) Loss of bladder and bowel control, alteration in sexual function

2) Thoracic injury: Partial or complete paraplegia

a) Loss of bladder and bowel control, alteration in sexual function

b) Partial or complete paralysis of lower extremities and major control of body trunk

c) Potential complication of autonomic dysreflexia—injury above T6

d) Respiratory complications

3) Lumbar

a) Partial or complete paralysis of lower extremities

b) Loss of bladder and bowel control, alteration in sexual function

✗ prevent OUT urinary retention, constipation, skin breakdn

d. Collaborative Care

1) **Nursing Interventions**

—VS
—bladder/bowel program
—safety

a) Immobilize the client.

(1) Spinal board

(2) Halo traction

(3) Gardner-Wells traction or Crutchfield tongs

(4) Cervical collar

b) Maintain and monitor respiratory function.

c) Monitor for spinal shock (loss of sensation, flaccid paralysis, and reflexes below the level of injury).

d) Monitor for neurogenic shock (decreased blood pressure, heart rate, and cardiac output; venous pooling).

e) Monitor for autonomic dysreflexia, a life-threatening syndrome with sudden, severe hypertension triggered by noxious stimuli below damage of cord. Can be caused by impaction, bladder distension, pressure points or ulcers, or pain.

★ still damn assess!
Injury T6 & above

(1) Manifestations

(a) Hypertension with bradycardia

(b) Headache, flushing *above level of injury*

(c) Piloerection ("goose bumps"), sweating

(d) Nasal congestion *cold & clammy below*

(2) **Nursing Interventions**

(a) Place the client in the high-Fowler's position to help decrease blood pressure.

(b) Determine and remove causative stimuli.

(c) Implement bowel and bladder management.

(d) Administer medications as prescribed.

(3) Therapeutic measures

(a) Surgical management

(4) Client Education and Referral

(a) Occupational and physical therapy

9. **Multiple sclerosis (MS)**: Chronic, progressive immune-mediated disease of the CNS, characterized by patches of demyelination in the brain and spinal cord in which symptoms occur in relapse and remission type pattern (exact cause unknown)

a. Contributing factors

1) Age 20 to 40 years

2) Female gender

3) Geographic: Europe, New Zealand, southern Australia, northern U.S., southern Canada

4) Genetic predisposition

quadriplegia paralysis 4 limbs

b. Manifestations vary in relation to location of lesion (plague).

1) MRI shows sclerotic patches through the brain and spinal cord

2) Fatigue

3) Visual disturbances: nystagmus, blurred vision, diplopia

4) Slurred speech

5) Spasticity and/or weakness of extremities, paresthesia, numbness, and pain

6) Emotional lability, depression

7) Intention tremors

8) Spastic bladder

c. Management

1) Currently there is no cure. Treatment is aimed at relieving symptoms and decreasing the frequency and severity of relapses.

2) During exacerbation, administer corticosteroids as prescribed.

3) Stress management techniques can be helpful to prevent exacerbations.

d. Collaborative Care

1) **Nursing Interventions**

a) Promote independence and maintaining an active, normal lifestyle as possible.

b) Can require education for self-catheterization.

c) Promote daily exercise with fall precautions.

d) Client should avoid stressors that exacerbate the condition (infections).

e) Prevent injury.

2) Medications

a) Immunosuppressants to reduced the frequency and duration of relapses: interferon beta-1a (Avonex) IM weekly, interferon beta-1b (Betaseron) subcutaneously, glatiramer acetate (Copaxone) subcutaneously daily

b) Muscle spasticity and tremors: baclofen (Lioresal), gabapentin (Neurontin), clonazepam (Klonopin)

c) Urinary problems and constipation: oxybutynin (Ditropan), tolterodine (Detrol), propantheline, psyllium (Metamucil)

d) Depression: amitriptyline, sertraline (Zoloft), fluoxetine (Prozac)

e) Sexual difficulties: sildenafil (Viagra)

f) Fatigue: amantadine (Symmetrel), modafinil (Provigil)

3) Client education and referrals

a) Referrals to occupational, physical, and speech therapy

b) Proper medication administration to include self-injection

c) Prevention of relapse

d) Self-catheterization if needed

10. **Parkinson's disease:** Chronic, progressive neurological disorder caused by loss of pigmented cells of substantia nigra and depletion of dopamine

a. Manifestations

1) Bradykinesia with rigidity

2) Resting tremor

3) Postural and gait disturbances

4) Expressionless, fixed gaze; masklike

5) Depression

6) Drooling and slurred speech

b. Collaborative Care

1) **Nursing Interventions**

a) Implement fall precautions.

b) Encourage clothing that fosters independence (no snaps, buttons, or zippers).

c) Encourage a high-fiber diet.

2) Medications

a) Antiparkinsonian agent: levodopa (Larodopa)

b) Dopamine agonist: bromocriptine mesylate (Parlodel)

c) Anticholinergic: benztropine (Cogentin)

d) Antiviral: amantadine hydrochloride (Symmetrel); side effects include tremor, rigidity, and bradykinesia

e) Antihistamine: diphenhydramine

3) Therapeutic measures

a) Thalamotomy and pallidotomy

b) Neural transplantation

c) Deep brain stimulation

4) Client education and referral

a) Injury prevention

b) Medication regimen

c) Promotion of adequate nutrition (may need supplementation)

d) Strategies to improve bowel and bladder function

e) Use of assistive devices

f) Referral to occupational, physical, and speech therapy

11. **Amyotrophic lateral sclerosis (ALS):** Progressive, invariably fatal neurological disease that attacks nerve cells (neurons) that control voluntary muscles; also known as Lou Gehrig's disease

a. Manifestations

1) Fasciculations (twitching), cramping, and muscle weakness

2) Fatigue

3) Slurred or nasal speech with difficulty forming words (dysarthria)

4) Difficulty chewing and swallowing (dysphagia)

5) Overactive deep-tendon reflex

6) Fatigue

7) Some experience cognitive impairment.

8) Eventual respiratory compromise. Death usually occurs from respiratory failure, infection, or aspiration.

b. Etiology unknown; no known cure; treatment is symptomatic

c. Collaborative care

  1) **Nursing Interventions**

    a) Reinforce client education.

    b) Provide information and support. Collect data about home support systems.

    c) Implement aspiration precautions and alternate methods of communication if needed.

    d) Support respiratory function (mechanical ventilation or noninvasive positive-pressure ventilation).

    e) Administer medications to provide relief from excessive salivation, pain, muscle cramps, constipation, and depression.

    f) Provide supportive services to the client and family with anticipatory grieving.

  2) Medications

    a) Glutamate antagonist: riluzole (Rilutek) can have a neuroprotective effect in early stages

    b) Manage spasticity: baclofen (Lioresal), dantrolene sodium (Dantrium), diazepam (Valium)

    c) Client education and referral

      (1) Disease progression and prognosis.

      (2) Complete advance directive

      (3) Interventions to maximize respiratory function and prevent infection

      (4) Strategies to prevent aspiration

      (5) Alternate communication methods

      (6) Referral to occupational, physical, speech therapy, home care, and hospice when needed

12. **Myasthenia gravis:** Autoimmune disorder in which antibodies are produced, it is thought by the thymus gland, which damages the acetylcholine receptor sites leading to impaired transmission at the myoneural junction. This results in voluntary muscle weakness that increases with activity, improves with rest, and is characterized by periods of exacerbation and remission.

a. Manifestations

  1) Muscular weakness that increases with activity and improves with rest.

  2) Early manifestations involve the ocular muscles leading to an increased risk of aspiration. Symptoms include diplopia, ptosis, dysphagia, and dysphonia.

  3) Progressive deterioration, particularly the respiratory system, and muscle wasting.

b. Diagnostic Procedures

  1) Edrophonium chloride (Tensilon): An acetylcholinesterase inhibitor is injected IV. Immediate improvement of symptoms that lasts approximately 5 min is considered a positive test and diagnostic of myasthenia gravis. May be used to differentiate between cholinergic and myasthenic crisis. The antidote atropine should be available to counteract possible side effects such as bradycardia, sweating, and cramping.

  2) Serum acetylcholine receptor antibodies

  3) MRI of thymus gland

  4) EMG

c. Types of Crisis

  1) Cholinergic: Usually from overmedication; muscle fasciculations, which can lead to respiratory distress, increased GI motility, hypersecretion, hypotension. No improvement or worsening of symptoms with Tensilon test.

  2) Myasthenic: Can be caused by a exacerbation trigger or inadequate medication. Characterized by varying degrees of respiratory distress, dysphagia, dysarthria, ptosis, diplopia, hypertension, and increased muscle weakness. Symptoms improve during Tensilon test.

d. Factors contributing to exacerbations

  1) Infections

  2) Pregnancy

  3) Stress, emotional distress, fatigue

  4) Increases in body temperature

  5) Inconsistency with medication administration

e. Collaborative Care

  1) **Nursing Interventions**

    a) Maintain patent airway.

      (1) Prevent aspiration.

      (2) Keep suction and manual ventilation equipment at bedside.

    b) Plan activities for the client early in the day to avoid fatigue.

    c) Provide small, frequent, high-calorie meals during the peak time for medications (within 45 min of administration).

    d) Administer medications on time.

    e) Provide eye care (instilling artificial tears and/or taping the eye shut at intervals as prescribed).

  2) Medications

    a) Anticholinesterase medications increase the amount of acetylcholine in the neuromuscular function.

      (1) Pyridostigmine (Mestinon): first-line therapy

      (2) Atropine is the antidote for anticholinesterase medications

    b) Immunosuppressants

      (1) Steroids: prednisone

      (2) Cytotoxic medications: azathioprine (Imuran)

  3) Therapeutic Measures

    a) Thymectomy (excision of the thymus)

    b) Intravenous immunoglobulin (IVIG)

    c) Plasmapheresis

  4) Client education and referral

    a) Importance of appropriate medication administration

    b) Prevention of aspiration (meals need to be timed with peak action of medication, head flexed forward, foods with thickened consistency, suction available in home)

    c) Energy conservation strategies

    d) Factors that contribute to exacerbations and actions to take if an exacerbation occurs

    e) Referral to speech therapy and Myasthenia Gravis Foundation of America

13. **Guillain-Barré syndrome**: Acute, autoimmune attack on the peripheral nerve and some cranial nerve myelin.

   a. Manifestations

      1) Usually preceded by an infection (respiratory or gastrointestinal)

      2) Usually presents with ascending weakness, which can progress to paralysis, leading to acute respiratory failure

      3) Hyporeflexia

      4) Recovery takes several months to 2 years

      5) Paresthesia and pain

   b. Collaborative Management

      1) **Nursing Interventions**

         a) Monitor respiratory status. Provide respiratory support as indicated.

         b) Monitor vital signs and ECG.

         c) Provide nutrition and prevent aspiration; can need parenteral supplementation.

         d) Manage bowel and bladder problems.

         e) Collaborate with physical therapy to maintain muscle strength, flexibility, and contractures.

         f) Prevent complications of immobility: pneumonia, DVT, urinary tract infection atelectasis, and skin breakdown.

         g) Decrease anxiety by providing information and support.

      2) Therapeutic Measures

         a) Respiratory support (can need mechanical ventilation)

         b) Plasmapheresis

         c) Intravenous immunoglobulin (IVIG)

      3) Client education and referral

         a) Verify client referrals to occupational, physical, speech, and respiratory therapy.

         b) Reinforce teaching of strategies to prevent complications of immobility.

         c) Inform that recovery can take up to 2 years.

D. **Common Surgical Procedures**

   1. **Laminectomy**: A surgical procedure to remove a portion of vertebrae for the treatment of severe pain and disability resulting from compression of spinal nerves by a ruptured disk or bony compression. Also an option to relieve persistent pain or to treat progressive neurological problems due to nerve compression

   2. **Diskectomy**: Surgical procedure to remove a herniated disk

   3. **Spinal Fusion**: Surgical fusion of the vertebral spinous process with a bone graft (either autologous or banked), which provides stabilization of the spine and decreases the risk of recurrence

      a. Collaborative Care (interventions for all procedures)

         1) Monitor vital signs.

         2) Monitor for neurological deficits.

         3) Monitor the dressing for spinal fluid, bleeding, or signs of infection.

         4) Log roll the client. Reinforce teaching with client to maintain proper alignment and decrease stress on the spine.

         5) Address sexual concerns.

         6) Manage pain.

         7) Verify referral for rehabilitation if indicated.

E. **Sensory Assessment**

   1. Ocular assessment

      a. Assessment of visual acuity with the use of the Snellen chart. The client stands 20 feet from the chart and is asked to read the smallest line. Corrective lenses for distance vision should be worn during test.

         1) Manifestation

            a) Myopia (nearsightedness): Distant objects appear blurred.

            b) Hyperopia (farsightedness): Close objects appear blurred.

            c) Presbyopia (farsightedness associated with aging): A progressive condition in which the lens of the eye loses its ability to focus.

            d) Macular degeneration: A progressive disorder of the retina causing the loss of central vision.

            e) Legal blindness: Vision in the better eye does not exceed 20/200 or whose widest visual field diameter is 20° or less.

      b. External eye exam

      c. Direct and indirect ophthalmoscopy

      d. Tonometry: measures intraocular pressure

   2. Treatment of visual acuity problems

      a. Abnormal refractory findings are typically treated with corrective lenses.

      b. Laser eye surgery (Lasik): This procedure changes the shape of the cornea with the goal of restoring 20/20 vision.

   3. Common optical problems

      a. Detached retina: Occurs when the sensory retina separates from the pigment epithelium of the retina. Vitreous humor fluid flows between the layers when a tear occurs in the retina. Can be related to age or trauma.

         1) Manifestations

            a) Sudden visual disturbances

            b) Flashes of light

            c) Blurred vision with floaters

            d) Curtain or shadow over visual field across one eye

         2) **Nursing Interventions** (preoperative)

            a) Maintain bed rest with patch to affected eye.

            b) Client should avoid coughing, sneezing, and straining.

            c) Surgical intervention includes scleral buckling, photocoagulation, cryosurgery, vitrectomy, and pneumatic retinopexy.

3) **Nursing Interventions** (postoperative)

   a) Maintain bed rest in prescribed position with eye patch and shield in place.

   b) Avoid jarring, bumping head, straining, or coughing.

   c) Administer medications as prescribed (antiemetic, antibiotic, anti-inflammatory).

   d) Reinforce education about importance of self-administration of eye drops on schedule.

b. Cataract: Slow, progressive clouding of the lens

1) Manifestations

   a) Painless diplopia, blurred vision

   b) Decreased visual acuity

   c) Frequent change in eyeglasses prescription

   d) Perception of surroundings being dimmer

2) **Nursing Interventions** (preoperative: dilate the eye)

   a) Administer medications as prescribed.

     (1) Mydriatics

     (2) Antibiotics

     (3) Corticosteroids

3) **Nursing Interventions** (postoperative)

   a) Keep the operative eye covered.

   b) Elevate head of bed 30° to 45°. Do not turn the client onto operative side.

   c) Client should avoid bending at the waist, lifting, sneezing, and coughing, and not touch the eye area.

   d) Prevent vomiting or straining.

   e) Client should report severe pain immediately.

4) Therapeutic Measures

   a) Surgical treatment: removal of the lens usually under local anesthesia, with intraocular lens implant

c. Glaucoma: Group of ocular conditions characterized by optic nerve damage, which can be caused by increased intraocular pressure (IOP)

1) Manifestations

   a) Acute (closed-angle) ocular emergency

     (1) Results from an obstruction to the outflow of aqueous humor resulting in increased intraocular pressure (IOP)

     (2) Rapidly progressive visual impairment

     (3) Severe pain in and around the eye

     (4) Reduced central visual acuity

     (5) Blurred vision with dilated pupils

     (6) Nausea and vomiting

   b) Open angle

     (1) Insidious onset with slowly decreasing visual acuity

     (2) Usually bilateral, but one eye can be more affected

     (3) Halos around lights

     (4) Fluctuating intraocular pressures

     (5) Can be asymptomatic

2) Collaborative Care

   a) **Nursing Interventions**

     (1) Administer medications consistently on time.

     (2) Avoid anticholinergic medications.

   b) Medications to promote pupils to contract

     (1) Cholinergics: miotics (pilocarpine, carbachol)

     (2) Adrenergic agonists: dipivefrin, epinephrine

     (3) Beta-blockers: betaxolol, timolol

     (4) Carbonic anhydrase inhibitors: acetazolamide

     (5) Prostaglandin analogues: latanoprost, bimatoprost

     (6) Alpha-adrenergic agonists: apraclonidine, brimonidine

   c) Therapeutic Measures

     (1) Laser trabeculoplasty

     (2) Iridotomy

     (3) Drainage implants or shunts

   d) Client Education

     (1) Reinforce teaching about appropriate administration of medications.

     (2) Discuss importance of avoiding activities that can increase IOP.

     (3) Inform of importance of follow-up appointments.

F. **Auditory Assessment**

1. Auditory Assessment

   a. Inspection of external ear

   b. Otoscopic examination

   c. Evaluation of gross auditory acuity

   d. Audiometry

2. Disorders

   a. **Ménière's disease:** Abnormal inner ear fluid balance, which can lead to disabling symptoms

     1) Manifestations

       a) Vertigo

       b) Tinnitus

       c) Pressure in the ear

3. Collaborative Care

   a. **Nursing Interventions**

     1) Provide with small, frequent meals low in sodium.

     2) Initiate and teach fall precautions.

     3) Maintain a quiet environment.

   b. Medications

     1) Antihistamines: meclizine (Antivert)

     2) Tranquilizers to control acute vertigo: diazepam (Valium)

     3) Antiemetics to control nausea, vomiting, and vertigo: promethazine

     4) Diuretics to reduce pressure from fluid

   c. Client Education

     1) Encourage a low-sodium diet.

     2) Encourage the client to drink plenty of fluids but to avoid caffeine and alcohol.

     3) Avoid monosodium glutamate (MSG), aspirin, and aspirin-containing medications, which can increase symptoms.

NEUROSENSORY END-OF-SECTION REVIEW

1. A client is scheduled for a CT with contrast. It is important to verify allergies to _____ and shellfish prior to a client receiving contrast dye.

2. A client should avoid any stimulant or depressive medications, as well as _____, prior to a scheduled for an electroencephalogram (EEG).

3. A PN is caring for a client who has a head injury. It is very important to monitor _____.

4. A PN is caring for a client who has a history of seizures. When caring for this client, it is important to place the bed in the _____ position and _____ the side rails.

5. A client is taking phenytoin (Dilantin) daily. This client should avoid consumption of _____.

6. A PN is caring for a client who has had a stroke and is experiencing dysphagia. During meals, the PN needs to have the client flex her head slightly _____ and place food on the _____ side.

7. A PN is caring for a client who has a spinal cord injury at T3. This client is at risk for autonomic dysreflexia, which is characterized by severe hypertension. Priority interventions include raising the head of bed, identifying and _____ the causative stimuli, and administering _____ medications as prescribed.

8. Priority care for a client who has myasthenia gravis includes administering medications at their _____ time of action (usually given within 45 min of meals) to prevent aspiration.

9. A client who has cataracts returns to the room following an intraocular lens implant. The client should avoid bending at the waist, _____, and _____.

10. A client who has Meniere's disease should follow a low-_____ diet. Due to this client's potential for vertigo, it is important to maintain _____ precautions.

Answer Key: 1. Iodine; 2. Caffeine; 3. Level of consciousness; 4. Lowest, Pad; 5. Alcohol;
6. Forward, Unaffected; 7. Removing, Antihypertensive; 8. Peak; 9. Sneezing, Coughing; 10. Fall

WORD BANK

Affected

Alcohol

Antihypertensive

Backward

Caffeine

Coughing

Fall

Forward

Highest

Iodine

Level of consciousness (LOC)

Lowest

Pad

Peak

Protein

Removing

Sneezing

Sodium

Unaffected

SECTION 11

Oncology Nursing

A. **Overview of Cancer**

1. Healthy cells transform into malignant cells upon exposure to certain etiological agents (viruses, chemicals, and physical agents).

2. Malignant cells metastasize and extend directly into adjacent tissue, moving through the lymph system, entering the blood circulation, and diffusing into body cavities.

B. **Risk Factors**

1. Age

   a. Older adult women most commonly develop colorectal, breast, lung, pancreatic, and ovarian cancers.

   b. Older adult men most commonly develop lung, colorectal, prostate, pancreatic and gastric cancers.

2. Race

3. Genetic disposition

4. Exposure to chemicals, viruses, tobacco, alcohol

5. Exposure to certain viruses, bacteria

6. Sun exposure

7. Diet high in red meat and fat and low in fiber

C. **General Disease-Related Consequences of Cancer**

1. Decreased immunity and blood-producing function

   a. Occurs most often with leukemia and lymphoma or any cancer that invades the bone marrow and reduces the production of WBCs, RBCs, and platelets, causing thrombocytopenia.

   b. Clients are at increased risk for infection.

   c. Changes are caused by the cancer or chemotherapy.

   d. Clients can experience weakness, fatigue, and bleeding.

2. Altered GI structure and function

   a. Impaired absorption and elimination related to tumor obstruction or compression.

   b. Tumors increase the metabolic rate, increasing the need for proteins, fats, and carbohydrates.

   c. Liver tumors reduce function and lead to malnutrition.

3. Motor and sensory deficits

   a. Occur when cancers invade the bone or brain, or compress nerves.

   b. Bone metastases cause pain, fractures, spinal cord obstruction, and hypercalcemia, which decreases mobility.

   c. Sensory changes occur if the spinal cord is damaged by tumor pressure or compression.

   d. Sensory, motor, and cognitive functions are impaired when cancer is in the brain.

   e. Pain is often significant, especially in the terminal stages of the disease process.

4. Decreased respiratory function

    a. Disrupts respiratory function and gas exchange (i.e., tumors in an airway cause an obstruction).

    b. Lung capacity is decreased; gas exchange is impaired.

    c. Tumors can compress blood and lymph vessels in the chest, blocking blood flow through the chest and lungs, causing pulmonary edema and dyspnea.

D. **Cancers/Tumors**

1. Classified according to type of tissue from which they evolve.

2. Carcinomas begin in epithelial tissue (skin, gastrointestinal tract lining, lung, breast, uterus).

3. Sarcomas begin in nonepithelial tissue (bone, muscle, fat, lymph system).

4. Adenocarcinomas arise from glandular organs.

5. Leukemias are malignancies of the blood-forming cells.

6. Lymphomas arise from the lymph tissue.

7. Multiple myeloma arises from plasma cells and affects the bone.

E. **Manifestations Suggesting Malignant Disease**

1. American Cancer Society Seven Warning Signs

    a. **C** – Change in bowel or bladder habits

    b. **A** – A sore that does not heal

    c. **U** – Unusual bleeding or discharge

    d. **T** – Thickening or lumps in breast or elsewhere

    e. **I** – Indigestion or difficulty swallowing

    f. **O** – Obvious change in wart or mole

    g. **N** – Nagging cough or hoarseness

2. Other manifestations

    a. Weight loss

    b. Fatigue/weakness

    c. Pain (might not occur until late in the disease process)

    d. Nausea/anorexia

F. **Cancer Management:** Purpose is to prolong survival time or improve the quality of life. Therapies include chemotherapy, radiation, surgery, hormonal manipulation, photodynamic therapy, immunotherapy, gene therapy, and a variety of alternative therapies.

1. Chemotherapy

    a. Systemic or local cytotoxic medications that damage a cell's DNA or destroy rapidly dividing cells. Combination of medications usually given.

    b. Classification (all cause bone marrow depression)

        1) Alkylating agents: uracil mustard (nitrogen mustard), cyclophosphamide (Cytoxan), cisplatin (Platinol)

        2) Antimetabolite: fluorouracil (5-FU, Efudex), methotrexate (MTX, Trexall)

        3) Antibiotics: doxorubicin hydrochloride, bleomycin (Blenoxane), dactinomycin (Actinomycin D)

        4) Antimitotics: vincristine (Oncovin), vinblastine (Velban)

        5) Hormones: estrogen, progesterone, tamoxifen citrate (Tamofen), peclitaxel (Taxol)

        6) Biological modifiers: epoetin alfa (Procrit), filgrastim (Neupogen)

    c. Common side effects and interventions to counteract

        1) Bone marrow suppression: neutropenia and leukopenia

            a) Interventions to enhance the immune system include a balanced diet, rest, and hand hygiene.

            b) Interventions to avoid infections

                (1) Limit visitors who might be ill.

                (2) Avoid fresh fruits, vegetables, and plants.

            c) Monitor temperature. Consider any temperature elevation in a client who has neutropenia as a possible sign of infection and report to provider.

            d) Implement protective isolation during hospitalization.

        2) Anemia

            a) Administer oxygen therapy.

            b) Provide iron-rich foods.

            c) Monitor CBC and blood transfusions as needed.

            d) Administer erythropoietin (Epogen) and epoetin alfa (Procrit) to increase RBCs.

        3) Thrombocytopenia

            a) Administer prescribed platelet transfusions, oprelvekin (Neumega) to increase platelets.

            b) Implement bleeding precautions. Avoid use of aspirin.

        4) Alopecia (hair loss 2 weeks after start of treatment)

            a) Apply ice to the scalp during chemotherapy to slow hair loss. Use gentle shampoo, hats, scarves, and sunscreen.

            b) Refer client to the American Cancer Society, which provides wigs and supportive services.

        5) Anorexia, nausea, vomiting, and GI issues

            a) Administer antiemetic prior to therapy: ondansetron (Zofran), dolasetron (Anzemet).

            b) Administer loperamide (Imodium A-D) to manage diarrhea.

            c) The client should drink cool beverages and eat small, favorite meals high in potassium with high-calorie supplements. Avoid unpleasant odors.

            d) Provide soft, bland, high-protein foods at room temperature for stomatitis. Use a straw for fluids. Rinse mouth with a topical anesthetic. Can need topical steroids and zinc supplements.

        6) Elevated uric acid, crystal, and urate stone formation

            a) Administer allopurinol (Zyloprim).

            b) Increase fluid intake.

        7) Mucositis: Often develops in the GI tract, especially in the mouth (stomatitis). Mucous membranes, because they undergo rapid cell division, are killed more rapidly than the cells are replaced.

            a) Inspect mouth and provide frequent oral hygiene, including teeth cleaning and mouth rinsing.

            b) Avoid traumatizing oral mucosa due to risk of bleeding. Use soft-bristled toothbrush or swabs.

            c) Use plain water or saline for oral rinses.

8) Specific medications have specific toxic effects.

   a) Doxorubicin hydrochloride: irreversible cardiomyopathy

   b) Anzemet (Platinol), methotrexate (Trexall): renal toxicity

   c) Vincristine sulfate (Oncovin): peripheral neuropathy

2. Radiation: Therapy destroys cancer cells with minimal exposure of normal cells to the damaging actions of radiation. Cells damaged by radiation either die or become unable to divide. Gamma rays are used most commonly because of their ability to penetrate tissues and damage cells.

  a. Radiation Delivery

   1) Teletherapy: distance treatment; the radiation source is external to the client.

   2) Brachytherapy: short or close therapy. Radiation comes into direct, continuous contact with the tumor tissues. Provides a high dose of radiation with a limited amount to surrounding tissues. (With brachytherapy, the radiation source is within the client who emits radiation and is a hazard to those around for a period of time.)

  b. **Nursing Interventions**

   1) Client must always be in the same position for all radiation treatments. Ensure that the client can get into and maintain the same position during treatment. Fixing devices and markings must be in the correct position for each treatment.

   2) Monitor condition of skin. Cleanse the area gently each day with water or mild soap.

   3) Wet reaction: skin's response to radiation. Skin becomes dry or develops blisters that may break, causing pain and the potential for infection. If dry reaction, keep clean and lubricated. If wet reaction, clean and cover to prevent infection.

   4) Client should not remove skin markings. Avoid powders, lotions, and creams unless prescribed.

   5) Client should wear soft, loose clothing and avoid exposure to the sun.

   6) For clients who have sealed implants of radioactive sources

    a) Assign client to a private room.

    b) Place "Caution: Radioactive Material" sign on the client's door in hospital setting.

    c) Wear a lead apron while providing care. Pregnant nurses should not care for these clients.

    d) Limit visitors to 30 min/day, and instruct to remain at least 6 feet from the source.

    e) Do not touch the radioactive source with bare hands.

    f) Save all radioactive dressings and linens until the radioactive source is removed.

    g) Follow institution guidelines for radiation containment.

3. Managing Cancer Pain: Adequate pain control can make a significant difference in improving the client's quality of life. Oncology clients are often undertreated for pain. As a client advocate, it is the nurse's responsibility to ensure that the client is receiving adequate pain control. (See Opioid Analgesics in Unit Four: Pharmacology in Nursing.)

4. Psychosocial support: Nursing support of the client who has cancer is very important. Issues include disturbed body image, and change in appearance, function, and role, which can affect the client's ability to deal with the diagnosis and treatment.

SECTION 12

Immunologic Disorders

> **KEY POINT:** The Centers for Disease Control and Prevention (CDC) is the best source for the most up-to-date information regarding HIV and AIDS.

A. **Acquired Immune Deficiency Syndrome (AIDS)**

1. Human immunodeficiency virus (HIV) can progress to AIDS. HIV is a viral infection that is transmitted via blood and other body fluids. It affects the ability of the immune system to fight infection, specifically, CD4 cells.

  a. HIV infection is divided into four stages.

   1) *Stage 1, Acute infection*: Described as the "worst flu ever." Retroviral syndrome usually occurs 2 to 4 weeks after the infection is acquired.

   2) *Stage 2, Latency*: Sometimes called asymptomatic HIV infection or chronic HIV infection. During this phase, HIV reproduces at very low levels, although it is still active. CD4 counts can remain at healthy levels. This stage can last 8 years or longer.

   3) *Stage 3, AIDS*: CD4 counts drop below 200 cells/mm^3. The body becomes susceptible to opportunistic infections. Survival in this stage is usually 1 to 3 years.

   4) *Stage 4, HIV Infection, Stage Unknown*: No information available on CD4+ T-lymphocyte count or percentage and no information available on AIDS-defining conditions.

2. Contributing Factors

  a. Unprotected sexual contact

  b. IV drug use; use of contaminated needles

  c. Multiple sexual partners

  d. Pregnancy and breastfeeding: transmission from mother to baby

  e. Blood transfusion (very small risk: 0.02%)

3. Manifestations

   a. Stages

      1) Stage 1: Acute infection

         a) Fever

         b) Lymph adenopathy

         c) Pharyngitis

         d) Rash

         e) Arthralgia, myalgia

         f) High HIV viral load; can test positive for antibodies.

         g) CD4 count is greater than 500 cells/mm^3

         h) Virus is transmissible to others

      2) Stage 2: Latency

         a) Lymphadenopathy, but can be asymptomatic

         b) Will test positive for HIV antibodies

         c) CD4 count is 200 to 499 cells/mm^3

      3) Stage 3: AIDS

         a) Opportunistic infections occur

           (1) Respiratory: pneumocystis carinii pneumonia, tuberculosis, Kaposi's sarcoma

           (2) GI: cryptosporidiosis, candida, cytomegalovirus (CMV), isosporiasis, Kaposi's sarcoma

           (3) Neuro: cytomegalovirus, toxoplasmosis, cryptococcosis, non- Hodgkin's lymphoma, varicella zoster (shingles), herpes simplex

           (4) Skin: shingles, herpes simplex, Kaposi's sarcoma

KAPOSI'S SARCOMA

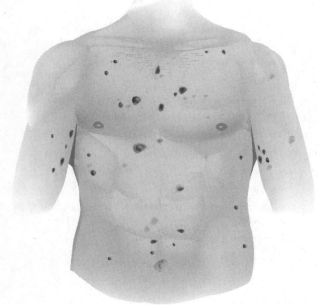

ALLEN CROSWHITE
ASSESSMENT TECHNOLOGIES INSTITUTE

   b) Wasting syndrome

   c) AIDS dementia

   d) Weakness and malaise

   e) Psychosocial: anxiety, depression, poor self-image

   f) CD4 count drops below 200 cells/mm^3

4. Diagnostic Procedures

   a. ELISA (antibody assay): Positive within 3 weeks to 3 months following infection. Most common and least expensive.

   b. Plasma HIV-1 RNA viral load is greater than 1,500 copies.

   c. CD4+ cell count: Decreased less than 750 cells/mm^3. Clients who have values less than 200 cells/mm^3 have an 85% likelihood of progressing to AIDS within 3 years.

   d. CBC and platelets are decreased.

   e. Brain, lung, or CT scans can be abnormal.

5. Collaborative Care

   a. **Nursing Interventions**

      1) Prevention

         a) Reinforce teaching about transmission routes.

         b) Emphasize need to use condoms with sexual encounters.

         c) Explain that risk is reduced by limiting sexual partners.

         d) Reinforce teaching with IV drug users to use clean needles or, if they reuse, to clean between each use with water and bleach.

         e) Emphasize need for pregnant women who are HIV-positive to begin or remain on antiviral therapy. Infants should NOT be breastfed.

         f) Ensure consistent use of standard precautions by health care workers in clinical settings.

      2) Stages 1 and 2

         a) Reinforce teaching about risk of transmission of HIV to others and ways to prevent.

         b) Emphasize importance of compliance with antiviral therapy, once initiated.

         c) Encourage healthy lifestyle habits.

         d) Provide psychological support.

      3) Stage 3

         a) Prevent infection.

         b) Enhance oxygenation.

         c) Provide comfort measures.

         d) Monitor weight, I&O, and calorie count. Encourage high-calorie foods.

         e) Perform frequent oral care.

         f) Provide scrupulous skin care.

         g) Monitor mental status. Reorient PRN. Maintain consistent environment.

         h) Provide psychosocial support. Include significant others.

b. Medications

  1) Medication therapy: highly active antiretroviral therapy guidelines (HAART) are devised by the World Health Organization and are updated as new research findings become available.

KEY POINT: Once a client begins HAART therapy, it is crucial that doses are NOT missed. Doing so contributes to medication resistance and reduces medication treatment options.

  2) Efavirenz (Sustiva), azidothymidine (AZT), and lamivudine (Epivir)

    a) Common adverse effects: neutropenia, gastrointestinal distress, anemia, insomnia

  3) Zidovudine (AZT): recommended for protecting the unborn fetus of women who are HIV-positive

  4) Interferon (Roferon)

  5) Pneumocystis pneumonia prophylaxis : pentamidine (Pentam 300)

  6) Antifungals: metronidazole (Flagyl) and amphotericin B (Fungizone)

  7) Antituberculosis medications as needed

  8) Acyclovir (Zovirax) herpes treatment

  9) Protease inhibitors: saquinavir (Fortovase), ritonavir (Norvir)

  10) Antivirals: zalcitabine, dideoxycytidine (Hivid)

c. Client Education

  1) Transmission, control measures, and safe sex practices

  2) Nutritional needs, self-medication of prescribed medications, and potential adverse effects

  3) Symptoms that need to be reported immediately (infection, bleeding)

  4) Need for follow-up monitoring CD4+ and viral load counts

B. **Systemic Lupus Erythematosus (SLE):** A chronic inflammatory disease that occurs when the body's immune system attacks the tissues and organs. Inflammation caused by lupus can affect multiple organ systems such as the joints, skin, kidneys, blood cells, heart, and lungs.

  1. Contributing Factors

    a. Female gender

    b. Age between 15 and 40 years

    c. African American, Latino, or Asian ethnicity

    d. Exposure to sunlight

    e. Long-term use of certain medications

      1) Chlorpromazine

      2) Hydralazine (Apresoline)

      3) Isoniazid

      4) Procainamide (Pronestyl, Procanbid)

    f. Exposure to mercury or silica

  2. Manifestations

    a. Insidious onset characterized by remissions and exacerbations

    b. Erythematosus "butterfly rash" on both cheeks and across the bridge of the nose; rash deepens on exposure to sunlight

ERYTHEMATOSUS "BUTTERFLY RASH"

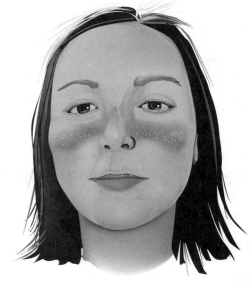

ALLEN CROSWHITE
ASSESSMENT TECHNOLOGIES INSTITUTE

    c. Polyarthralgia

    d. Fever, malaise, and weight loss

    e. Alopecia

    f. Anemia, lymphadenopathy

    g. Positive for antinuclear antibodies

    h. Depression

    i. Coin-like lesions (in discoid lupus)

    j. Pleural effusion, pneumonia

    k. Pericarditis

    l. Raynaud's phenomenon

    m. Neurological: psychosis, paresis, seizures, migraines

    n. Abdominal pain

    o. Edema

    p. Nephritis

  3. Collaborative Care

    a. **Nursing Interventions**

      1) Monitor vital signs, especially related to cardiovascular function.

      2) Monitor urinary function.

      3) Provide comfort measures.

      4) Encourage rest periods during the day.

      5) Provide measures that promote restful sleep.

      6) Cleanse skin with mild soap and pat to dry. Apply moisturizer.

      7) Monitor for infection, and teach measures to avoid.

b. Medications

    1) NSAIDs to reduce inflammation: contraindicated for clients who have renal compromise

    2) Corticosteroids for immunosuppression and to reduce inflammation

    3) Immunosuppressant agents: methotrexate (Rheumatrex), azathioprine (Imuran)

    4) Antimalarial (hydroxychloroquine [Plaquenil]) for suppression of synovitis, fever, and fatigue

c. Client Education and Referral

    1) Client should use sunscreen and wear protective clothing.

    2) Encourage small, frequent meals if anorexia is present.

    3) Limit salt intake for fluid retention secondary to steroid therapy and renal involvement.

    4) Refer to support groups as appropriate.

SECTION 13

Burns

A. **Overview**

1. Thermal, chemical, electrical, and radioactive agents can cause burns, resulting in cellular destruction of the skin layers and underlying tissue. The type and severity of the burn affect the treatment plan.

2. Burn injuries can result in the loss of temperature regulation, sweat and sebaceous gland function, and sensory and organ function.

3. Burn assessment and severity are based upon the following.

    a. Percentage of total body surface area (TBSA)

    b. Depth of the burn

    c. Body location

    d. Client's age

    e. Causative agent

    f. Presence of other injuries

    g. Respiratory involvement and overall health of the client

B. **Burn Assessment**

1. Extent of body surface (see "Rule of Nines" below)

2. Depth of burn and manifestations (see "Burn Descriptions" below)

❗ Point to Remember

The Rule of Nines assesses the percentage of burn and is used to help guide treatment decisions, including fluid resuscitation. It is part of the guidelines to determine burn management.

RULE OF NINES

Estimating TBSA Affected by Burns

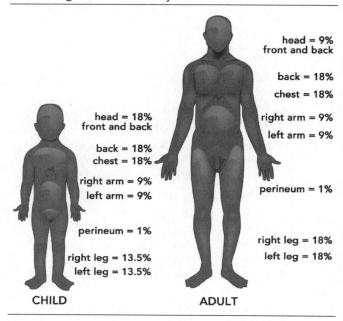

head = 9% front and back

back = 18%

chest = 18%

right arm = 9%

left arm = 9%

perineum = 1%

right leg = 18%

left leg = 18%

ADULT

head = 18% front and back

back = 18%

chest = 18%

right arm = 9%

left arm = 9%

perineum = 1%

right leg = 13.5%

left leg = 13.5%

CHILD

Example

An adult client weighing 165 lb is brought to the emergency department with second-degree burns covering the anterior and posterior surfaces of both legs.

Calculate the % of burn.

Anterior/posterior of right leg = 18%

Anterior/posterior of left leg = 18%

18% + 18% = 36%

BURN DESCRIPTIONS

CLASSIFICATION	DEGREE (OLD TERM)	LAYER INVOLVED	APPEARANCE	EXAMPLES	PAIN
Superficial	First degree	Epidermis	Pink to red, tender, no blisters, mild edema, no eschar	Sunburn, flash burns	Yes
Superficial Partial Thickness	Second degree	Epidermis and parts of dermis	Red to white with blisters, mild to moderate edema, no eschar	Flame or burn scalds	Yes
Deep Partial Thickness	Third degree	Epidermis and deep into dermis	Red to white with moderate edema, no blisters, soft/dry eschar	Flame and burn scalds; grease, tar, or chemical burns; exposure to hot objects for prolonged time	Yes
Full-Thickness	Third degree	Same as partial—may extend into subcutaneous tissue; nerve damage	Red to tan, black, brown, white. No blisters; severe edema, hard inelastic eschar	Burn scalds; grease, tar, chemical, or electrical burns; exposure to hot objects for prolonged time	May or may not be painful
Deep Full-Thickness	Fourth degree	All layers plus muscles, tendons, bones	Black with no edema	Chemical	None

3. Diagnostic testing
   a. CBC, serum electrolytes, BUN, ABGs, fasting blood glucose, liver studies, urinalysis, clotting studies, and chest x-ray. Add creatinine and myoglobin for deep burns.
      1) Initial fluid shift (first 24 hr after injury)
         a) Hct/Hgb elevated due to fluid shifts into interstitial spacing and fluid loss
         b) Sodium decreased secondary to third spacing
         c) Potassium increased due to disruption of sodium-potassium pump, tissue destruction, and RBC hemolysis
      2) Fluid mobilization (48 to 72 hr after injury)
         a) Hct/Hgb decrease due to fluid shift from interstitial back into vascular fluid
         b) Sodium remains decreased; potassium increases due to renal loss and movement back into the cells
   b. WBC count: initial increase then decrease with a shift to the left (an increase in the percentage of neutrophils having only one or a few lobes)
         a) Blood glucose: elevated due to stress response
         b) ABGs: slight hypoxemia and metabolic acidosis
         c) Total protein and albumin: low due to fluid loss

C. **Collaborative Care**
   1. **Nursing Interventions** for moderate and major burns
      a. Maintain airway and ventilation.
      b. Provide humidified oxygen as prescribed.
      c. Monitor vital signs.
      d. Maintain cardiac output by IV fluid replacement. (Parkland formula may be used)
         1) Give 4 mL/kg/% burn.
         2) Give half of total fluids in first 8 hr.
         3) Give second half over remaining 16 hr.
         4) Deduct any fluid given prehospital from the amount to be infused in the first 8 hr.
      e. Maintain urine output of 30 to 50 mL/hr for a burn client.
      f. Monitor for manifestations of shock.
      g. Provide pain management.
      h. Monitor for and prevent infection.
      i. Provide nutritional support.
         1) Client with a large burn injury will be in a hypermetabolic state and may need up to 5,000 calories/day.
         2) Increase protein intake to prevent tissue breakdown and promote healing.
         3) Enteral or total parenteral therapy is often necessary.
      j. Promote restoration of mobility.
      k. Provide psychological support to both client and family members.

[handwritten margin notes: ABC's • Head-Toe assessment • Fluid resuscitation • Pain • Wound]

2. Medications
   a. Antimicrobial creams
      1) Silver nitrate 0.5% soaks
      2) Silver sulfadiazine 1% (Silvadene) cream: broad-spectrum coverage, water-soluble
      3) Mafenide acetate (Sulfamylon) cream: broad-spectrum coverage; penetrates tissue wall; never use a dressing; breakdown of medication causes a heavy acid load, which can cause acidosis; painful
      4) Bacitracin
   b. Pain management
      1) PCA infusion pump for continuous dosing
      2) Intravenous opioid analgesics: morphine sulfate, hydromorphone (Dilaudid), and fentanyl (Sublimaze)

3. Treatments
   a. Wound care
   b. Biologic skin coverings
   c. Permanent skin coverings

4. Methods of Treating Burns
   a. Open-exposure method
      1) Allows for drainage of burn exudate
      2) Eschar forms hardened crust (can constrict circulation, requiring escharotomy)
      3) Use of topical therapy; asepsis crucial
      4) Skin easily visualized and monitored
      5) Range of motion easier
      6) Disadvantages
         a) Increases pain and heat loss
         b) Difficult to manage burns of hands and feet
   b. Closed method
      1) Gauze dressing wrapped distal to proximal
      2) Decreased fluid and heat loss
      3) Limited mobility can result in contractures
      4) Wound assessment only during dressing changes
   c. Topical antimicrobials (see "Medications" above)
   d. Biologic dressings and tissue grafts
      1) Homograft or allograft (human tissue donors)
      2) Xenograft or heterograft (animal sources)
      3) Amniotic membrane
      4) Biosynthetic (Biobrane) or synthetic (transparent film)

5. Client Education
   a. Skin care following discharge
      1) Wear pressure garment 23.5 hr/day to reduce scarring and control swelling.
      2) Engage in regular exercise per physical therapy.
      3) Elevate affected areas as much as possible.
      4) Keep skin moisturized.
      5) Control itching with cool baths and loose, cotton fabric.
      6) Avoid sun exposure.
      7) Change in appearance of skin as scars fade from red to near-natural coloration.
      8) Encourage the client to consume extra calories and protein.

End-of-Life Care

A. **Definition:** Care and management of the client and caregivers facing end-of-life care issues with the outcome of providing "good death"

B. **Contributing Factors**

1. Chronic terminal illness
2. Hospice care
3. Palliative care

C. **Manifestations**

1. Anorexia
2. Decreased peripheral circulation (mottled skin)
3. Disorientation and somnolence
4. Cheyne-Stokes respirations
5. Increased respiratory secretions
6. Decreased metabolic function
7. Incontinence
8. Restlessness
9. Weakness and fatigue

D. **Collaborative Care**

1. **Nursing Interventions**

   a. Collect data about an end-of-life care plan, advanced directives, and caregiver support.
   b. Do not force client to eat or drink.
   c. Talk to the client even if the client does not respond.
   d. Keep perineal area clean and dry.
   e. Position for comfort.
   f. Elevate head of bed.
   g. Administer medications to manage pain, restlessness, and excess secretions.
   h. Avoid noxious stimuli.

2. Symptom Management

   a. Pain is the symptom dying clients fear the most.
      1) Long-acting opioid narcotics
      2) Massage
      3) Music therapy
      4) Aromatherapy
   b. Dyspnea and gurgling are the "most distressing" symptoms noted by caregivers.
      1) Morphine elixir
      2) Scopolamine (transdermal or parenteral)
      3) Oxygen via nasal cannula
      4) Avoid deep suctioning
   c. Restlessness and agitation
      1) Lorazepam (Ativan)
      2) Haloperidol (Haldol)
   d. Nausea and vomiting
      1) Prochlorperazine (Compazine)
   e. Incontinence
      1) Keep perianal area clean and dry.
      2) Use disposable underpads or paper undergarments.
      3) Client might be more comfortable with urinary catheter.

E. **Referral and Follow-up**

1. Hospice care
2. Chaplain
3. Social services

F. **Postmortem Care**

1. Notify provider, chaplain, and mortuary as defined by end-of-life care plan.
2. If no autopsy is planned, remove any tubes or lines.
3. Clean and prepare client for immediate viewing as desired by family or significant other.
4. Provide family or significant other the opportunity to participate in care as desired.
5. Verify the completion of death certificate and required facility documents.
6. Prepare client for transport to morgue, funeral home, or mortuary per facility protocol (ensure client identification tags are present).

Nutrition: Therapeutic Diets

I Overview

A. To a large degree, nutrients absorbed and used by the body determine the health of the body.

B. The process of ingestion, digestion, absorption, and metabolism of food and fluids is essential for life. Disease processes and altered clinical conditions involving the GI tract can prevent all or some of these processes from taking place.

C. The nurse reviews the medical history and conducts nutritional data collection to determine the possibility of increased metabolic needs, and sources of potential problems with ingestion, digestion, or absorption.

D. Contributing factors can include chronic disease, trauma, recent surgery of the GI tract, drug and alcohol abuse, and altered cognitive and functional processes that affect nutritional status.

E. The nurse should check for

1. Decreased appetite; weight loss
2. History of recent illness
3. Poor-fitting or no dentures, or poor dental health
4. Poor eyesight; dry mouth or mucous membranes
5. Cognitive or functional decline; chronic physical illness
6. Acute or chronic pain; history of substance abuse
7. Altered mental health conditions, economic, or environmental factors that can affect nutritional requirements
8. Weight gain or subjective reports of lack of satiety

F. Older adults in any health care or community setting are at increased risk for altered nutrition due to the physiologic changes of aging, cognitive and functional decline, environmental factors, and social isolation.

II Guidelines for Healthy Eating

A. **Protein:** 10% to 35% of total kcal/day

B. **Fat:** 20% to 35% of total kcal/day

C. **Carbohydrates:** 40% to 65% of total kcal/day

D. **Fluid recommendations:** 2 to 3 L/day for women; 3 to 4 L/day for men

E. **Fiber recommendations:** 25 g/day for women; 38 g/day for men.

F. **Sodium recommendations:** 1,500 mg/day or less for adults older than 50 years, African Americans, and clients who have a history of diabetes mellitus, hypertension, or chronic kidney disease.

G. Recommendations differ for pregnant/lactating women, children, and teens.

FOODS WITH INCREASED LEVELS OF FAT AND WATER-SOLUBLE VITAMINS

Foods Rich in Fat-Soluble Vitamins

Vitamin A	Liver, egg yolk, whole milk, butter, green and yellow vegetables
Vitamin D	Fish oils, fortified milk and margarine, sunlight
Vitamin K	Egg yolks, liver, cheese, green leafy vegetables

Foods Rich in Water-Soluble Vitamins

Vitamin C	Citrus fruits, tomatoes, broccoli, cabbage
Thiamine (B_1)	Lean meats (beef, pork, liver), whole grain cereals, legumes
Riboflavin (B_2)	Milk, organ meats, enriched grains, green leafy vegetables
Niacin (B_3)	Meat, beans, peas, peanuts, enriched grains
Pyridoxine (B_6)	Products containing yeast, wheat, corn, organ meats
Cobalamin (B_{12})	Lean meats, liver, kidneys
Folic acid (B_9)	Leafy green vegetables, eggs, liver

III Therapeutic and Modified Diets

A. **Overview**

1. Therapeutic nutrition is often an essential component in the treatment of disease and clinical disorders.

2. A diet becomes therapeutic when modifications are made to meet client needs. Modifications can include increasing or decreasing caloric intake, fiber, or other specific nutrients; omitting specific foods; and modifying the consistency of foods.

3. Nurses often collaborate with or refer clients to the dietitian for nutritional or dietary concerns.

B. **Clear-Liquid Diet**

1. Indications

   a. Resting GI tract

   b. Maintaining fluid balance

   c. Immediate postoperative period

   d. Nausea, vomiting, diarrhea

   e. Preparation for diagnostic testing

   f. Short-term basis only; nutritionally inadequate

2. Consists of products that are liquid at room temperature

   a. Primarily water

   b. Tea and coffee

   c. Broth

   d. Carbonated beverages

   e. Clear juices

   f. Gelatin

   g. Limited caffeine due to risk of dehydration

C. **Full-Liquid Diet**

1. Indications

   a. Advanced to this if tolerates clear liquids

   b. Intolerance to solid foods

   c. Febrile illness

   d. Acute gastritis

2. Consists of

   a. Clear liquids

   b. Milk products

      1) Milk

      2) Custard

      3) Pudding

      4) Creamed soups

      5) Ice cream/sherbet

   c. Strained fruits, vegetables, and cereal

D. **Pureed Diet**

1. Indications

   a. Transition from full liquid to regular diet

   b. Swallowing or chewing difficulties; oral/facial surgery

2. Consists of

   a. Food and fluids that have been pureed to a thick liquid form (e.g., scrambled eggs; pureed meats, vegetables, fruits)

   b. Consistency varies with client needs

   c. Nutritional content varies with client needs

E. **Soft Diet (Bland or Low-Fiber)**

1. Indications

   a. Transition from liquid to regular diet

   b. Acute infections

   c. Chewing difficulties

   d. Gastric or duodenal ulcers by eliminating irritating foods

2. Consists of the following foods

   a. Low in fiber

   b. Lightly seasoned

   c. Easily digested

   d. Smooth and creamy

   e. Non-gas-forming: avoid cereals, beans, fruits and vegetables

F. **Mechanical Soft Diet**

1. Indications
   a. Chewing or swallowing difficulty
   b. Head, neck, or mouth surgery
   c. Intestinal stricture
   d. Post CVA
2. Consist of foods that require minimal chewing
   a. Ground or finely diced meat
   b. Canned fruits
   c. Softly cooked vegetables
   d. Cheese
   e. Rice
   f. Light bread
3. Foods to exclude
   a. Dried fruits
   b. Most raw fruits and vegetables
   c. Nuts and food with seeds

G. **Low-Protein Diet**

1. Indications
   a. Hepatic encephalopathy
   b. Hepatic coma
   c. Renal impairment
2. High-protein foods to limit
   a. Meats
   b. Eggs
   c. Milk and milk products
   d. Beans
3. Other dietary considerations
   a. Increase carbohydrates to meet nutritional needs.
   b. Limit sodium in presence of edema or ascites.

H. **High-Protein Diet**

1. Indications
   a. Tissue repair and building
   b. Burns
   c. Malabsorption syndromes
   d. Pregnancy
2. Encourage high biological value (HBV) protein
   a. Egg whites (gold standard)
   b. Soy products
   c. Milk products
   d. Fish and fowl
   e. Organ and meat sources
3. Encourage oral fluids to decrease damage to renal capillaries as a result of increased protein.

I. **Diet for Alteration in Amino-Acid Metabolism**

1. Use for phenylketonuria (PKU), galactosemia, and lactose intolerance.
2. Dietary restrictions are aimed at reducing or eliminating the offending enzyme.
3. Avoid milk and milk products for all three diets. Include soy-based supplements.
4. For PKU, avoid high-protein foods such as meats, dairy products, and eggs. In addition, avoid aspartame (NutraSweet), which contains phenylalanine.
5. For galactosemia, the simple sugar in lactose must be avoided. Educate families to read labels carefully, as galactosemia can be life-threatening.
6. Supplement calcium and vitamin D in those with lactose-restricted or -eliminated diets.

J. **Low-Cholesterol Diet**

1. Indications
   a. Cardiovascular disease
   b. Diabetes mellitus
   c. Hyperlipidemia
2. Limit animal products that are high in low-density lipoproteins, saturated fats, and trans fats
   a. Egg yolks
   b. Organ meats
   c. Fatty meats (bacon)
   d. Whole milk, butter
3. Encourage high-density lipoproteins, omega-3 fatty acids, and unsaturated fats
   a. Sardines and salmon
   b. Olive and flaxseed oils
   c. Shellfish
   d. Walnuts
   e. Fruits and vegetables
   f. Lean meats
   g. Skinless fowl

K. **Modified-Fat Diet**

1. Indications
   a. Gallbladder disease
   b. Hepatic disorders
   c. Cystic fibrosis
   d. Malabsorption syndrome
2. Foods to avoid
   a. Whole-milk products
   b. Gravies, creams
   c. Fatty meat and fish
   d. Nuts and chocolate
   e. Polyunsaturated oils
3. Foods allowed
   a. Two to three eggs per week
   b. Lean meat, fowl, fish
   c. Fruits and vegetables
   d. Bread and cereal

L. **Potassium-Modified Diets**

1. High-potassium foods

   a. Bananas

   b. Oranges

   c. Apples

   d. Milk

   e. Spinach

   f. Apricots and prunes

   g. Soy, lima, and kidney beans

   h. Baked potatoes (white and sweet)

2. Low-potassium foods

   a. Breads

   b. Cereals

   c. Asparagus

   d. Cabbage

   e. Cherries

   f. Blackberries and blueberries

M. **Sodium-Restricted Diets**

1. Indications

   a. Hypertension: DASH diet recommended, which emphasizes whole grains, fruits and vegetables, low-fat or fat-free dairy, fish, poultry, beans, seeds and nuts

   b. Heart failure

   c. Myocardial infarction

   d. Adrenal cortical diseases

   e. Kidney disease

   f. Lithium carbonate therapy

   g. Cystic fibrosis

   h. Liver cirrhosis

   i. Preeclampsia

2. High-sodium foods

   a. Salty snack foods (potato chips)

   b. Canned soups and vegetables

   c. Baked goods that contain baking powder or baking soda

   d. Processed meats, such as bologna, ham, and bacon

   e. Dairy products, especially cheese

   f. Pickles, olives

   g. Soy sauce, steak sauce

   h. Salad dressings

3. Encourage clients to become "label savvy" for sodium.

N. **Iron Alterations**

1. Increased iron intake is indicated for correction or prevention of iron deficiency anemia, which is most likely to occur in infants, toddlers, adolescents, and pregnant women.

2. Food sources high in iron include fish; meats (particularly organ meats); green leafy vegetables; enriched breads, cereals, and macaroni products; whole-grain products; dried fruits, such as raisins and apricots; and egg yolks.

3. Vitamin C enhances absorption of iron from the gastrointestinal tract.

4. Oral iron supplementation can cause constipation and GI distress, so adequate iron intake through foods is ideal.

O. **Calcium Alterations**

1. Increased calcium intake is indicated for growing children and adolescents, pregnant and lactating women, and postmenopausal women (to help prevent osteoporosis and osteopenia).

2. Food sources high in calcium include milk and milk products such as yogurt and cheese; dark green vegetables such as collard greens, kale, and broccoli; dried beans and peas; shellfish and canned salmon; and antacids such as Tums, Rolaids, and Titralac.

3. No more than 600 mg calcium can be absorbed at one time, so supplements should be taken 3 times daily; no more than 2,500 mg/day of calcium should be consumed.

4. Vitamin D is required for absorption of calcium from the gastrointestinal tract.

NUTRITION: THERAPEUTIC DIETS END-OF-SECTION REVIEW

Match the disease process with the most appropriate diet.

1. Impaired swallowing	A.	High-fiber
2. Constipation	B.	Low-fiber
3. Diarrhea	C.	Pureed food
4. Inflammatory bowel disease	D.	Avoid gluten
5. Celiac disease	E.	Clear liquids
6. Immediate postoperative period	F.	High-protein
7. Wounds	G.	Increase fluids

Answer Key: 1. C; 2. A; 3. G; 4. B; 5. D; 6. E; 7. F

SECTION 16

"Need to Know" Laboratory Values

I Serum Electrolytes

A. **Sodium (Na⁺):** 136 to 145 mEq/L

B. **Potassium (K⁺):** 3.5 to 5 mEq/L

C. **Calcium total (Ca⁺⁺):** 9.0 to 10.5 mg/dL

D. **Magnesium (Mg⁺⁺):** 1.3 to 2.1 mEq/L

E. **Phosphorus (PO₄):** 3.0 to 4.5 mg/dL

F. **Chloride (Cl):** 98 to 106 mEq/L

II Arterial Blood Gases (ABGs)

A. **pH:** 7.35 to 7.45

B. **PaCO₂:** 35 to 45 mm Hg

C. **PaO₂:** 80 to 100 mm Hg

D. **HCO₃ (bicarbonate):** 21 to 28 mEq/L

III CBC

A. **RBCs:** males 4.7 to 6.1 million/uL; females 4.2 to 5.4 million/uL

B. **Hgb males:** 14 to 18 g/dL; females: 12 to 16 g/dL

C. **Hct males:** 42% to 52%; females 37% to 47%

D. **WBCs:** 5,000 to 10,000 mm³

E. **Erythrocyte sedimentation rate (ESR):** less than 20 mm/hr

IV Blood Lipid Levels

A. **Total serum cholesterol:** desirable less than 200 mg/dL; risk for cardiac or stroke event with levels greater than 150 mg/dL (target range for therapy and has been shown to be the cut point to decrease cerebrovascular or arterial incidences)

B. **LDL (low-density lipids):** desirable less than 130 mg/dL

C. **HDL (high-density lipids):** males 35 to 65 mg/dL; females 35 to 80 mg/dL

D. **Triglycerides:** desirable less than 150 mg/dL; males 40 to 160 mg/dL; females 35 to 135 mg/dL

V Anticoagulant Therapy Coagulation Times

A. **PT:** 11 to 12.5 seconds. Therapeutic range for anticoagulant therapy is 1.5 to 2 times the normal or control value.

B. **Partial thromboplastin time (aPTT):** 30 to 40 seconds. Therapeutic range for anticoagulant therapy is 1.5 to 2 times the normal or control value.

C. **INR**

1. Normal INR is 0.7 to 1.8. Therapeutic INR is 2.0 to 3.0 for anticoagulant therapy.

2. The INR is a corrected ratio of a client's prothrombin time to normal.

3. Universal test is not affected by variations in laboratory norms.

4. If the client requires anticoagulation, the desired value is increased to approximately 2 to 3.

D. **Platelets:** 150,000 to 400,000/mm3

VI Liver Function Tests

A. **Albumin:** 3.5 to 5 g/dL

B. **Ammonia:** 15 to 45 mcg/dL

C. **Total bilirubin:** 0.1 to 1.0 mg/dL

D. **Total protein:** 6 to 8 g/dL

VII Urinalysis

A. **Specific gravity:** 1.005 to 1.025   *↑ Concentrated / more dilute*

B. **Protein:** 0.8 mg/dL

C. **Glucose:** less than 0.5 g/day

D. **Ketones:** none

E. **pH:** 4.6 to 8

F. **WBC:** males 0 to 3 per high-power field; females 0 to 5 per high-power field

VIII Renal Function

A. **Serum creatinine:** males 0.6 to 1.2 mg/dL; females 0.5 to 1.1 mg/dL

B. **BUN:** 10 to 20 mg/dL

C. **Creatinine clearance test:** males 90 to 139 mL/min; females 80 to 125 mL/min. This is a calculation of glomerular filtration rate (GFR) and is the best indicator of overall renal function.

IX Blood Glucose Levels

A. **Glucose (fasting):** 70 to 105 mg/dL

B. **Glycosylated hemoglobin (HbA1c):** 4% to 6% is within the expected reference range. Greater than 8% indicates poor diabetes mellitus control.

X Therapeutic Medication Levels

A. **Aminophylline:** 10 to 20 mcg/mL

B. **Carbamazepine:** 5 to 12 mcg/mL

C. **Digoxin:** 0.8 to 2.0 ng/mL

D. **Gentamicin:** 0.5 to 0.8 ng/mL

E. **Lidocaine:** 1.5 to 5.0 mcg/mL

F. **Lithium:** 0.4 to 1.4 mEq/L

G. **Magnesium sulfate:** 4 to 8 mg/dL

H. **Phenobarbital:** 10 to 30 mcg/mL

I. **Phenytoin:** 10 to 20 mcg/mL

J. **Quinidine:** 2 to 5 mcg/mL

K. **Salicylate:** 100 to 250 mcg/mL

L. **Theophylline:** 10 to 20 mcg/mL

M. **Tobramycin:** 5 to 10 mcg/mL

XI Toxic Medication Levels

A. **Acetaminophen:** greater than 250 mcg/mL

B. **Aminophylline:** greater than 20 mcg/mL

C. **Amitriptyline:** greater than 500 ng/mL

D. **Digoxin:** greater than 2.4 ng/mL

E. **Gentamicin:** greater than 12 mcg/mL

F. **Lidocaine:** greater than 5 mcg/mL

G. **Lithium:** greater than 2.0 mEq/L

H. **Magnesium sulfate:** greater than 9 mg/dL

I. **Methotrexate:** greater than 10 mcmol over 24 hr

J. **Phenobarbital:** greater than 40 mcg/mL

K. **Phenytoin:** greater than 30 mcg/mL

L. **Quinidine:** greater than 10 mcg/mL

M. **Salicylate:** greater than 300 mcg/mL

N. **Theophylline:** greater than 20 mcg/mL

O. **Tobramycin:** greater than 12 mcg/mL

NOTE: Normal laboratory value reference ranges can have slight variations depending on the facility or organization. To recognize deviations, candidates should know the laboratory value ranges. It is important to recognize values that are elevated or low.

Mental Health Nursing

Overview

I Mental Health

A state of well-being in which each individual is able to realize his own potential, cope with the normal stresses of life, work productively and fruitfully, and contribute to the community.

II Mental Illness

A clinically significant behavioral or psychological syndrome marked by the client's distress, disability, or the risk of suffering disability or loss of freedom.

III Mental Health Nursing

This type of nursing employs a purposeful use of self as its art, and a wide range of nursing, psychosocial, and neurobiological theories and research evidence as its science.

MENTAL HEALTH-ILLNESS CONTINUUM

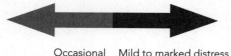

Occasional stress with no impairment.	Mild to marked distress with moderate to chronic impairment.

A. **Theoretical Models**
   1. Psychoanalytic
      a. Sigmund Freud
         1) Id, ego, superego
         2) 5 Stages of Development
            a) Oral: 0 to 1 year
            b) Anal: 1 to 3 years
            c) Phallic: 3 to 6 years
            d) Latency: 6 to 12 years
            e) Genital: 12 years to young adult
         3) Transference
         4) Countertransference

   b. Erik Erikson
      1) 8 Stages of Growth and Development
         a) Infancy: 0 to 1 year
            Trust vs. Mistrust
         b) Early Childhood: 1 to 3 years
            Autonomy vs. Shame and Doubt
         c) Preschooler: 3 to 6 years
            Initiative vs. Guilt
         d) School Age: 6 to 12 years
            Industry vs. Inferiority
         e) Adolescence: 12 to 20 years
            Identity vs. Role Confusion
         f) Young Adult: 20 to 35 years
            Intimacy vs. Isolation
         g) Middle Adult: 35 to 65 years
            Generativity vs. Stagnation
         h) Older Adult: 65 years and older
            Integrity vs. Despair

   2. Behavioral
      a. Ivan Pavlov
         Classical Conditioning
      b. B. F. Skinner
         Operant Conditioning

   3. Humanistic
      a. Abraham Maslow
         Hierarchy of Needs

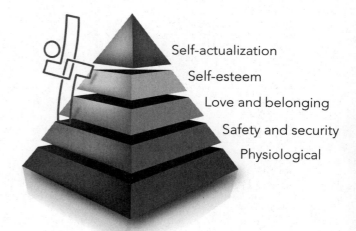

Self-actualization
Self-esteem
Love and belonging
Safety and security
Physiological

THEORISTS

MAJOR THEORETICAL CONTRIBUTIONS	MAJOR CONTRIBUTIONS USED IN NURSING

Psychoanalyst: Sigmund Freud

Interactive systems of the personality: Id, ego, and superego **5 Stages of Development**: Oral, anal, phallic, latency, and genital Erik Erikson later expanded upon these stages.	**Transference** develops when the client experiences feelings toward the nurse or therapist that were originally held toward significant others. **Countertransference** is the health care worker's unconscious, personal response to the client.

Psychoanalyst: Erik Erickson

8 Stages of Growth and Development	Erikson's developmental framework helps the nurse identify age appropriate behaviors during assessment.
Infancy (0 to 1 year): Trust vs. Mistrust Behavior: Hopefulness, trusting vs. withdrawn, alienated	Success: Trust should be seen with the primary caregiver. Crisis: Infant is withdrawn and unresponsive.
Early Childhood (1 to 3 years): Autonomy vs. Shame and Doubt Behavior: Self-control and using willpower vs. uncertainty of doing anything at all	Success: A toddler shows signs of self-control as in toilet training. Crisis: A toddler shows signs of doubt in being able to toilet train.
Preschooler (3 to 6 years): Initiative vs. Guilt Behavior: Ability to initiate activities vs. feeling conflicted about what was initiated	Success: A preschooler may initiate helping set the table for dinner. Crisis: A preschooler took candy without paying for it and knew it was wrong.
School Age (6 to 12 years): Industry vs. Inferiority Behavior: Feeling competent in activities and work vs. feelings of low self-esteem	Success: "I'm getting really good at piano since I started taking lessons." Crisis: "I'm dumb because I can't read as fast as everyone else."
Adolescence (12 to 20 years): Identity vs. Role Confusion Behavior: A sense of self vs. becoming confused about self	Success: "I am fine with who I am." Crisis: "I belong to a gang because I am nothing without them."
Young Adult (20 to 35 years): Intimacy vs. Isolation Behavior: Ability to love deeply and commit oneself in relationships vs. remaining uncommitted and alone	Success: "My partner has been my best friend for 10 years." Crisis: "No one is worthy of being in a relationship with me."
Middle Adult (35 to 65 years): Generativity vs. Stagnation Behavior: Ability to give and care for others vs. self-absorption and inability to grow as a person	Success: "I will be taking a leave of absence for 3 months to stay with my mother who is terminally ill." Crisis: "This old scar on my face is worse than having cancer."
Older Adult (65 years and older): Integrity vs. Despair Behavior: Sense of accomplishment in life vs. feeling dissatisfied with life	Success: "I have led a happy and productive life." Crisis: "I'm not ready to die. The doctors are wrong."

Behaviorist: Ivan Pavlov

Classical Conditioning: Pavlov discovered when a neutral stimulus (a bell) was repeatedly paired with another stimulus (food that triggered salivation), eventually the sound of the bell alone could elicit salivation in the dogs.	Humans can also experience classical conditioned responses that are involuntary and not spontaneous choices.

Behaviorist: B.F. Skinner

Operant Conditioning: Voluntary behaviors are learned through consequences and behavioral responses are elicited through reinforcement, which causes a behavior to occur more frequently.	Positive behavior can be encouraged to continue through positive reinforcement such as offering a reward or returning a privilege.

Humanistic: Abraham Maslow

The Hierarchy of Needs Pyramid

	Self-actualization	People strive to become everything they are capable of.
	Self-esteem	People need to have a high self-regard, and have it reflected to them from others.
	Love and belonging	This involves the need for intimate relationships, and experiencing love and affection.
	Safety and security	Once physiological needs are met, safety needs emerge. These include security, protection, freedom from fear, and a need for law and order.
	Physiological	The most basic needs are food, oxygen, water, sleep, sex, and a constant body temperature. If all needs were deprived, this level would take priority.

THEORY REVIEW

List Erikson's (E) stage of growth and development and Maslow's (M) priority need for the following scenarios.

1. A teenager is admitted to the emergency department following a MVA related to alcohol intoxication.

E:

M:

2. An older adult client who lives alone is being discharged following a total knee replacement.

E:

M:

3. An infant is born weighing 1.2 kg (2.6 lb).

E:

M:

4. A young college graduate who recently became engaged receives a diagnosis of tinea corporis.

E:

M:

5. A fourth-grader is admitted to a psychiatric hospital for depression and suicidal ideation due to bullying at school.

E:

M:

Answer Key: 1. Identity vs. Role Confusion, Physiological (The basic needs to sustain life are priority due to the injuries.); 2. Integrity vs. Despair, Physiological (The basic needs to maintain life is priority because the client lives alone and is physically compromised.); 3. Trust vs. Mistrust, Physiological (The basic needs to maintain life is priority.); 4. Intimacy vs. Isolation, Love and Belonging (Physiological and Safety are not priority with tinea corporis because neither are threatened with this diagnosis. However, intimacy and love and belonging are priority needs.); 5. Industry vs. Inferiority, Safety (This pediatric client must have protective/safe measures taken to maintain life.).

B. **Nursing Process**

1. *Assess* using the Mental Status Examination (MSE)

2. *Appearance*: Grooming, dress, hygiene, facial expression

   a. *Behavior*: Excessive or reduced body movements, level of eye contact

   b. *Speech*: Slow, rapid, normal, loud, soft, disorganized

   c. *Mood*: Sad; labile; euphoric; flat, bland affect

   d. *Thoughts*: Disorganized, flight of ideas

   e. *Perceptual Disturbances*: Hallucinations, delusions

   f. *Cognition*: Orientation to time, place and person, level of consciousness, remote and recent memory, judgment

   g. *Ideas of Harming Self or Others*: Presence of a plan, means and opportunity to carry out the plan

3. *Diagnose* with input from the treatment team.

   a. This should include the problem with the probable cause and supporting data.

   b. Example: Hopelessness (problem) related to multiple losses (probable cause) as evidenced by lack of motivation to care for self (supporting data).

4. *Plan* interventions based on the following criteria:

   a. Safe for client, other clients, staff, and family.

   b. Compatible with other therapies, client's personal goals, and cultural values.

   c. Realistic and individualized with consideration given to the client's age, physical condition, willingness to change, and community resources.

   d. Evidence-based when available.

5. *Implementation* should include:

   a. Coordination of care with all members of the treatment team.

   b. Health teaching and promotion.

   c. Milieu therapy.

   d. Pharmacological and integrative therapies.

6. *Evaluation* should be based on:

   a. Ongoing assessment of data for consideration of revisions in the treatment plan.

   b. Evidence-based criteria.

C. **Nurse-Client Relationship**

1. Orientation Phase: This phase can last for a few meetings or longer.

   a. Rapport and trust is established.

   b. The nurse's role is clarified, and all roles are defined.

   c. Confidentiality is established.

   d. The terms of termination are introduced.

   e. The nurse becomes aware of transference and countertransference issues.

   f. Client problems are articulated, and mutually agreed-upon goals are established.

2. Working Phase: This allows for a strong working relationship.
    a. Maintain client relationship.
    b. Gather further data.
    c. Promote client's problem-solving skills.
    d. Facilitate behavioral change.
    e. Overcome resistance behaviors.
    f. Evaluate problems and goals.
    g. Promote practice and expression of alternative adaptive behaviors.
3. Termination Phase: This is the final phase of the nurse-patient relationship.
    a. Summarize the goals achieved.
    b. Discuss new coping strategies.
    c. Review situations that occurred during the relationship.
    d. Exchange memories and validate experiences of the relationship to promote closure.
4. Factors that Promote Client Growth
    a. Communicating genuineness
    b. Expressing empathy
    c. Having positive regard for client
D. **Communication Techniques**
1. Therapeutic
    a. *Active listening* includes:
        1) Observing the client's nonverbal behaviors.
        2) Understanding and reflecting on the client's verbal message.
    b. *Clarifying* techniques
        1) *Restating* allows the nurse to mirror overt and covert messages.
        Client: "I can't focus."
        Nurse: "You are having problems focusing?"
        2) *Reflecting* provides a means to assist the client to better understand his thoughts and feelings.
        Client: "What should I do about my son's addiction?"
        Nurse: "What do you think you should do?"
        3) *Exploring* allows the nurse to examine ideas and experiences in more depth.
        "Tell me more about..."
    c. *Ask open-ended questions* to elicit client responses. "What do you perceive as your biggest stressor right now?"
    d. *Offer Self*
    "I would like to spend time talking with you."
    e. *Offer General Leads*
    "And then?"
    f. *Focus*
    "You've mentioned many events. Let's talk about your wanting to end it all again."
2. Nontherapeutic
    a. *Giving Premature Advice*
    "You should leave your home immediately."
    b. *Minimizing Feelings*
    "Things often get worse before they get better."
    c. *False Reassurance*
    "Everything is going to be fine."
    d. *Disapproval*
    "I disagree with that."
    e. *Making Value Judgments*
    "You wife is dying of lung cancer, and you smoke?"

COMMUNICATION REVIEW

Analyze the following communication scenarios and determine whether the nurse's responses are therapeutic or nontherapeutic and which communication technique is used.

Scenario	Therapeutic / Nontherapeutic	Communication Technique
1. Client: "I wish I were dead." Nurse: "I know what you mean."	☐ THERAPEUTIC ☐ NONTHERAPEUTIC	COMMUNICATION TECHNIQUE:
2. Client: "I am so worried." Nurse: "What specifically are you worried about?"	☐ THERAPEUTIC ☐ NONTHERAPEUTIC	COMMUNICATION TECHNIQUE:
3. Client: "If I could just make move closer to my family." Nurse: "Tell me more about that."	☐ THERAPEUTIC ☐ NONTHERAPEUTIC	COMMUNICATION TECHNIQUE:
4. Client: "I wish everyone would leave me alone." Nurse: "You are going to do fine, you'll see."	☐ THERAPEUTIC ☐ NONTHERAPEUTIC	COMMUNICATION TECHNIQUE:

Answer Key: 1. Nontherapeutic/minimizing feelings; 2. Therapeutic/clarifying with reflection; 3. Therapeutic/exploring; 4. Nontherapeutic/false reassurance

3. **Group Therapy:** A group of individuals interacting together with a shared purpose.

4. Phases of Group Development

   a. Orientation phase defines the purpose of the group.

   b. Working phase allows for a focus on problem-solving.

   c. Termination phase promotes reflection on the progress that has been made.

5. Types of Groups

   a. Medication Education

      1) These groups are designed to teach clients about their medications and allow for questions and concerns to be discussed.

   b. Dual Diagnosis

      1) These groups engage clients in treatment, and their use of substances following a systematic process.

   c. Symptom Management

      1) These groups assist clients with a common symptom that results in a disorder such as anger or anxiety.

   d. Stress Management

      1) These groups focus on teaching relaxation techniques.

   e. Support/Self-Help

      1) These groups are designed to maintain or enhance personal and social functioning through life's challenges. Examples can include bereavement and survivors of cancer.

SECTION 2

Anxiety and Anxiety Disorders

A. **Anxiety**

1. Definition: A universal human emotion that is considered the most basic of human emotions. Mild anxiety provides needed energy to achieve life's goals.

2. Levels of Anxiety

   a. Mild: occurs in normal experience of everyday life, and promotes a sharp focus of reality.

   b. Moderate: narrows the perceptual field, and some details become excluded.

   c. Severe: severely narrows the perceptual field, and right amount of focus on detail is lost.

   d. Panic: the extreme level of anxiety, and leaves a person unable to process the environment.

LEVELS OF ANXIETY

	SIGNS AND SYMPTOMS	NURSING INTERVENTIONS
Mild	Heightened perceptual field, alert and can grasp what is going on, restlessness, irritability or impatience, foot or finger tapping	Help the client identify the anxiety. Anticipate anxiety-provoking situations. Demonstrate interest in client by leaning forward and maintaining eye contact. Ask questions to clarify what is said. Encourage problem-solving.
Moderate	Narrow perceptual field, voice tremors, difficulty concentrating, increased respiratory and heart rate, pacing, banging hands on table	
Severe	Greatly reduced perceptual field, attention scattered, feelings of dread, confusion, hyperventilation, tachycardia, threats and demands	Maintain calm manner. Remain with client. Minimize environmental stimuli. Use clear, simple statements. Use low-pitched voice. Listen for themes in communication. Attend to physical and safety needs.
Panic	Unable to focus on the environment, feelings of "ceasing to exist," sleeplessness, can have hallucinations or delusions	

B. **Defense Mechanisms**

1. Definition: Automatic coping styles that protect individuals from anxiety and maintain self-image.

2. Adaptive Use: Allows anxiety to be lowered and goals to be achieved.

3. Maladaptive Use: Occurs when one or several are used in excess, disallowing goals to be achieved.

4. Defense Mechanisms

   a. Denial: Unconscious attempt to escape unpleasant realities.

      1) Adaptive Use: Client states, "I don't believe you" when hearing news that a loved one died.

      2) Maladaptive Use: A woman who lost her husband 3 years ago keeps his clothes hanging in the closet and talks about him in the present tense.

   b. Projection: Blaming one's thoughts or actions on another.

      1) Adaptive Use: A woman who is unconsciously attracted to another man teases her husband about flirting.

      2) Maladaptive: A woman who has repressed an attraction toward other women refuses to socialize, fearing other women will make homosexual advances.

   c. Regression: Reverting to an earlier developmental level

      1) Adaptive: A 5-year-old begins sucking his thumb when a new sibling is born.

      2) Maladaptive: An employee who is not promoted begins missing appointments and showing up late for meetings.

   d. Sublimation: Directing unacceptable behaviors into a socially acceptable area. This is always adaptive.

      1) Example: A student who is angry with a faculty member writes a short story of a hero.

C. **Anxiety Disorders**

1. Clients who have anxiety disorders use ineffective behaviors to try to control their anxiety.

2. Types of Anxiety Disorders

   a. Phobias

      1) Definition: Persistent, irrational fear of a specific object, activity or situation that leads to avoidance

      2) Examples:

         a) Acrophobia: Fear of heights

         b) Hematophobia: Fear of blood

         c) Claustrophobia: Fear of closed spaces

   b. Panic

      1) Definition: Panic attacks are the most commonly seen feature of this disorder. Panic attacks are characterized as a sudden onset of extreme apprehension or fear usually associated with impending doom.

   c. Obsessive-Compulsive Disorder (OCD)

      1) Definition: Obsessions are thoughts, impulses, or images that persist and cannot be dismissed from the mind. Compulsions are ritualistic behaviors an individual feels driven to perform to attempt a reduction of anxiety. Obsessions and compulsions often occur together. The rituals become time-consuming, interfering with normal routines and relationships.

   d. Generalized Anxiety Disorder (GAD)

      1) Definition: Characterized by excessive anxiety or worry about numerous situations, and the anxiety is out of proportion to the true impact of the event.

   e. Posttraumatic Stress Disorder (PTSD)

      1) Definition: Persistent re-experiencing of a highly traumatic event that involved actual or threatened death or serious injury to self or others to which the individual responded with intense fear, helplessness, or horror.

ANXIETY DISORDERS

	SIGNS AND SYMPTOMS
Phobias	Irrational fear of an object or situation that persists. Example: Agoraphobia is fear of being alone in open or public places. The client might not leave home.
Panic disorder	Recurrent episodes of panic attacks that can include palpitations, chest pain, breathing difficulties, nausea, feelings of choking.
Obsessive-compulsive disorder (OCD)	Obsessions: persistent intrusive thoughts. Compulsions: repetitive behaviors that a client feels driven to perform (handwashing).
Generalized anxiety disorder (GAD)	Excessive anxiety/worry more days than not over 6 months associated with restlessness, fatigue, difficulty concentrating, sleep disturbances, and irritability.
Posttraumatic stress disorder (PTSD)	Persistent re-experiencing of a highly traumatic event through dreams, flashbacks, thoughts, and images

3. Medications for Anxiety Disorders

   a. Antidepressants

      1) Selective Serotonin Reuptake Inhibitors (SSRIs)

         a) Citalopram (Celexa)

         b) Escitalopram (Lexapro)

         c) Fluoxetine (Prozac)

      2) Serotonin-Norepinephrine Reuptake Inhibitors (SNRIs)

         a) Duloxetine (Cymbalta)

         b) Venlafaxine (Effexor)

      3) Tricyclics

         a) Imipramine (Tofranil)

   b. Antianxiety Agents

      1) Benzodiazepines

         a) Alprazolam (Xanax)

         b) Clonazepam (Klonopin)

         c) Diazepam (Valium)

      2) Nonbenzodiazepine

         a) Buspirone

   c. Anticonvulsants

      1) Gabapentin (Neurontin)

      2) Valproic acid (Depakote)

ANXIETY DISORDER REVIEW

Match the disorder with the correct nursing communication.

____ 1. Phobias

____ 2. Panic disorder

____ 3. Generalized anxiety disorder (GAD)

____ 4. Obsessive-compulsive disorder (OCD)

____ 5. Posttraumatic stress disorder (PTSD)

a. "You are having difficulty sleeping due to nightmares since the tornado?"

b. "Tell me more about your partner's response when you must wash your hands 8 to 10 times before preparing meals."

c. "Where would you like to begin our discussion regarding your fear of attending a concert?"

d. "What do you believe brings on your episodes of chest pain and rapid breathing?"

e. "You have mentioned a lot of stressors that have been occurring for several months. Which situation is causing the greatest stress for you?"

Answer Key: 1. C; 2. D; 3. E; 4. B; 5. A

Schizophrenia

A. Schizophrenia

1. Definition: Potentially devastating brain disorder that affects a person's thinking, language, emotions, social behavior, and ability to perceive reality accurately.

2. Phases

   a. Acute: Onset or exacerbation of symptoms with loss of functional abilities.

   b. Stabilization: Symptoms diminish and client progresses toward previous level of functioning.

   c. Maintenance: The client is at or near baseline functioning.

3. Types

   a. Paranoid: Strong irrational suspicion with dominant symptoms of hallucinations and delusions.

   b. Disorganized: The most socially impaired form, with dominant symptoms of disorganized speech and behavior, as well as inappropriate affect.

   c. Catatonic: The essential feature is abnormal levels of motor behavior, either extreme motor agitation or retardation.

4. Assessment

   a. *Positive symptoms* are the presence of something that is not normally present, such as:

      1) Hallucinations are based on the senses (auditory, tactile, olfactory, visual).

      2) Delusions are false fixed beliefs and can be persecutory, grandiose, somatic, or religious.

      3) Bizarre behavior can be seen in inappropriate clothing, aggressive, or repetitive behavior.

   b. *Negative symptoms* refer to diminished or absent characteristics of normal function such as a blunted affect, social withdrawal, or loss of motivation.

   c. *Cognitive symptoms* are revealed through the client's thought process that interferes with performing daily functions. This could manifest as impaired judgment, impaired memory, or illogical thinking.

5. Treatment

   a. Atypical antipsychotics

      1) Aripiprazole (Abilify)

      2) Olanzapine (Zyprexa)

      3) Quetiapine (Seroquel)

      4) Risperidone (Risperdal)

   b. Conventional antipsychotics

      1) Chlorpromazine

      2) Thioridazine (Mellaril)

      3) Fluphenazine

      4) Haloperidol (Haldol)

   c. Therapy

      1) Cognitive behavioral therapy can assist in controlling symptoms.

TYPES OF SCHIZOPHRENIA

TYPES	DESCRIPTION	SIGNS AND SYMPTOMS	AGE OF ONSET	NURSING INTERVENTIONS
Paranoid	Any intense and strongly defended suspicion can be regarded as paranoia.	Clients are usually frightened, guarded, and untrusting, and can behave defensively. A delusion can include someone trying to kill them. The most common defense mechanism used is projection. If the client feels angry, she might state, "I'm not angry, you are." Ideas of reference can be used. If a client sees a nurse speaking with a psychiatrist, the client may believe the discussion is about her.	Late 20s to 30s	Provide a safe, secure environment. Maintain a therapeutic, objective communicative approach. If delusions exist with food being poisoned, provide commercially sealed packages when possible.
Disorganized	This subtype is the most regressed and socially impaired due to the disorganization of thoughts.	Associative looseness, inappropriate affect, bizarre mannerisms, incoherence of speech, and extreme social withdrawal. Poorly organized hallucinations and delusions. Often live in the homeless population.	Early to middle teens	Communication should be concise, clear and concrete. Tasks should be taken one at a time. Repeated focusing may be required to keep the client on topic.
Catatonic	Either abnormal levels of motor retardation (withdrawn phase) or motor agitation (excited phase) are seen.	Withdrawn › Stuporous or comatose appearance › Mute for hours, days, or weeks › Acutely aware of environment, though appear detached › Unable or refuse to participate in activities Excited › Talk or shout continually and incoherently › Hyperactive behavior	Abrupt	Withdrawn › Remain objective. › Avert frustration and anger when client does not participate in activities. Excited (similar to mania) › Use clear, direct communication. › Use stimulation reduction. › Monitor for adequate caloric intake and rest.

SCHIZOPHRENIA REVIEW

Determine whether the following symptoms are positive or negative.

1. The client shows a flattened affect.	☐ POSITIVE ☐ NEGATIVE
2. The client states the CIA is spying on his every move.	☐ POSITIVE ☐ NEGATIVE
3. The client stops speaking to everyone.	☐ POSITIVE ☐ NEGATIVE
4. The client does not complete a task.	☐ POSITIVE ☐ NEGATIVE
5. The client states she feels spiders crawling all over her body.	☐ POSITIVE ☐ NEGATIVE

Answer Key: 1. Negative; 2. Positive; 3. Negative; 4. Negative; 5. Positive

SECTION 4

Disorders of Children and Adolescents

A. **Pervasive Developmental Disorders**

1. Autistic Disorder

   a. Definition: A complex neurobiological and developmental disability that typically appears before age 3 years.

   b. Presenting Symptoms

      1) Impaired language development

      2) Impaired behavior development

      3) Impaired social interaction development

   c. Medications

      1) Antipsychotics

      2) Selective serotonin reuptake inhibitors (SSRIs)

2. Asperger's Syndrome

   a. Definition: Developmental disorder that affects the ability to effectively socialize and communicate with others. Social awkwardness and intense obsession in specific topics are noted in childhood.

3. Rett Syndrome

   a. Definition: A disorder that is diagnosed exclusively in girls before age 4 years.

   b. Presenting Symptoms

      1) Impairment in communication

      2) Seizure disorder

      3) Abnormal gait

      4) Impaired head growth

      5) Severe or profound mental retardation

 4. **Nursing Interventions**

   a. Assess for developmental delays.

   b. Assess caregiver-child relationship.

   c. Assess for family coping skills (risk for child abuse).

B. **Attention Deficit Disorder (ADD)**
   Attention Deficit Hyperactivity Disorder (ADHD)

1. Definition: Children who have ADD show an inappropriate degree of inattention and impulsiveness. These symptoms are present for children who have ADHD with the addition of hyperactivity.

 2. **Nursing Interventions**

   a. Observe relationship between the child and caregivers.

   b. Monitor the caregiver's parenting practices for rules and responsibilities within the family.

   c. Monitor the child's cognitive and psychosocial development including social skills.

   d. Check school history for strengths and disciplinary problems.

3. Medications

   a. Stimulants

      1) Methylphenidate (Ritalin)

      2) Amphetamine and dextroamphetamine (Adderall)

   b. Antidepressants

      1) Nortriptyline (Aventyl)

      2) Bupropion (Wellbutrin)

C. **Behavior Disorders**

1. Oppositional Defiant Disorder

   a. Definition: Recurrent pattern of negative, disobedient, hostile, defiant behavior toward authority figures without violating the basic rights of others.

   b. Presenting Symptoms

      1) Persistent stubbornness

      2) Argumentativeness

      3) Limit testing

      4) Unwillingness to negotiate

      5) Quick annoyance

      6) Refusal to accept blame

   c. **Nursing Interventions**

      1) Identify issues that result in power struggles and triggers for outbursts.

      2) Monitor the child's view of her behavior and its effect on others.

      3) Explore how the child can exercise control and take responsibility and problem-solve for future situations.

2. Conduct Disorder

   a. Definition: Persistent pattern of behavior in which the rights of others are violated and age-appropriate societal norms or rules are disregarded.

   b. Complications

      1) Academic failure

      2) School suspensions and dropouts

      3) Juvenile delinquency

      4) Substance abuse and dependency

c. **Nursing Interventions**

  1) Monitor for seriousness, types, and initiation of disruptive behavior, and how it has been managed.

  2) Monitor anxiety, aggression and anger levels, motivation, and the ability to control impulses.

  3) Monitor moral development to understand the impact of hurtful behavior on others.

  4) Monitor the ability to form a therapeutic relationship and engage in honest and committed therapeutic work.

  5) Monitor for substance use.

d. Medications

  1) Antipsychotics

    a) Risperidone (Risperdal)

  2) Stimulants

    a) Methylphenidate (Ritalin)

  3) Antidepressants

    a) Bupropion (Wellbutrin)

  4) Mood Stabilizers

    a) Carbamazepine (Tegretol)

DISORDERS OF CHILDREN AND ADOLESCENTS REVIEW

Match the following disorder with the correct nursing assessment.

____ 1. Rett syndrome	a. A nurse observes a child defiantly communicating to the caregiver.	
____ 2. Conduct disorder	b. A nurse obtains drug screen results for an adolescent who has been in juvenile detention.	
____ 3. ADHD		
____ 4. Autistic disorder	c. A nurse observes and documents a child's lack of speech.	
____ 5. Oppositional defiant disorder (ODD)	d. A nurse observes a child fidgeting and not paying attention during an interview.	
	e. A nurse monitors for impaired head growth and notes a seizure disorder in the client's history.	

Answer Key: 1. E; 2. B; 3. D; 4. C; 5. A

SECTION 5

Depressive/Bipolar Disorders

A. **Major Depressive Disorder (MDD)**

1. Definition: Represents a change in previous functions, and symptoms include distress or impaired social, occupational, or other important areas of functioning.

2. Symptoms

  a. Depressed mood most of the day

  b. Anhedonia

  c. Greater than 5% of weight loss or gain in 1 month

  d. Insomnia or hypersomnia

  e. Anergia

  f. Feelings of worthlessness

  g. Decreased concentration

3. Primary Risk Factors

  a. Female gender

  b. Unmarried status

  c. Low socioeconomic class

  d. Early childhood trauma

  e. Family history of depression

  f. Postpartum period

  g. Medical illness

4. Three Phases of Treatment and Recovery

  a. Acute is focused on reducing depressive symptoms and lasts 6 to 12 weeks.

  b. Continuation is focused on prevention of a relapse through pharmacotherapy, education and psychotherapy and lasts 4 to 9 months.

  c. Maintenance is focused on prevention of further episodes and lasts 1 year or more.

5. **Nursing Interventions**

  a. Monitor for symptoms. Depressed mood, anhedonia, and anergia are most common.

  b. Monitor the client's risk of harm to self or others.

  c. Monitor the client's use of drugs and alcohol.

  d. Monitor client's history of depression.

  e. Monitor client's support systems.

  f. Encourage activities that raise self-esteem.

  g. Encourage exercise.

  h. Work with client to identify cognitive distortions.

6. Medications

  a. Selective Serotonin Reuptake Inhibitors (SSRIs)

    1) Citalopram (Celexa)

    2) Escitalopram (Lexapro)

  b. Serotonin Norepinephrine Reuptake Inhibitors (SNRIs)

    1) Venlafaxine (Effexor)

    2) Duloxetine (Cymbalta)

  c. Norepinephrine Dopamine Reuptake Inhibitor (NDRI)

    1) Bupropion (Wellbutrin)

  d. Tricyclic Antidepressants (TCAs)

    1) Imipramine (Tofranil)

  e. Monoamine Oxidase Inhibitors (MAOIs)

    1) Phenelzine (Nardil)

    2) Tranylcypromine (Parnate)

7. Electroconvulsive Therapy (ECT)

  a. Induced seizure activity found to be helpful in treating clients who have MDD. Clients can experience temporary short-term memory loss after several ECT treatments.

B. **Suicide**

1. Definition: Self-imposed death manifested through inner pain, hopelessness, and helplessness, often accompanied by a psychiatric disorder.

2. **Nursing Interventions**

   a. Monitor for suicidal ideation with intent.

   b. Monitor for lethal suicide plan.

   c. Monitor for coexisting psychiatric or medical illness.

   d. Monitor for family history of suicide.

   e. Monitor for recent lack of support.

   f. Monitor for feelings of hopelessness and helplessness.

   g. Monitor for covert statements such as "Things will never work out."

   h. Monitor for overt statements such as "I can't take it anymore."

3. Environmental Guidelines for Suicide Prevention

   a. Plastic eating utensils

   b. Unbreakable glass windows

   c. Locked doors on unit

   d. Screening of all potentially harmful gifts (flowers in a glass vase)

   e. Injury-proof rooms and bathrooms

   f. Remove all possessions from client that could lead to injury

   g. One-on-one constant supervision

C. **Bipolar Disorder**

1. Definitions

   a. Bipolar I: At least one episode of mania alternating with major depression. Psychosis can accompany mania.

   b. Bipolar II: Hypomanic episodes associated with euphoria alternate with major depression with higher risk of suicide. Psychosis is not present.

   c. Hypomania is characterized by a disturbance in mood observed by others and does not require hospitalization.

   d. Mania is severe enough to cause marked impairment in activities or relationships and can necessitate hospitalization to prevent harm to self or others.

2. Presenting Symptoms

   a. Inflated self-esteem or grandiosity

   b. Decreased need for sleep

   c. More talkative than usual

   d. Flight of ideas

   e. Increase in goal directed activity

   f. Excessive involvement in unrestrained buying sprees, poor business investments, or sexual indiscretions due to loss of impulse control.

3. **Nursing Interventions**

   a. Identify whether client is a danger to self or others.

   b. Identify the need to protect client from uninhibited behaviors.

   c. Monitor for coexisting medical conditions such as substance use disorder.

4. Medications

   a. Lithium (Lithobid)

   b. Anticonvulsants: valproic acid (Depakote)

   c. Atypical Antipsychotics

      1) Aripiprazole (Abilify)

      2) Risperidone (Risperdal)

   d. Antianxiety Agents: clonazepam (Klonopin)

REVIEW OF DEPRESSIVE/BIPOLAR DISORDERS

Place a check by the nursing interventions that are considered therapeutic for a client experiencing the following.

Depression

☐ 1. Encourage exercise.

☐ 2. Encourage overgeneralizations.

☐ 3. Encourage problem-solving.

☐ 4. Encourage formation of supportive relationships.

Mania

☐ 1. Provide short explanations.

☐ 2. Use firm calm approach.

☐ 3. Provide frequent high-calorie fluids.

☐ 4. Monitor.

Answer Key:
Depression/Therapeutic: 1, 3, 4. Overgeneralizations such as "She always" or "He never" lead to negative appraisals, making 2 incorrect. Mania/Therapeutic: 1, 2, 3. Client will need decreased stimuli and cannot maintain focus to watch a movie.

SECTION 6

Personality Disorders

A. **Personality Disorders**

1. All personality disorders share characteristics of inflexibility and difficulties in interpersonal relationships that impair social or occupational functioning.

2. Cluster A

   a. Paranoid

   b. Schizoid

   c. Schizotypal

3. Cluster B

   a. Antisocial

   b. Borderline

   c. Narcissistic

   d. Histrionic

4. Cluster C

   a. Dependent

   b. Obsessive-compulsive

   c. Avoidant

B. **Medications**

1. Depending on the disorder:

   a. Antidepressants

   b. Antianxiety agents

   c. Antipsychotics

PERSONALITY DISORDERS

DISORDER	NURSING INTERVENTIONS
Cluster A (Odd/Eccentric)	
Paranoid Distrust and suspiciousness of others	Avoid being too nice or too friendly. Give clear explanations. Warn about any changes and reasons for delays.
Schizoid Pattern of detachment from social relationships, often choosing solitary activities	Avoid being too nice or too friendly. Try not to increase socialization.
Schizotypal Pattern of social and interpersonal deficits marked by discomfort with close relationships and perceptual distortions	Respect client's need for social isolation. Be aware of client's suspiciousness.
Cluster B (Dramatic/Emotional)	
Antisocial Pattern of disregard for and violation of the rights of others	Set clear limits on specific behavior. Be aware of guilt and manipulation the client will attempt when not getting what he wants.
Borderline Pattern of instability of interpersonal relationships, self-image, and affect	Provide clear and consistent boundaries. Use clear communication. Be aware of manipulative behaviors. Assess for self-mutilating behaviors.
Narcissistic Pattern of grandiosity, need for admiration, and lack of empathy	Remain neutral and avoid power struggles. Convey unassuming self-confidence.
Histrionic Pattern of excessive emotionality and attention-seeking	Understand seductive behavior as a response to distress. Model concrete, descriptive vs. vague language.
Cluster C (Anxious/Fearful)	
Dependent Excessive need to be taken care of that leads to submissive behavior	Be aware of countertransference that can occur due to client's clinging behavior. Identify current stresses. Satisfy client's needs with limits.
Obsessive-Compulsive Pattern of preoccupation with orderliness, perfectionism, and control at the expense of flexibility	Guard against power struggles with client as the need to control is high. Monitor client's use of intellectualization, rationalization, and reaction formation as defense mechanisms.
Avoidant Pattern of social inhibition, feelings of inadequacy, and hypersensitivity to negative evaluation	Maintain a friendly, accepting, reassuring approach. Do not push client into social situations.

PERSONALITY DISORDER REVIEW

Select whether the following nursing interventions are therapeutic or nontherapeutic:

1. Communicate behavioral expectations that are easily understood and nonpunitive.	☐ THERAPEUTIC ☐ NONTHERAPEUTIC
2. Discuss concerns about behavior with client.	☐ THERAPEUTIC ☐ NONTHERAPEUTIC
3. Assist client to identify consequences and benefits of her behavior.	☐ THERAPEUTIC ☐ NONTHERAPEUTIC
4. Bargain with client to establish behavioral expectations.	☐ THERAPEUTIC ☐ NONTHERAPEUTIC
5. Encourage client to participate in problem-solving.	☐ THERAPEUTIC ☐ NONTHERAPEUTIC

Answer Key: 1. T/Helps establish trust and a positive rapport with client; 2. T/Allows the client to reflect on behavior; 3. T/Allows the client to reflect on behavior; 4. NT/Client behavioral expectations should be achievable and mutually agreed upon. A manipulative personality will seek to bargain, and the nurse must not participate; 5. T/The client should consistently participate in problem-solving with professional guidance.

SECTION 7

Addictive Disorders

A. **Definitions**

1. **Substance Abuse:** Maladaptive pattern of substance use that negatively affects obligations (work, school, parenting), judgment (driving), or relationships, and/or continued use despite personal problems.

2. **Substance Dependence:** Maladaptive pattern of substance use, leading to distress manifested by tolerance to the drug, withdrawal syndrome, or lack of success at controlling use.

3. **Codependent Behaviors:** These behaviors include attempting to control someone else's drug use, finding excuses for the person's substance abuse, or destroying the person's drug or alcohol supply.

CENTRAL NERVOUS SYSTEM DEPRESSANTS

DRUG	Barbiturates Benzodiazepines Alcohol
INTOXICATION	Slurred speech, unsteady gait, drowsiness, impaired judgment
WITHDRAWAL	Nausea and vomiting, tachycardia, diaphoresis, tremors, grand mal seizures

CENTRAL NERVOUS SYSTEM STIMULANTS

DRUG	Cocaine Amphetamines
INTOXICATION	Tachycardia, dilated pupils, elevated blood pressure, grandiosity, impaired judgment, paranoia with delusions
WITHDRAWAL	Fatigue, depression, agitation, apathy, anxiety, craving

OPIATES

DRUG	Heroin Meperidine (Demerol) Fentanyl (Sublimaze) Hydromorphone (Dilaudid)
INTOXICATION	Constricted pupils, decreased respirations, decreased blood pressure, initial euphoria followed by dysphoria
WITHDRAWAL	Yawning, insomnia, panic, diaphoresis, cramps, nausea and vomiting, chills, fever, diarrhea

B. **Nursing Interventions**

1. Monitor vital signs.
2. Monitor for dehydration.
3. Monitor for low self-worth.
4. Monitor for client safety.
5. Monitor toxicology screen/blood alcohol level.
6. Monitor for severe withdrawal syndrome.
7. Monitor for an overdose that warrants immediate medical attention.
8. Monitor for suicidal thoughts and behaviors.
9. Monitor family members for codependency.
10. Explore the client's interests in participating in a 12-step program such as Alcoholics Anonymous or Narcotics Anonymous.
11. Explore the family's interest in participating in self-help groups, such as Al-Anon or Alateen.

SECTION 8

Cognitive Disorders

A. **Delirium and Dementia**

1. *Delirium* is characterized by a disturbance of consciousness and a change in cognition that develop over a short period of time.
2. *Dementia* is a progressive deterioration of cognitive functioning and global impairment of intellect with no change in consciousness.

COGNITIVE DISORDERS

	Delirium	Dementia
ONSET	Sudden, over hours to days	Slowly, over months to years
CONTRIBUTING FACTORS	Fever, hypotension, infection, hypoglycemia, adverse drug reaction, head injury, emotional stress, seizures	Alzheimer's disease, neurological disease, vascular disease, alcohol use disorder, head trauma
COGNITION	Impaired memory, judgment, and attention span that can fluctuate	Impaired memory, judgment, and attention span; abstract thinking
SPEECH	Rapid, inappropriate, incoherent	Incoherent, slow, inappropriate
PROGNOSIS	Reversible with treatment	Not reversible

3. Alzheimer's disease is the most common cause of dementia in older adults. It is marked by impaired memory and thinking skills. This disease is classified into four stages.

   a. Stage 1: Mild

   1) The loss of intellectual ability is insidious. The client loses energy, drive, and initiative, and has difficulty learning.

   b. Stage 2: Moderate

   1) Deterioration becomes evident, and the client cannot remember a home address or date. Memory gaps occur, hygiene suffers, and clothing might be put on incorrectly. Mood swings occur, and the client can have moments of paranoia, anger, jealousy, and apathy. Care and supervision become a full-time job.

   c. Stage 3: Moderate to Severe

   1) The client becomes unable to identify familiar objects or people. Repeated instructions are needed to perform simple tasks. Wandering begins to occur, and the client becomes a danger to self. Total care is necessary.

   d. Stage 4: Late

   1) The client becomes unable to read or write, has blunted emotions, cannot recognize familiar objects, and loses the ability to talk and walk. This stage is often recognized by stupor and coma. Death is frequently secondary to infection or choking.

4. Medications for Clients who have Alzheimer's Disease

   a. Cholinesterase Inhibitors

   1) Donepezil (Aricept)

   2) Galantamine (Razadyne)

   b. NMDA Antagonist

   1) Memantine (Namenda)

   c. Selective Serotonin Reuptake Inhibitors (SSRI)

   1) Citalopram (Celexa)

   2) Paroxetine (Paxil)

   d. Antianxiety Agents

   1) Lorazepam (Ativan)

   2) Oxazepam (Serax)

5. **Nursing Interventions** for Dementia

   a. Evaluate the client's level of cognitive and daily functioning.
   b. Identify any threats to client's safety.
   c. Review all medications the client is taking.
   d. Interview family members to obtain a full history.
   e. Use short, simple words and phrases.
   f. Speak slowly.
   g. Have clocks, calendars, and personal items in clear view.
   h. Explore how well the family understands the disease progression.
   i. Review resources available to the family.

6. **Nursing Interventions** for Delirium
   a. Establish the client's baseline level of consciousness by interviewing family members.
   b. Monitor vital signs and perform neurological checks.
   c. Monitor for acute onset and fluctuating levels of consciousness.
   d. Monitor the client's ability to function in the immediate environment.
   e. Determine the physiologic reason delirium is occurring.
   f. Maintain comfort measures.

COGNITIVE DISORDER REVIEW

Place a check next to the nursing interventions that could be used for a client who has Alzheimer's disease.

☐	1. Keep client in a locked setting.
☐	2. Monitor for physiological reason for confusion.
☐	3. Give step-by-step instructions.
☐	4. Perform neurological checks.
☐	5. Administer donepezil (Aricept) as prescribed.

Answer Key:
Correct: 1. Wandering begins to occur in stage 3, and a locked setting is needed; 3. Clear, simple instructions can be needed as early as stage 1; 5. This is a commonly prescribed medication for a client who has Alzheimer's.
Incorrect: 2. This intervention is best for a client who has delirium.
4. Neurological checks are used for clients who have delirium, not dementia.

SECTION 9

Eating Disorders

A. **Anorexia Nervosa**
1. An eating disorder characterized by an extreme fear of obesity and altered perception of one's own body weight.
2. *Restricting*: Client drastically restricts food intake and does not binge or purge.
3. *Binge eating-purging*: Client engages in binge eating and purging behaviors.
4. Presenting Signs and Symptoms
   a. Terror of gaining weight
   b. Preoccupation with thoughts of food
   c. Judges self-worth by body weight
   d. Low body weight
   e. Amenorrhea
   f. Cold extremities
   g. Constipation
   h. Hypotension, bradycardia
   i. Impaired renal function
   j. Hypokalemia

5. **Nursing Interventions**
   a. Develop a supportive relationship with client.
   b. Monitor electrolytes and vital signs.
   c. Monitor food and fluid intake.
   d. Set achievable weight goals.
   e. Limit exercise regimen to promote weight gain.
   f. Explore client's feelings of self-worth.
   g. Assist in the development of effective coping strategies.
   h. Encourage client attendance in behavior modification therapy.
   i. Encourage family support groups.
   j. Administer antidepressants as prescribed.
   k. Provide positive reinforcement for weight gain.

B. **Bulimia Nervosa**
1. An uncontrollable compulsion to consume large amounts of food in a short period (binge eating), followed by a compensatory need to rid the body of the calories consumed.
   a. Purging: Client uses self-induced vomiting, laxatives, diuretics, and enemas to lose or maintain weight.
   b. Nonpurging: Client may also compensate for binge eating through other means, such as excessive exercise.
      1) Presenting Signs and Symptoms
         a) Bradycardia, hypotension
         b) Electrolyte imbalances
         c) Erosion of teeth
         d) Esophageal tears from vomiting
         e) Normal to slightly low body weight
         f) Muscle weakening
         g) Calluses/scars on hand from self-induced vomiting
      2) **Nursing Interventions**
         a) Develop a supportive relationship with client.
         b) Monitor electrolytes and vital signs.
         c) Monitor food and fluid intake.
         d) Monitor the client 30 to 60 min after a meal.
         e) Monitor exercise regimen.
         f) Explore client's feelings of self-worth.
         g) Observe teeth for erosion and caries.
         h) Observe room for food hoarding.
         i) Encourage client attendance in behavior modification therapy.
         j) Encourage family support groups.
         k) Administer antidepressants as prescribed.

REVIEW OF EATING DISORDERS

Determine whether the following nursing interventions support restricting anorexia, purging bulimia, or both.

1. Monitor dental erosion.	☐ ANOREXIA	☐ BULIMIA
2. Monitor ECG for arrhythmias.	☐ ANOREXIA	☐ BULIMIA
3. Monitor exercise regimen.	☐ ANOREXIA	☐ BULIMIA
4. Check for calluses on hands.	☐ ANOREXIA	☐ BULIMIA
5. Monitor for significant weight loss.	☐ ANOREXIA	☐ BULIMIA

Answer Key: 1. Bulimia due to self-induced vomiting; 2. Both have electrolyte imbalances that can lead to arrhythmias; 3. Both. Clients who have anorexia have a weight gain goal and exercise should be monitored. Clients who have bulimia will use exercise as a way to purge calories; 4. Bulimia due to self-induced vomiting; 5. Anorexia. Clients who have bulimia have normal to slightly low body weight.

SECTION 10

Anger/Violence, Abuse, and Assault

A. **Anger and Violence**

1. Definitions

   a. Anger is an emotional response to frustration of desires and can be expressed in a healthy way. Problems begin to occur when anger is expressed through violence.

   b. Feelings that can precipitate anger: Discounted, embarrassed, guilty, humiliated, hurt, ignored, unheard, rejected, threatened, tired, and vulnerable.

   c. Violence is always an objectionable act that involves intentional use of force that can result in injury or death.

2. Predictors of Violence

   a. Stone silence

   b. Alcohol or drug intoxication

   c. Pacing and restlessness

   d. Jaw clenching, rigid posture

   e. Verbal abuse

   f. Loud voice

   g. Intense or avoidance of eye contact

3. Cycle of Violence

   a. *Tension-Building Stage* is characterized by minor incidents such as pushing and verbal abuse. The victim often accepts blame.

   b. *Battering Stage* is characterized by the abuser releasing built-up tension by beating the victim brutally. The victim might try to cover the injury.

   c. *Honeymoon Stage* is characterized by kindness and loving behaviors, such as flowers, and the victim wants to believe the abuser will change.

CYCLE OF VIOLENCE

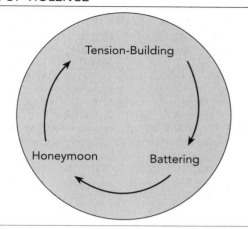

4. **Nursing Interventions**

   a. De-escalation

      1) Maintain a calm approach.

      2) Use short, simple sentences.

      3) Avoid verbal struggles/conflict.

      4) Monitor for stressors.

      5) Use a nonaggressive posture.

      6) Maintain client's self-esteem/dignity.

      7) Maintain a large personal space.

   b. Medications

      1) Antianxiety Agents

         a) Lorazepam (Ativan)

         b) Alprazolam (Xanax)

         c) Diazepam (Valium)

      2) Antipsychotics

         a) Haloperidol (Haldol)

         b) Chlorpromazine

   c. Restraints and Seclusion

      1) Restraints are a manual method to prevent client movement with the intention to protect the client from self-harm or assaulting others.

      2) Seclusion is the involuntary confinement of a client alone in a room. The goal is always centered around the safety of the client and others, and is never punitive.

B. **Abuse**

1. *Physical abuse* is the infliction of physical pain or bodily harm such as hitting or choking.

2. *Sexual abuse* is any form of sexual contact or exposure without consent. This is often referred to assault when referring to adults.

3. *Emotional abuse* is the infliction of mental anguish, such as threatening or intimidating.

4. *Neglect* can be physical or emotional in providing basic needs, educational in failing to make provisions for a child, and medical in failing to provide needed care.

5. *Economic abuse* is the withholding of financial support or illegal use of funds for one's personal gain.

6. The victim interview:

DO'S	DO NOT'S
Conduct the interview in private.	Try to prove abuse.
Be direct, honest, and professional.	Display horror, anger, or shock.
Be understanding and attentive.	Place blame or make judgments.
Observe for client safety.	Force anyone to remove clothing.

C. **Sexual Assault**

1. Any type of sexual activity to which the victim does not consent, ranging from inappropriate touching to penetration.

2. Rape is nonconsensual vaginal, anal, or oral penetration obtained by force or by threat of bodily harm, or when consent is unobtainable.

   a. Drugs associated with date rape

      1) Gamma-hydroxybutyrate (GHB) produces relaxation, euphoria, and disinhibition.

      2) Flunitrazepam (Rohypnol) causes sedation, muscle relaxation, and amnesia.

3. Rape Trauma Syndrome

   a. This is a variant of PTSD that can lasts for weeks following rape. Symptoms can include feelings of numbness, disbelief, fear, denial, flashbacks, and emotional lability.

4. **Nursing Interventions**

   a. Use a nonjudgmental and empathic approach.

   b. Identify, treat, and document all injuries.

   c. Provide a private environment and limit personnel who examine the client.

   d. Monitor client emotions and provide support.

REVIEW FOR ANGER/VIOLENCE, ABUSE, AND ASSAULT

Match the following.

____ 1. A nonpunitive intervention used to protect the client from harming self or others	a. Lorazepam (Ativan)
____ 2. A stage of violence in which gifts and apologies are administered	b. Seclusion
____ 3. Antianxiety agent	c. Predictor of violence
____ 4. The failure to make educational provisions for a child	d. Honeymoon
____ 5. Intense eye contact	e. Haloperidol (Haldol)
____ 6. Antipsychotic	f. Neglect

Answer Key: 1. B; 2. D; 3. A; 4. F; 5. C; 6. E

Legal Aspects of Mental Health Nursing

A nurse who works in a mental health setting is responsible for providing ethical, competent, and safe care consistent with local, state, and federal laws.

A. **Types of Admissions**

   1. Voluntary

      a. Admits self

      b. Consents to all treatment

      c. Can refuse treatment, including medications, unless a danger to self or others

      d. Can demand and receive discharge

   2. Involuntary

      a. Client deemed by lawful authority to be a danger to self or others

      b. At the end of a specified time, the client must have a hearing or be released

B. **Informed Consent Required for:**

   1. Electroconvulsive therapy

   2. Medications

   3. Seclusion

   4. Restraints

C. **Client Rights**

   1. Clients who receive a diagnosis of or are hospitalized with a mental health disorder are guaranteed the same civil rights as any other citizens.

      a. Right to receive or refuse treatment

      b. Access to stationery and postage

      c. Receipt of unopened mail

      d. Visits by health care provider, attorney, or clergy

      e. Daily interaction with visitors or phone access

      f. Right to have and/or spend money

      g. Storage space for personal items

      h. Right to own property, vote, and marry

      i. Right to make wills and contracts

      j. Access to educational resources

      k. Right to sue, or be sued, including challenging one's hospitalization

! Point to Remember

A nurse's priority is to promote and provide care to a client in the least restrictive environment possible.

Maternal and Newborn Nursing

SECTION 1

Female Reproductive System

I Reproduction

A. **Reproductive Organs**

1. Ovaries
2. Fallopian tubes
3. Uterus
4. Cervix
5. Vagina

B. **Fertilization and Fetal Development**

1. Conception (fertilization): union of sperm and ovum
2. Conditions necessary for fertilization

   a. Mature egg and sperm

   b. Timing

      1) Lifetime of ovum is 24 hr.

      2) Lifetime of sperm in female genital tract is 72 hr.

      3) Menstruation begins approximately 14 days after ovulation if conception has not occurred.

   c. Vaginal and cervical secretions

      1) Less acidic during ovulation (sperm cannot survive in a highly acidic environment)

      2) Thinner during ovulation (sperm can penetrate more easily)

   d. Process of fertilization (7 to 10 days)

      1) Ovulation occurs.

      2) Ovum travels to fallopian tube.

      3) Sperm travels to fallopian tube.

      4) One sperm penetrates the ovum.

      5) Zygote forms (fertilized egg).

      6) Zygote migrates to uterus.

      7) Zygote implants in uterine wall.

      8) Progesterone and estrogen are secreted by the corpus luteum to maintain the lining of the uterus and prevent menstruation until the placenta starts producing these hormones. (Progesterone is a thermogenic hormone that raises body temperature, an objective sign that ovulation has occurred.)

3. Placental development

   a. Chorionic villi

      1) Secrete human chorionic gonadotropin (hCG), which stimulates production of estrogen and progesterone from the corpus luteum.

      2) Production of hCG begins on the day of implantation and can be detected by day 6.

      3) Burrow into the endometrium, forming the placenta.

   b. Placental hormones

      1) hCG

      2) Human chorionic somatomammotropin (hCS), previously called human placental lactogen (hPL): acts as growth hormone and insulin antagonist

      3) Estrogen and progesterone

4. Fetal membranes develop and surround the fetus.

   a. Amnion: inner membrane

   b. Chorion: outer membrane

5. Umbilical cord

   a. Two arteries carry deoxygenated blood to the placenta.

   b. One vein carries oxygenated blood to the fetus.

   c. No pain receptors .

   d. Encased in Wharton's jelly (thick substance that surrounds the umbilical cord and acts as a buffer, preventing pressure on the vein and arteries in the umbilical cord).

   e. Covered by chorionic membrane.

6. Amniotic fluid

   a. Replaced every 3 hr

   b. 800 to 1,200 mL at end of pregnancy

   c. Functions: temperature regulation, protection, and promotes musculoskeletal development of the fetus

SECTION 2

Pregnancy

I Prenatal period

Begins with conception and ends before birth.

A. **Anatomy and Physiology**

1. **Female Anatomy:** Hormones, ovulation, organs

2. **Male Anatomy:** Sperm, vas deferens, seminal fluid

3. **Fetal/Maternal Circulation:** Fetal and maternal blood do not mix

PSYCHOLOGICAL AND PHYSIOLOGICAL ADAPTATIONS OF PREGNANCY

TRIMESTER	NURSING INTERVENTIONS/CLIENT EDUCATION
Ambivalence	
1st	Collect data about meaning of pregnancy to the client/partner and socioeconomic supports. Refer if needed.
Accepting	
2nd	Collect data to determine if ambivalence is increased and how the client views the fetus.
Preparing for birth	
3rd	Reinforce teaching about manifestations of onset of labor, newborn care, feeding methods, birth control, and home preparations for baby. Review birthing plan.
Skin: striae, linea nigra, chloasma	
2nd, 3rd	Discuss that commercial treatments are not useful; pigmentation usually disappears after pregnancy; striae can fade.

TRIMESTER	NURSING INTERVENTIONS/CLIENT EDUCATION

Breasts: size, striae, tenderness

1st	Fullness and sensitivity are hormone-related. Client should wear supportive bra. OTC products do not reduce stretch marks.

Breasts: colostrum

2nd, 3rd	Colostrum can be expressed as early as 16 weeks. Review breast care, pads, nipple care, and to keep dry.

Respiratory: dyspnea

2nd, 3rd	Sleep propped or sitting up. Lightening (fetus begins descent into pelvis) between 38 to 40 weeks. Can breathe easier.

Cardiovascular: faintness and syncope

2nd	Moderate exercise, deep breathing, avoid sudden changes in position. Side-lying position.

Cardiovascular: varicose veins

2nd, 3rd	Monitor activity: sitting/standing; constrictive clothing; crossing legs. Review leg elevation, position changes, support hose, and exercise.

GI: nausea/vomiting

1st	Review diet: dry crackers, 5 to 6 small meals, ginger, raspberry. Avoid fried, odorous, spicy foods and foods with strong smells. Monitor weight, UO, and signs of hyperemesis. Client should call provider if cannot eat/drink for more than 24 hr, urine becomes scant and dark, heart pounds, or she becomes dizzy.

GI: constipation

2nd, 3rd	Reinforce teaching about activity, fluids, and fiber.

GI: heartburn

2nd, 3rd	Encourage small meals; sit upright for 30 min or more after eating; avoid spicy, fatty foods. Drink hot herbal tea.

GU: frequency

1st, 3rd	Monitor for UTI. Encourage frequent voiding; do not decrease fluids. Urinate after intercourse. Call provider if dysuria, cloudy or foul-smelling urine, or flank pain. Kegel exercises.

GU: leukorrhea

2nd, 3rd	Presence is normal. Do not douche. Maintain good hygiene. Wear perineal pads. Report if accompanied by pruritus, foul odor, or change in character.

GU: Braxton Hicks

2nd, 3rd	Difference between Braxton Hicks and true labor. See Table: False vs. True Labor.

Nutrition

1st, 2nd, 3rd	Monitor and reinforce teaching about weight gain patterns; average weight gain 25 to 35 lb; caloric increase 300 to 400 kcal/day; protein increase by 25 g/day; iron intake 30 mg/day; folate intake 600 mcg/day; prenatal vitamins. Limit caffeine intake.

SIGNS/SYMPTOMS OF PREGNANCY

Presumptive — Subjective signs/symptoms

Amenorrhea

Fatigue

Nausea and vomiting

Urinary frequency

Breast changes: Darkened areola, enlarged Montgomery's tubules

Quickening: slight fluttering movements of the fetus felt by the client, usually between 16 to 20 weeks of gestation

Probable — Objective signs

Cervical changes

Hegar's sign: softening and compressibility of lower uterus

Chadwick's sign: deepened violet-bluish color of vaginal mucosa secondary to increased vascularity of the area

Goodell's sign: softening of cervical tip

Ballottement: rebound of unengaged fetus

Braxton Hicks contractions – false contractions, painless, irregular, and usually relieved by walking

Positive pregnancy test

Positive — Attributable only to presence of fetus

Fetal heart tones

Visualization of fetus by ultrasound

Fetal movement palpated by an experienced examiner

B. **Verifying Pregnancy**

1. Serum and urine tests provide an accurate assessment for the presence of hCG.

2. hCG can be detected 6 to 11 days in serum and 26 days in urine after conception following implantation.

   a. Production begins with implantation, peaks at about 60 to 70 days of gestation, and then declines until around 80 days of pregnancy, when it begins to gradually increase until term.

   b. Higher levels can indicate multifetal pregnancy, ectopic pregnancy, hydatidiform mole (gestational trophoblastic disease), or a genetic abnormality such as Down syndrome.

   c. Lower blood levels of hCG can suggest a miscarriage or ectopic pregnancy. Some medications (anticonvulsants, diuretics, tranquilizers) can cause false-positive or false-negative pregnancy results.

C. **Calculating Delivery Date**

1. Nagele's rule: Formula for calculating estimated date of confinement (EDC) or estimated date of birth (EDB). To calculate EDB, subtract 3 months and add 7 days to the first day of the last menstrual period.

2. McDonald's method: Measure uterine fundal height in centimeters from the symphysis pubis to the top of the uterine fundus. Between 18 and 30 weeks gestation, the fundal height measurement should approximate gestational age.

D. **Antepartal Fetal Assessment**

1. Ultrasound

   a. Indications for use

      1) Confirm pregnancy and location (uterine vs. ectopic).

      2) Evaluate fetus: number, heart beat, gestational age, abnormalities, growth and development, activity (BPP).

      3) Evaluate placenta: location (previa or abruptio), grading.

      4) Evaluate amniotic fluid volume.

   b. **Nursing Interventions**

      1) Preparation of a client

         a) Explain the procedure.

         b) Ensure client has a full bladder.

2. Non-stress test (NST)

   a. Most widely used test for evaluating fetal well-being

   b. Noninvasive

   c. Monitors response of the fetal heart rate (FHR) to fetal movement

   d. Indications for use

      1) Monitor for fetal well-being and an intact CNS during the third trimester.

      2) Monitor fetus of clients who have high-risk pregnancies such as those who have maternal diabetes mellitus, hypertension, heart disease, IUGR, post dates, history of previous stillbirth, or decreased fetal movement.

e. Interpretation of findings

   1) Reactive NST (normal)

      a) Two or more fetal heart rate accelerations (increase in FHR of at least 15/min above the baseline and last 15 seconds) within a 20-min period.

      b) Before 32 weeks gestation, acceleration is defined as increase of at least 10/min lasting at least 10 seconds in FHR.

   2) Non-reactive NST (abnormal)

      a) Does not produce two or more qualifying accelerations in 20 min.

      b) If does not meet criteria in 40 min, additional testing is indicated: contraction stress test (CST) or biophysical profile (BPP).

f. **Nursing Interventions**

   1) Seat the client in a reclining chair or place in a semi-Fowler's or left-lateral position.

   2) Apply two belts and transducers to the client's abdomen.

REACTIVE NST

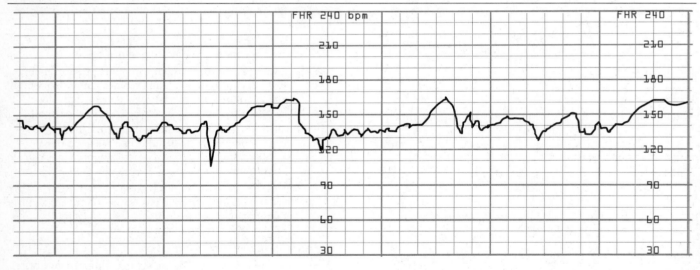

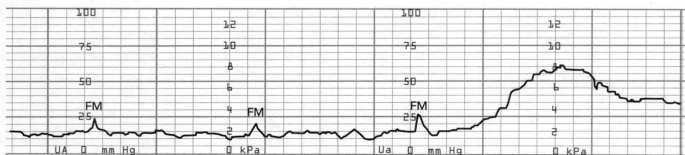

3. Contraction stress test (CST)

  a. Method

    1) Nipple stimulation

    2) Oxytocin (Pitocin) IV

  b. Indications for use

    1) Non-reactive NST

    2) High-risk pregnancies; same as indications for NST

  c. **Nursing Interventions**

    1) Explain procedure and obtain informed consent.

    2) Obtain baseline FHR, fetal movement, and contraction pattern 10 to 20 min before and 30 min after.

    3) Initiate method and observe for tachysystole (hyperstimulation).

    4) Obtain at least three contractions in a 10-min period, each lasting 40 to 60 seconds.

    5) Maintain bed rest during the procedure.

  d. Interpretation of findings

    1) Test results are negative, positive, equivocal, suspicious, or unsatisfactory.

    2) Negative CST (normal)

      a) At least three uterine contractions in 10 min, with no late decelerations

      b) Reassuring finding

    3) Positive CST (abnormal)

      a) Late decelerations occur with 50% or more of contractions

      b) Nonreassuring finding

      c) Suggestive of uteroplacental insufficiency.

4. Biophysical profile (BPP)

  a. Uses real-time ultrasound to visualize physiological characteristics of the fetus.

  b. Assesses five variables: fetal breathing movements, gross body movements, fetal heart rate, reactive FHR (NST), amniotic fluid volume.

  c. Award score of 0 (abnormal finding) or 2 (normal finding) to each variable.

5. Amniocentesis

  a. Early pregnancy

    1) Genetic work-up for fetal anomalies (e.g., Down syndrome, Trisomy 18, Trisomy 13)

    2) Detect presence of AChE in NTD

    3) Performed at 14 to 16 weeks

  b. Late in pregnancy

    1) Monitor fetal lung maturity and fetal well-being.

    2) L:S ratio of 2:1 indicates fetal lung maturity.

  c. **Nursing Interventions** for amniocentesis

    1) Preprocedure: Explain procedure and risks to client and obtain informed consent.

    2) Ensure client has a patent IV.

    3) Postprocedure

      a) Monitor FHR, fetal activity.

      b) Monitor for signs of labor.

      c) Monitor for vaginal bleeding or hemorrhage.

      d) Rho(D) immune globulin (Rhogam) is administered if client is Rh-negative.

    4) Education on complications to report

      a) Bleeding

      b) Contractions

      c) Manifestations of infection

NOTE: According to the NCLEX® scope of practice, only RNs may administer Rhogam IM. It is a blood product!

6. Percutaneous umbilical blood sampling (PUBS)

  a. Also referred to as cordocentesis

  b. Direct access to fetal circulation

  c. Used for fetal blood sampling and transfusion

  d. Performed in high-risk centers

7. Chorionic villi sampling

  a. Obtain sample of chorionic villi (placental) tissue.

  b. Check for fetal genetic abnormalities.

  c. Performed transcervical or transabdominal.

  d. Performed between 8 to 12 weeks.

  e. Similar risk and nursing interventions as amniocentesis.

8. Maternal serum alpha-fetoprotein screening (MSAFP)

  a. Screening tool for neural tube defects (NTDs)

  b. Ideally performed at 16 to 18 weeks

  c. Lower than normal levels—follow up for Down syndrome

  d. Higher than normal levels—follow up for neural tube defects

E. **Fetal Assessment**

  1. FHR expected reference range is 110 to 160/min.

  2. Fundal height used to evaluate gestational age and growth of fetus.

  3. Fetal activity: kick counts or daily fetal movement counts.

    a. Contact provider if fetal movement decreases or ceases entirely for 12 hr.

    b. Contact if less than 10 kicks/2 hr.

    c. Try to do at the same time each day.

    d. Most active after meals and in the evening.

    e. Fetal movement may be decreased by drugs including alcohol and cigarette smoke.

    f. Obesity can hinder the sensation of fetal activity.

II Obstetrical Terminology

A. **Pregnancy Outcome**

1. Gravidity: number of pregnancies

2. Parity: number of pregnancies in which the fetus or fetuses reach viability (20 weeks), regardless of whether the fetus is born alive or stillborn.

3. Five-digit system (GTPAL)

    a. G – Gravidity (number of pregnancies including this pregnancy)

    b. T – Term births (38 weeks or more)

    c. P – Preterm births (from 20 weeks up to 37 completed weeks)

    d. A – Abortions/miscarriages (prior to viability)

    e. L – Living children

4. Fetal age

    a. Preterm

    b. Term

    c. Postterm

III Collaborative Care

A. **Prenatal Care**

1. Initial exam

    a. Psychosocial assessment

    b. Complete history including medications; pertinent history from partner; family history of genetic concerns

    c. Complete physical

    d. Baseline laboratory values

        1) CBC

        2) Blood type and Rh

        3) Urinalysis

        4) STI screen, including:

            a) HIV

            b) Rubella titer

            c) Hepatitis B

    e. Nutritional counseling (see the "Psychological and Physiological Adaptations of Pregnancy" table on page 184)

    f. Teratogens: Fetus especially vulnerable during first trimester.

        1) Drugs

            a) Category C and D medications such as coumadin, lithium, methimazole, phenytoin, tetracycline, and antipsychotics

            b) Illegal drugs

        2) Cigarettes and alcohol

            a) Smoking increases incidence of abortion, prematurity, SGA, and SIDS.

            b) Quantity of alcohol to produce fetal effects is unclear: IUGR, CNS malformation, neurologic problems.

        3) Thermal risks and radiation

            a) Avoid hot tubs, long baths, or excessively hot showers.

        4) Infections

            a) Group B Strep

                (1) Culture obtained at 35 to 36 weeks.

                (2) Treat positive culture with PCN IVBP every 4 hr during labor.

                (3) Monitor newborn for infection.

            b) TORCH

                (1) T – Toxoplasmosis

                (2) O – Other (GBS, hepatitis, HIV, syphilis, varicella)

                (3) R – Rubella

                (4) C – Cytomegalovirus

                (5) H – Herpes infections

            c) See the "Sexually Transmitted Infections" table on page 215.

2. Initial and subsequent exams

    a. Weight

    b. Fundal height

    c. FHR

    d. Fetal activity (include date of quickening)

    e. Urine check for glucose and protein

    f. Anticipatory guidance. See "Psychological and Physiological Adaptations of Pregnancy" table on page 184. Review when to contact provider.

        1) Rupture of membranes prior to 37 weeks

        2) Abdominal or back pain (contractions) before 37 weeks

        3) Vaginal bleeding

        4) Elevated temperature

        5) Dysuria, oliguria

        6) Severe headache with vision changes

3. 16 weeks

    a. Screen for NTDs with maternal serum alpha fetoprotein.

4. 28 weeks

    a. Screen for diabetes mellitus.

    b. Rho(D) immune globulin (Rhogam) is administered if Rh-negative.

    c. Begin NST testing twice a week for any pregnancy at risk for intrauterine fetal death.

5. 35 weeks

    a. Test for group B strep.

B. **Anticipatory Care:** Do not assume symptoms are normal adaptations of pregnancy. See "Psychological and Physiological Adaptations of Pregnancy" table on page 184.

1. Physiological changes

    a. Physiologic changes in pregnancy are the result of hormone production and the enlarging uterus.

PHYSIOLOGIC CHANGES

SYSTEM	CHANGES
Reproductive	Uterus increases in size, shape, position
	Ovulation and menses cease
Cardiovascular	Increased cardiac output and blood volume (45% to 50% at term)
	Increased heart rate
	Increased coagulation
Respiratory	Increased maternal oxygen needs
	Uterine enlargement displaces diaphragm, causing increased respiratory rate and decreased total lung capacity
Musculoskeletal	Pelvic joint relaxation
	Body alterations require adjustment in posture
	Separation of rectus abdominis muscles
Gastrointestinal	Nausea and vomiting
	Slowed digestive processes, constipation
Renal	Increased glomerular filtration, urinary frequency
Endocrine/ Metabolic	Increased hormone production (hCG, progesterone, estrogen, hPL and prostaglandins)
	Increased thyroid and parathyroid activity
	Insulin resistance
Integument	Hyperpigmentation causing chloasma, linea nigra, striae gravidarum, and palmar erythema

   b. Changes in physical appearance can lead to a negative body image. The client might make statements of resentment toward the pregnancy and express anxiousness for the pregnancy to be over soon.

   2. Expected vital signs

   a. Blood pressure

      1) Within the prepregnancy range during first trimester

      2) Decreases 5 to 10 mm Hg during second trimester

      3) Returns to prepregnancy at 20 weeks

      4) Position affects blood pressure; supine position can cause supine hypotensive syndrome or vena cava syndrome. Manifestations include dizziness, lightheadedness, and pale, clammy skin. Interventions include left-lateral side, semi-Fowler's position, or wedge under one hip if supine.

   b. Pulse

      1) Increases by 10 to 15/min around 20 weeks

   c. Respirations

      1) Increases by 1 to 2/min due to elevation of the diaphragm

   3. Fetal heart tones

   a. Normal baseline rate 110 to 160/min

   b. Accelerations are reassuring, indicate intact fetal CNS

Complications of Pregnancy

Medical Problems

Preexisting conditions can complicate pregnancy. Some medical conditions develop during pregnancy and cause complications.

NOTE: Remember that only the RN may care for or assess high-risk or unstable clients, according to the NCLEX® scope of practice.

A. **Cardiac Disease**

   1. Contributing Factors

   a. Preexisting heart condition

   b. Increased maternal plasma volume

   2. Greatest risks for heart failure

   a. End of second trimester (28 to 32 weeks)

   b. During labor

   c. After delivery (first 48 hr)

   3. Manifestations

   a. Client will exhibit manifestations of right or left heart failure (see unit 6, section 8)

   b. Changes specific to pregnancy

      1) Intrauterine growth restriction

      2) Decreased amniotic fluid

      3) FHR with decreased variability

      4) Mild to moderate high blood pressure (140 to 159 mm Hg systolic or 90 to 159 mm Hg diastolic measured on two occasions at least 4 hr apart)

   c. Diagnostic testing specific to pregnancy

      1) Laboratory Testing

      2) Ultrasound

      3) NST

      4) Biophysical profile

   4. Collaborative Care

   a. **Nursing Interventions**

      1) Monitor for manifestations of fatigue, anemia, weight gain more than 1 to 2 lb/week, pulmonary edema, peripheral edema, palpitations, tachycardia, and angina.

      2) Recognize and report change in client condition.

      3) Prevent infection.

      4) Provide nutritional counseling.

b. **Medications:** Pharmacological management is determined by the client's cardiac diagnoses and clinical presentation.

　1) Propranolol (Inderal): beta blocker; used to treat tachyarrhythmias and to lower maternal blood pressure

　2) Ampicillin (Polycillin): antibiotic; prophylaxis given to prevent endocarditis

　3) Heparin sodium: anticoagulant used in treating clients with pulmonary embolus, deep-vein thrombosis, prosthetic valves, cyanotic heart defects, and rheumatic heart disease

　4) Digoxin (Lanoxin): cardiac glycoside; used to increase cardiac output during pregnancy; may be prescribed if fetal tachycardia is present

　5) Anticoagulant therapy (heparin)

B. **Hypertension in Pregnancy:** Hypertensive disease in pregnancy is divided into clinical subsets: gestational hypertension; mild and severe preeclampsia; eclampsia; and hemolysis, elevated liver enzymes, and low platelets (HELLP) syndrome.

1. **Vasospasm** contributing to poor tissue perfusion is the underlying mechanism for the signs and symptoms of pregnancy hypertensive disorders.

2. **Gestational hypertension (GH)**

　a. Begins after the 20th week of pregnancy.

　b. Presents with elevated blood pressure of 140/90 mm Hg or greater.

　c. Proteinuria can be present (not required for diagnosis)

　d. Blood pressure returns to baseline by 12 weeks postpartum.

3. **Severe preeclampsia**

　a. Blood pressure 160/110 mm Hg or greater on two separate occasions 6 hr apart on bed rest

　b. Proteinuria is present (not used to confirm severity)

　c. Oliguria

　d. Cerebral or visual disturbances (headache and blurred vision)

　e. Hyperreflexia with possible ankle clonus

　f. Pulmonary or cardiac involvement

　g. Extensive peripheral edema

　h. Hepatic dysfunction (elevated liver function tests)

　i. Epigastric and right upper-quadrant pain

　j. Thrombocytopenia

4. **Eclampsia**

　a. Severe preeclampsia plus seizure activity

　b. Usually preceded by persistent headache, blurred vision, severe epigastric or right upper quadrant abdominal pain, and altered mental status

5. **HELLP** syndrome is a variant of GH in which hematologic conditions coexist with severe preeclampsia involving hepatic dysfunction. HELLP syndrome is diagnosed by laboratory tests, not clinically.

　a. H – hemolysis resulting in anemia and jaundice

　b. EL – elevated liver enzymes resulting in elevated ALT and AST, epigastric pain, and nausea and vomiting

　c. LP – low platelets (less than 100,000/mm3), resulting in thrombocytopenia, abnormal bleeding and clotting time, bleeding gums, petechiae, and possibly DIC

NOTE: Gestational hypertensive disease and chronic hypertension can occur simultaneously. Gestational hypertensive diseases are associated with placental abruption, acute kidney failure, hepatic rupture, preterm birth, and fetal and maternal death.

6. Contributing Factors

　a. No single profile identifies risks for gestational hypertensive disorders, but some high risks include:

　　1) Maternal age younger than 20 or older than 40

　　2) First pregnancy

　　3) Morbid obesity

　　4) Multifetal gestation

　　5) Chronic kidney disease

　　6) Chronic hypertension

　　7) Familiar history of preeclampsia

　　8) Diabetes mellitus

　　9) Rh incompatibility

　　10) Molar pregnancy

　　11) Previous history of GH

7. Lab and Diagnostic Testing

　a. Blood pressure elevation

　b. Urine studies: urinalysis for proteinuria; 24-hr urine protein

　c. Liver enzymes, serum creatinine, BUN, uric acid

8. Collaborative Care

　a. **Nursing Interventions**

　　1) Monitor blood pressure.

　　2) Administer medications.

　　3) Discuss nutrition (balanced diet; 60 to 70 g protein, 1,200 mg calcium, 400 mcg folic acid; limit salty foods; eat foods with roughage; avoid alcohol and tobacco; and limit caffeine intake).

　　4) Perform maternal assessments: daily weight, I&O, reflexes, CNS.

　　5) Obtain fetal assessments: serial ultrasound, Doppler blood flow analysis; NST, CST, BPP; fetal kick count.

　　6) Encourage bed rest on left side.

　　7) Initiate seizure precautions (preeclampsia/eclampsia).

　　8) Provide quiet environment: private room not next to nurses' station, dim lights.

　　9) Monitor and report changes in client's condition (risk for HELLP and DIC with severe preeclampsia).

b. Medications

1) Magnesium sulfate: anticonvulsant

a) Magnesium sulfate is the medication of choice for prophylaxis or treatment. Reduces seizure threshold (depression of the CNS); secondary side effect is decreased blood pressure as it relaxes smooth muscles.

NOTE: If magnesium toxicity is suspected, discontinue magnesium infusion immediately. Administer calcium gluconate and notify provider. Take actions to prevent respiratory or cardiac arrest.

C. **Diabetes Mellitus**

1. Types

a. Pregestational diabetes mellitus: Client had diabetes prior to pregnancy.

b. Gestational diabetes mellitus: An impaired tolerance to glucose with the first onset or recognition during pregnancy. The ideal blood glucose level during pregnancy is 70 to 110 mg/dL. Client develops diabetes mellitus during pregnancy, usually in the second or third trimester.

2. Contributing Factors

a. Obesity

b. Maternal age older than 25 years

c. Family history of diabetes mellitus

d. Previous delivery of an infant who was large or stillborn

3. Manifestations

a. Hyperglycemia

b. Insulin resistance

4. Laboratory Testing and Diagnostic Procedures

a. Routine urinalysis with glycosuria.

b. Glucose tolerance test (50 g oral glucose load, followed by plasma glucose analysis 1 hr later performed at 24 to 28 weeks of gestation—fasting not necessary; a positive blood glucose screening is 140 mg/dL or greater; additional testing with a 3-hr glucose tolerance test is indicated).

1) A 3-hr glucose tolerance test (following overnight fasting, avoidance of caffeine, and abstinence from smoking for 12 hr prior to testing; a fasting glucose is obtained, a 100 g glucose load is given, and serum glucose levels are determined at 1, 2, and 3 hr following glucose ingestion).

c. Monitor HbA1c.

d. Monitor for ketones.

e. BPP to ascertain fetal well-being.

f. Amniocentesis with alpha-fetoprotein.

g. NST to assess fetal well-being.

5. Collaborative Care

a. Risks to newborn increase with poor glucose control.

1) Congenital anomalies

2) Spontaneous abortions

3) Macrosomia: birth trauma and dystocia

4) Death

5) Hypoglycemia after birth

b. **Nursing Interventions**

1) Diet

2) Exercise

3) Blood glucose monitoring

4) Oral hypoglycemics are not used in pregnancy.

5) If medication is needed, insulin will be used.

a) Can need insulin if not already using.

b) Insulin needs decrease first trimester.

c) Insulin needs increase during the second and third trimester due to increase amount of hPL (insulin antagonist).

D. **Hyperemesis Gravidarum:** Excessive pregnancy-related nausea and/or vomiting. Hospitalization can be necessary because of dehydration and weight loss.

1. Begins first or second month of pregnancy

2. Contributing Factors

a. High levels of human chorionic gonadotropin (hCG)

b. At times may have a psychological cause

3. Manifestations

a. Loss of 5% or more of prepregnancy body weight

b. Dehydration, causing ketosis and constipation

c. Nutritional deficiencies

d. Metabolic imbalances

4. Collaborative Care

a. **Nursing Interventions**

1) Monitor psyche; refer as needed.

2) Monitor weight.

3) Monitor for dehydration, electrolyte imbalance, and metabolic alkalosis.

4) Monitor I&O.

5) Administer IV fluids.

6) Small meals per client preference.

b. Medications

1) Antiemetics such as ondansetron (Zofran)

2) Vitamin B₆ (no more than 100 mg daily)

c. Therapeutic Measures

1) Acupressure

2) Relaxation techniques

d. Client Education

1) Nausea and vomiting usually peak between 2 and 12 weeks of pregnancy and go away by the second half of pregnancy.

2) Eat small, frequent meals. Eating dry foods, such as crackers, can help relieve uncomplicated nausea.

3) Increase fluid intake to prevent dehydration. Reinforce teaching to increase fluids during the times of the day when the client feels the least nauseated. Seltzer, ginger ale, or other sparkling waters can be helpful.

II Placental and Cervical Problems

A. **Abruptio Placenta**

1. Contributing Factors
   a. Trauma
   b. Preeclampsia
   c. Multiparity
   d. Cocaine use

B. **Placenta Previa**

1. Contributing Factors
   a. Placenta implants completely or partially over cervical os

PLACENTA PREVIA AND ABRUPTIO PLACENTA

	PLACENTA PREVIA	ABRUPTIO PLACENTA
Vaginal bleeding	Usually bright red. Can range from minimal to severe and life-threatening. Color of bleeding bright red.	Can range from absent to moderate dependant on the grade of abruption. Blood usually dark red in color.
Pain	Often none	Abdomen "boardlike" and very tender
Maternal effect	Hemorrhage, shock, death	
Fetal effect	Anoxia, CNS trauma, death	
Treatment	Partial previa can be treated with bed rest. Complete previa will be treated as with abruptio placenta.	Emotional support; immediate cesarean birth; blood transfusions, monitor for DIC.

NOTE: Vaginal exams are contraindicated with vaginal bleeding.

C. **Hydatidiform Mole/Molar Pregnancy:** Benign abnormal growth of chorionic villi. Appears as avascular transparent grapelike clusters. Can develop choriocarcinoma (rare)

1. Contributing Factors
   a. Previous use of ovulation-stimulating drugs
   b. Age extremes: very young or over 40
   c. History of spontaneous abortion
   d. Poor nutrition
   e. Often unknown

2. Manifestations
   a. Vaginal bleeding; brown, grapelike clusters; anemia
   b. Rapid uterine growth (increase in fundal height); cramping
   c. Extreme nausea
   d. Hyperthyroidism
   e. Preeclampsia

3. Diagnostic Testing
   a. Ultrasound
   b. Persistent, high, hCG levels

4. Collaborative Care
   a. Monitor psyche
   b. Spontaneous expulsion

   c. Elective expulsion
   1) Curettage
   2) Induction not recommended
   3) Rhogam post-expulsion if Rh-negative
   4) Post-expulsion
      a) Follow postpartum protocol.
      b) Continue to monitor hCG levels.
      c) Follow up to rule out choriocarcinoma.
      d) Discuss contraception; should avoid pregnancy for 1 year or until hCG levels return to normal.

D. **Abortion:** Expulsion of the fetus prior to viability

1. Types
   a. Spontaneous
   b. Therapeutic
   c. Elective

2. Collaborative Care
   a. Provide psychological support.
   b. Assist with ultrasound.
   c. Save all passed tissue for examination.
   d. Monitor for signs of hemorrhage (perform pad count, monitor Hgb and Hct).
   e. Monitor for signs of shock.
   f. Prepare for D&C.
   g. Rho(D) immune globulin (Rhogam) is administered to Rh-negative clients.

3. Discharge Teaching
   a. Notify provider if signs of infection occur, bleeding increases, or signs of depression develop.
   b. Discuss future pregnancy plans, birth control.
   c. Provide follow-up exam.

E. **Cervical Insufficiency (Incompetent Cervix):** Premature dilation of the cervix, usually in second trimester

1. Contributing Factors
   a. Cervical trauma
   b. Previous spontaneous delivery in second trimester

2. Manifestations
   a. Increase in pelvic pressure
   b. Pink-stained vaginal discharge or bleeding
   c. Uterine contractions

3. Diagnostic and therapeutic procedures
   a. Ultrasound showing short cervix (less than 20 mm in length)
   b. Prophylactic cervical cerclage; removed at 37 weeks

4. Collaborative Care
   a. Emotional support
   b. If able to maintain pregnancy:
   1) Bed rest
   2) Monitor client and fetus
   3) Tocolytics
   4) Hydration
   5) Cerclage (purse string suture)

F. **Ectopic Pregnancy:** Fertilized egg implants outside of uterus (pelvis, abdomen, often fallopian tubes)

1. Contributing Factors

   a. Narrowing or scarring of fallopian tube: previous STI or PID; IUD; endometriosis; tubal surgery

2. Manifestations

   a. One or two missed menses

   b. Unilateral stabbing pain and tenderness in lower abdomen

   c. Bleeding

   d. Shock (hypotension, tachycardia, pallor).

3. Collaborative Care

   a. Provide psychological support.

   b. Replace fluids.

   c. Administer methotrexate (MTX).

   d. Prepare for surgery and postoperative care.

PRENATAL NURSING CARE WORKSHEET

Prioritize which of the following patients the nurse should see first and why. Which prioritization guideline is used?

A. A client who is 14 weeks gestation and has severe vomiting

B. A client who is 16 weeks gestation and states she has not felt fetal movement

C. A client who is 18 weeks gestation and exhibits total weight gain of 4.5 kg (10 lb)

D. A client who is 20 weeks gestation and reports a white vaginal discharge with pruritus

Answer: Apply Maslow's physiologic needs as the prioritizing guideline. The client who has severe vomiting has the highest physiological risk related to dehydration, electrolyte imbalance, and metabolic alkalosis. The other clients need additional follow-up but are not as high risk. First fetal movement (quickening) occurs during the second trimester and for some women is difficult to identify. A total weight gain of 4.5 kg falls within the average of 1 to 2 kg in the first trimester and approximately 0.5 kg/week during second and third trimesters. Pattern of weight gain is also important. White vaginal discharge with pruritus is typical of vaginal candidiasis that is common during pregnancy related to the change in the pH of the vagina.

Labor and Delivery

Labor and Delivery

Labor and delivery include the period during which the baby and placenta are delivered and up to 2 hr after delivery.

A. **Labor and Delivery Processes**—Six major factors ("P's") of labor and delivery process.

1. **Psyche**—The mother's psychological response to labor

2. **Powers**—Uterine contractions

   a. Uterine contractions: Act to dilate and efface the cervix

      1) Frequency—from the beginning of one contraction to the beginning of the next contraction. Contraction frequency closer than 2 min is considered hyperstimulation.

      2) Duration—from the beginning to end of the same contraction. Contraction duration greater than 90 seconds is considered hyperstimulation.

      3) Intensity—strength of the uterine contraction. Can only be accurately measured with an internal uterine pressure catheter (IUPC).

   b. Effacement—shortening and thinning of the cervix. The goal is 100% effacement.

   c. Dilation—opening of the cervix. The diameter of the cervix ranges from 0 cm (closed) to 10 cm (fully dilated).

3. **Passenger**—the fetus and placenta

4. **Presentation**—the part of the fetus that enters the pelvic inlet first

   a. The three primary presentations are cephalic, breech, and shoulder. Breech and shoulder presentations are indications for cesarean birth.

   b. Station—the relationship of the presenting part to the maternal ischial spines that measures the degree of descent of the fetus

      1) Negative stations are above ischial spines (-1, -2).

      2) Zero station is at the ischial spines, or engaged (0).

      3) Positive stations are below the ischial spines (+1, +2, +3). Delivery is typically sooner.

5. **Position**—relationship of presenting part (occiput, mentum, sacrum) to the maternal pelvic inlet. Clients with fetus in persistent occiput posterior position (POP) have increased back (labor) pain and longer labors.

6. **Passageway**—the birth canal, pelvis, cervix, pelvic floor and vagina

   a. Cephalopelvic disproportion—When the fetus has a head size, shape, or position that does not allow for passage through the pelvis. This also can occur secondary to maternal pelvic structure or associated problems.

B. **Manifestations of False vs. True Labor**

FALSE VS. TRUE LABOR

	FALSE LABOR	TRUE LABOR
Uterine contractions		
	Braxton Hicks, irregular, do not increase in frequency or intensity. Usually felt in the lower back or the abdomen above the umbilicus. Decrease with walking or position changes. Often cease with sleep, comfort measures, oral hydration, and emptying of bladder.	Can begin irregularly but become regular in frequency, become stronger and last longer. Walking can increase contraction intensity. Contractions continue despite comfort measures. Usually felt in the lower back radiating to the abdomen.
Cervical dilation and effacement		
	No significant change in dilation or effacement. Cervix often stays in posterior position.	Cervical dilation and effacement steadily progress
Bloody show		
	Usually not present	Present as cervix dilates
Fetus		
	Presenting part not engaged in pelvis	Presenting part engages in pelvis

C. **Nursing Care During Labor and Delivery**

1. Admission assessment includes prenatal and medical and surgical history.

2. Obtain informed consents.

3. Review birth plan.

4. Active labor is considered an emergency medical condition by the Emergency Medical Treatment and Active Labor Act (EMTALA).

5. Monitor maternal and fetal status:

   a. Vital signs and physical assessment

   b. FHR

      1) Normal rate is 110 to 160/min; varies with fetal age

      2) Variability best indicator of fetal well-being. Moderate = 6 to 25/min

      3) External: auscultation, ultrasound transducer

      4) Internal: spiral electrode

         a) Requires ruptured membranes

NOTE: Any internal monitoring increases the risk of infection.

   c. Uterine contractions

      1) External: manual or tocotransducer

      2) Internal: intrauterine pressure catheter (IUPC)

   d. Vaginal discharge

   e. Cervix

      1) Cervical exams are done with sterile gloves.

      2) Limit exams especially if a vaginal infection is suspected or if ROM has occurred.

NOTE: Try to limit the frequency of vaginal exams secondary to the risk of infection.

NURSING CARE: STAGES OF LABOR

First Stage

Cervix dilates from 0 to 10 cm.

Three phases:

› **Latent Phase: 0 to 3 cm**

  » Contractions

    › Irregular, mild-moderate

    › Frequency 5 to 30 min

    › Duration 30 to 45 seconds

  » Client talkative and excited

› **Active Phase: 4 to 7 cm**

  » Contractions

    › Regular, moderate-strong

    › Frequency 3 to 5 min

    › Duration 40 to 70 seconds

  » Client anxious and in pain

› **Transitional phase: 8 to 10 cm**

  » Contractions

    › Regular, very strong

    › Frequency 2 to 3 min

    › Duration 45 to 90 seconds

  » Client can have nausea/vomiting and can become irritable.

 NURSING INTERVENTIONS

Monitor maternal/fetal status.

Monitor amniotic fluid status. Nitrazine paper used if suspect ROM. It will turn blue in the presence of alkaline amniotic fluid (pH 6.5 to 7.5).

Assist with nonpharmacological pain management. Provide analgesia if requested.

Second Stage

Pushing stage. From complete dilation through delivery of baby.

 NURSING INTERVENTIONS

Monitor FHR at least every 15 min.

Assist with pushing, breathing (prevent hyperventilation), comfort.

Record delivery time, medications, and episiotomy/laceration.

Third Stage

After delivery of baby until delivery of placenta. Contractions are usually mild. Client is usually focused on her baby.

 NURSING INTERVENTIONS

Monitor vital signs, bleeding, and fundus.

Provide immediate care of newborn: ABC, Apgar score, warm environment, safety measures, and infection control.

Fourth Stage

1 to 2 hr after delivery of the placenta.

 NURSING INTERVENTIONS

Encourage breastfeeding and promote bonding.

Monitor vital signs, fundus, and lochia every 15 min x 4; every 30 min x 2; and in 60 min.

Hemorrhage is priority concern.

D. **Fetal Assessment During Labor**

1. Indications for assessment of FHR

   a. On admission and regular intervals as indicated by hospital protocol

   b. Before and after any procedure (medication, anesthesia, ROM, vaginal exam, ambulation)

   c. Throughout labor (high-risk pregnancy, use of oxytocic agents, fetal distress)

THREE-TIER FHR CLASSIFICATION SYSTEM

Category I (normal)

Baseline FHR of 110 to 160/min

Baseline FHR variability: moderate heart rate beat fluctuations (6 to 25/min)

Accelerations: present or absent

Early decelerations: present or absent

Variable or late decelerations: absent

Category II

All FHR tracings not categorized as Category I or III

Category III (abnormal)

Sinusoidal pattern

Absent baseline FHR variability and any of the following

› Recurrent variable decelerations

› Recurrent late decelerations

› Bradycardia

d. Periodic FHR changes

   1) Accelerations (reassuring) 15/min change lasting 15 seconds (term fetus)

   2) Decelerations; early, late, variable

PERIODIC FHR CHANGES

Name: VEAL	Cause: CHOP	Management: MINE
Variable	Cord compression	Move client
Early	Head compression	Identify labor progress
Acceleration	Other (okay)	No action needed
Late	Placental insufficiency	Execute actions immediately

EARLY DECELERATION

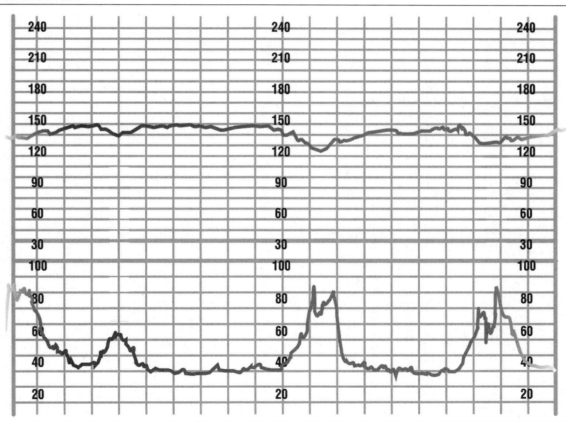

VARIABLE DECELERATION

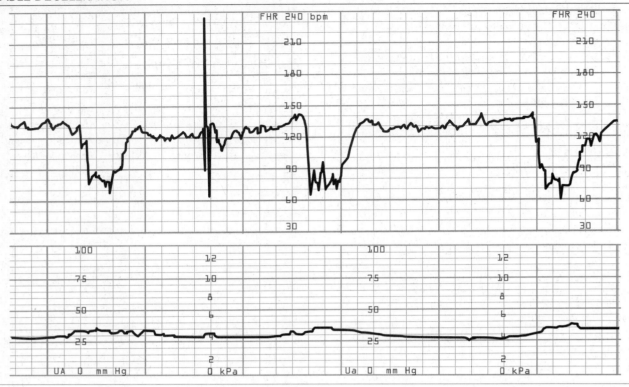

LATE DECELERATION

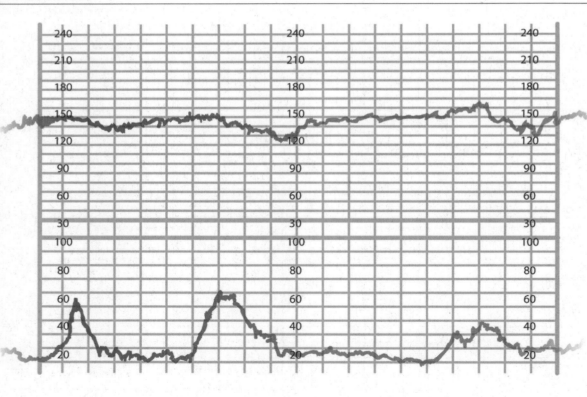

E. Medications used in labor and delivery

MEDICATIONS USED IN LABOR AND DELIVERY

MEDICATION	USE	NURSING INTERVENTIONS
Oxytocin (Pitocin)	Stimulate uterine contractions May be used in all stages of labor	Monitor contractions and FHR. Monitor vital signs. Administer by IV infusion pump through secondary line. Stop immediately for late decelerations or tachysystole (hyperstimulation). Have tocolytic (terbutaline) immediately available for tachysystole.
Methylergonovine maleate (Methergine)	Stimulate uterine contractions after delivery Treat postpartum hemorrhage	Monitor bleeding and uterine tone. Obtain baseline blood pressure. Massage fundus. Administer 0.2 mg IM or PO as prescribed.
Calcium gluconate (generic only)	Antidote for magnesium sulfate toxicity	Administer calcium gluconate 1 g (10 mL 10% solution) IV for signs of toxicity. Dilute with equal amounts of NS and administer 0.5 to 1 mL/min.
Terbutaline (Brethine), ritodrine HCl (Yutopar)	Tocolytic used for preterm labor	Monitor contractions and FHR. Monitor vital signs. Administer terbutaline subcutaneous 0.25 mg every 20 min as needed. Monitor for side effects: tremors, dizziness, headache, tachycardia, hypotension, anxiety. Do not administer if client complains of chest pain. Notify provider if: blood pressure less than 90/60 mm Hg; pulse rate greater than 130/min; signs of pulmonary edema; FHR greater than 180/min. Administer beta blocking agent as antidote.
Indomethacin (Indocin)	May be used as tocolytic for preterm labor	Monitor contractions and FHR. Monitor vital signs (can mask maternal fever) Administer with food to decrease side effect of GI distress. Only administer if gestational age is less than 32 weeks.
Magnesium sulfate	Tocolytic used for preterm labor CNS depressant to prevent seizure in preeclampsia	Preterm Labor › Monitor contractions and FHR. › Monitor fetal movement and FHR variability. › Monitor vital signs and urine output. Preeclampsia › Monitor vital signs, urine output, DTRs, and LOC. › Monitor magnesium levels (therapeutic range 4 to 8 mg/dL). › Administer via infusion pump in diluted form. › Use indwelling catheter to monitor urinary elimination. › Stop immediately if: respirations less than 12, altered LOC, magnesium levels above 10 mEq/L or 9 mg/dL. › Administer calcium gluconate 1 g (10 mL of 10% solution) for signs of toxicity. › Observe neonate for signs of respiratory depression, hypotonia, lethargy, and hypocalcemia. › Contraindicated for women with myasthenia gravis.
Naloxone HCl (Narcan)	Antidote for opioid induced respiratory depression Reverse pruritus from epidural opioid	Monitor respiratory effort. Do not administer if mother is opioid-dependent. Newborn: Administer 0.1 mg/kg IV, IM, SQ, or ET tube. Adult: Administer 0.4 to 2 mg IV, may repeat IV at 2 to 3 min intervals up to 10 mg, can also administer IM or SQ.
Betamethasone (Celestone)	Preterm labor (24 to 32 weeks) › Prevent or reduce neonatal respiratory distress syndrome in preterm infants › Stimulate production or release of lung surfactant in preterm fetus	Monitor for signs of preterm labor. Administer 12 mg deep IM for two doses 24 hr apart. Monitor blood glucose levels and lung sounds.
Prostaglandin (Cytotec, Cervidil, Prepidil)	Preinduction cervical ripening (Bishop score 4 or less)	Obtain informed consent. Monitor contractions and FHR. Monitor vital signs. Evaluate Bishop score. Use cautiously in women with history of asthma, glaucoma, renal, hepatic, or cardiovascular disorders. Contraindicated in presence of fetal distress or vaginal bleeding.

LABOR AND DELIVERY MEDICATIONS WORKSHEET

Match the medication in the first column with the related statement in second column.

_____ 1. oxytocin (Pitocin)

_____ 2. misoprostol (Cytotec)

_____ 3. penicillin G

_____ 4. methylergonovine (Methergine)

_____ 5. terbutaline sulfate

_____ 6. betamethasone (Celestone)

_____ 7. methotrexate (Amethopterin)

_____ 8. indomethacin (Indocin)

A. Contracts the uterus after delivery, used to treat postpartum hemorrhage. Need baseline blood pressure before administering.

B. Induces labor, or contracts the uterus after delivery. Stop immediately in the presence of late decelerations.

C. Stimulates fetal lung maturation between 24 to 32 weeks gestation.

D. Softens and thins the cervix.

E. Prostaglandin synthetase Inhibitor. Can be used as tocolytic in preterm labor.

F. Used during labor when client is positive for Group B *streptococcus*.

G. May be used with ectopic pregnancy to stop the growth of the embryo to save the tube.

H. Beta adrenergic agonist used as last resort for preterm labor. Call provider for heart rate greater than 130/min.

Answer key: 1. B; 2. D; 3. F; 4. A; 5. H; 6. C; 7. G; 8. E

F. **Pain Management in Labor and Delivery**

1. Nonpharmacologic pain management

   a. Childbirth preparation methods such as Lamaze, Bradley, Dick-Read, and/or pattern breathing methods are used to promote relaxation and pain relief.

   b. Sensory stimulation strategies (based on the gate-control theory) to promote relaxation and pain relief

      1) Aromatherapy

      2) Breathing relaxation techniques

      3) Visual imagery and use of focal points

      4) Music

   c. Cutaneous strategies (based on the gate-control theory) to promote relaxation and pain relief

      1) Back rubs and massage

      2) Effleurage: light, gentle, circular stroking of the client's abdomen with fingertips

      3) Sacral counterpressure

      4) Water therapy

   d. Frequent maternal position changes

      1) Semi-sitting

      2) Squatting

      3) Kneeling

      4) Rocking

      5) Supine (must have wedge under one hip to tilt the uterus to avoid supine hypotension syndrome)

2. Pharmacologic pain management: analgesia and anesthesia

   a. When given early in labor, can slow or stop labor

   b. Opioid analgesics given late in labor can cause newborn respiratory depression

   c. Butorphanol tartrate (Stadol) and nalbuphine hydrochloride should not be given to clients who have opioid dependency.

   d. Fentanyl citrate (Sublimaze) and sufentanil (Sufenta) have a short duration of action. Commonly administered with epidural and intrathecal anesthesia.

   e. Naloxone (Narcan) should be available as an antidote. Not given to client or newborn if woman is opioid-dependent.

f. **Regional blocks** are most commonly used. They include pudendal, epidural, and intrathecal blocks.

g. **Pudendal block** provides local anesthesia to the perineum, vulva, and rectal areas during delivery. It is administered 10 to 20 min before delivery.

h. **Epidural block** consists of a local anesthetic along with an analgesic morphine (Duramorph) or fentanyl (Sublimaze) injected into the epidural space at the level of the fourth or fifth vertebra. Continuous infusion or intermittent injections may be administered through an indwelling epidural catheter. Client-controlled epidural analgesia is a favored method of acute pain relief management for labor and birth. Hypotension is the most common side effect.

   1) **Nursing Interventions**

      a) Administer 1 liter IV fluid bolus before epidural anesthesia.

      b) Monitor platelet count prior to initiation of epidural.

      c) Assist in sitting or side-lying position.

      d) Monitor blood pressure frequently.

      e) Monitor for bladder distention.

      f) Continue to monitor level of pain.

      g) Assist client to turn side to side every hour.

      h) Promote safety.

      i) Keep catheter insertion site clean and dry.

      j) Monitor return of sensation in legs.

      k) Assist with standing and walking first time after sensation returns.

   2) Contraindications to subarachnoid and epidural blocks.

      a) Maternal hypotension

      b) Coagulopathy (receiving anticoagulant therapy, or history of bleeding disorder)

      c) Infection at injection site

      d) Increased intracranial pressure

      e) Maternal inability to cooperate

G. **Therapeutic Procedures to Assist with Labor and Delivery**

1. **Amniotomy**: The artificial rupture of the amniotic membranes (AROM) to initiate or improve contractions. Labor typically begins within 12 hr after the membranes rupture. The client is at an increased risk for cord prolapse or infection.

   a. **Nursing Interventions**

      1) Record baseline FHR prior to, continuously during, and after the procedure.

      2) Observe for changes in FHR: bradycardia, variable decelerations, or late decelerations (cord compression or prolapse).

      3) Monitor the amount, color, consistency, and odor of the amniotic fluid.

      4) Implement comfort measures such as perineal care and clean pads.

      5) Monitor temperature every 2 hr.

2. **Induction/Augmentation of Labor**: The process of chemically or mechanically initiating or strengthening uterine contractions

   a. Indications

      1) Maternal issues: history of rapid labors, preeclampsia, diabetes mellitus, severe Rh isoimmunization, chronic kidney disease, and pulmonary disease.

      2) Fetal/placental issues: IUGR, PROM, chorioamnionitis, postdates, fetal demise.

      3) Inadequate uterine contractions (Pitocin used to augment labor).

   b. Medications

      1) Chemical methods used to soften cervix

         a) Prostaglandin E2 (Cervidil)

         b) Prostaglandin E1 (Cytotec)

      2) Medication used to initiate induction

         a) IV oxytocin (Pitocin)

      3) **Nursing Interventions**

         a) Obtain informed consent. Monitor FHR and uterine activity every 15 min and with every change in dose.

         b) Observe for and report uterine tachysystole (more than 5 contractions in 10 min) or fetal distress.

         c) Obtain vital signs every 30 min and with every oxytocin change in dose.

         d) Oxytocin is discontinued with signs of fetal distress or uterine tachysystole (hyperstimulation):

            (1) Contraction frequency more often than every 2 min

            (2) Contraction duration longer than 90 seconds

            (3) Contraction intensity greater than 90 mm Hg with IUPC

            (4) Prepare to administer terbutaline (Brethine) 0.25 mg subcutaneously, to decrease uterine activity.

3. **Vacuum Extraction**: Attachment of a vacuum cup to the fetal head to assist in birth of the head

   a. Indications

      1) Maternal exhaustion and ineffective pushing

      2) Fetal distress during second stage of labor

   b. **Nursing Interventions**

      1) Place in lithotomy position and support with pushing.

      2) Monitor and record FHR before and during vacuum application.

      3) Monitor for bladder distention before application.

      4) Observe neonate for bruising and caput succedaneum. Inform parents caput should resolve within 24 hr.

4. **Forceps**: Obstetric instrument used to aid in delivery of the fetal head.

   a. Indications

      1) Poor progress

      2) Fetal distress

      3) Persistent occiput posterior position

      4) Abnormal presentation

   b. **Nursing Interventions**

      1) Monitor the neonate for intracranial hemorrhage, facial bruising, and facial palsy.

      2) Check FHR before traction is applied.

   c. Complications

      1) Lacerations to cervix or vagina

      2) Bladder or urethral injury

      3) Urine retention resulting from bladder or urethral injuries.

      4) Hematoma formation in the pelvic soft tissues

5. **Episiotomy**: An incision that is made into the perineum to enlarge the vaginal outlet during delivery

   a. **Nursing Interventions**

      1) Monitor for pain, healing, infection, laceration of the anal sphincter (fourth-degree tear), and hemorrhage.

      2) Encourage Kegel exercises to improve and restore perineal muscle tone.

      3) Apply ice packs.

      4) Educate client on perineal care.

6. **Cesarean Birth**: Birth of fetus through a transabdominal incision of the uterus.

   a. Types

      1) Low transverse: decrease chance of uterine rupture with future pregnancies; less bleeding after delivery

      2) Classic: rarely used

   b. Indications

      1) Previous cesarean birth

      2) Failure to progress in labor

      3) Fetal factors: malpresentation; fetal distress; cephalopelvic disproportion; multiple fetuses; macrosomia; prolapsed cord

      4) Maternal factors: positive HIV, active genital herpes

c. **Nursing Interventions**

   1) Obtain informed consent.

   2) Perform preoperative assessment and surgical checklist.

   3) Administer preoperative medications.

   4) Insert IV and Foley catheter.

   5) Perform postoperative and postpartum assessment.

   6) Monitor for bleeding at site and lochia.

   7) Obtain routine postoperative vital signs.

   8) Monitor effects of anesthesia.

   9) Monitor need for pain management.

   10) Monitor for thrombophlebitis.

NCLEX ALERT: LABOR AND DELIVERY

1. It is never good to be late. (Late decelerations are bad.)

2. Absent variability (a straight line) for FHR is critical.

3. Never place laboring client flat on her back (supine hypotension/vena cava syndrome).

4. Unexplained pain in a labor and delivery client is not good (preterm labor, abruptio placenta, amniotic fluid embolism, uterine rupture).

5. Never provide fundal pressure with shoulder dystocia (suprapubic pressure okay, also assist with McRoberts maneuver).

6. OB client with tachycardia: Think hemorrhage first.

7. Medications for postpartum hemorrhage include: oxytocin (Pitocin), methylergonovine (Methergine), and carboprost tromethamine (Hemabate).

8. Quick onset of epigastric pain is often the aura to seizure activity (implement safety precautions).

9. Oxygen administration should be via nonrebreather face mask.

10. Nonpharmacologic measures should be used in combination with pharmacologic interventions.

Complications During Labor and Delivery

A. **Preterm Labor:** Uterine contractions with cervical changes that occur between 20 and 37 weeks of gestation

  1. Contributing Factors

    a. Demographic factors

      1) Age less than 15 and greater than 35

      2) Low socioeconomic status

    b. Biophysical factors

      1) Previous preterm labor or birth

      2) Multifetal pregnancy

      3) Hydramnios

      4) Recurrent infection

    c. Behavioral factors

      1) Lack of prenatal care

      2) Poor nutrition

      3) Substance abuse

      4) Excessive exercise, physical or emotional stress

B. **Fetal Distress**

  1. FHR baseline below 110 or above 160/min

  2. Absent FHR variability

  3. Fetal blood pH less than 7.2

  4. Contributing Factors

    a. Uteroplacental insufficiency

      1) Acute uteroplacental insufficiency

        a) Excessive uterine activity associated with use of oxytocin (Pitocin)

        b) Maternal hypotension: epidural, vena caval compression, supine position, hemorrhage

        c) Placental separation: abruptio, placenta previa

      2) Chronic uteroplacental insufficiency

        a) Gestational hypertension

        b) Chronic hypertension

        c) Smoking or illicit drug use

        d) Diabetes mellitus

        e) Postmaturity

  5. **Nursing Interventions**

    a. Oxytocin must be discontinued.

    b. Administer oxygen at 8 to 10 L/min by nonrebreather face mask.

    c. Turn onto left side.

    d. Increase IV fluids.

    e. Notify the provider.

    f. Perform fetal scalp stimulation or vibroacoustic stimulation per protocol.

C. **Umbilical Cord Problems**

1. Contributing Factors

   a. Cord compression: pressure on the umbilical cord during pregnancy, labor, or delivery that reduces blood flow from the placenta to the fetus

      1) Causes: abnormal presentation, inadequate pelvis, presenting part at high station, multiple gestations, prematurity, premature rupture of membranes, and/or polyhydramnios

      2) Complications: fetal asphyxia

   b. Nuchal cord (cord around neck)

   c. Prolapsed cord

2. **Nursing Interventions**

   a. Prolapsed cord

      1) Call for assistance immediately.

      2) Notify provider.

      3) The provider or RN will use sterile-gloved hand, insert two fingers into the vagina, and apply finger pressure on either side of the cord to the fetal presenting part to elevate it off of the cord.

      4) Reposition in a knee-chest or Trendelenburg position.

      5) Administer oxygen at 8 to 10 L/min by nonrebreather face mask.

      6) If cord is protruding from the vagina, wrap it loosely in a sterile saline-soaked towel.

      7) Closely monitor FHR for variable decelerations and bradycardia.

      8) Prepare for immediate birth: vaginal or cesarean.

   b. Cord compression

      1) Position change is priority.

      2) Administer oxygen at 8 to 10 L/min by nonrebreather face mask.

      3) Prepare to assist with amnioinfusion.

D. **Emergency Childbirth**

1. Contributing Factors

   a. Precipitous delivery

2. **Nursing Interventions**

   a. Encourage mother to pant, unless the fetus is in breech presentation.

   b. Support the perineum.

   c. Rupture the membranes if they have not yet ruptured.

   d. Feel for the cord around the neonate's neck, and gently slip it over his head.

   e. Keep the neonate dry and warm.

   f. Do not cut the cord.

   g. Deliver the placenta. Expect a gush of blood and a lengthening of the cord.

   h. Save the placenta.

   i. Massage fundus. Encourage breastfeeding to contract uterus.

E. **Dystocia: Dysfunctional, Abnormal labor**

1. Contributing Factors

   a. Dysfunction of uterine contractions

   b. Abnormal position

   c. Cephalopelvic disproportion

   d. Maternal exhaustion

   e. Macrosomia

2. **Nursing Interventions**

   a. Monitor fetus and status of labor.

   b. Encourage to void and ambulate regularly.

   c. Assist in positioning and coaching during contractions.

   d. Prepare for a possible forceps, vacuum-assisted, or cesarean birth.

   e. Shoulder dystocia: McRoberts maneuver and suprapubic pressure (not fundal pressure).

SECTION 6

Postpartum

I Postpartum/Puerperium

A. **Approximate duration:** 6 weeks

B. **Main goal:** prevent postpartum hemorrhage

C. **Greatest risks:** hemorrhage, shock, and infection

D. **Includes:** physiological and psychological adjustments

E. **Changes after delivery of the placenta:** hormones (estrogen, progesterone, and placental enzyme insulinase [hPL]) decrease causing decreased blood glucose (hPL), diaphoresis and diuresis (estrogen). Oxytocin increases (contractions, breast milk and involution).

F. **Physical Assessment**

1. Vital signs, Hgb, Hct, CBC, estimated blood loss in delivery

2. Pain

   a. Monitor location, intensity of pain.

   b. Examine location of pain.

   c. Implement nonpharmaceutical measures.

   d. Implement pharmaceutical measures.

      1) Consider safety of medications related to breastfeeding.

         a) Hydrocodone/acetaminophen (Vicodin)

         b) Ibuprofen (Motrin, Advil)

         c) Acetaminophen/codeine (Tylenol #3)

         d) PCA such as morphine sulfate

3. Breasts

a. Colostrum

   1) Transitions to milk 48 to 96 hr

   2) High nutrition

b. Milk production occurs about day 2 or 3

   1) Sucking stimulates uterine contractions, promotes uterine involution and increased milk production.

   2) Supplementing with formula can decrease production.

   3) Breast milk actively supports the immune system. It protects against many bacterial, viral, and protozoal infections. IgA is major immunoglobulin in human milk that provides passive immunity.

c. Engorgement

   1) About 48 hr postpartum

   2) Can cause slight rise in temperature

   3) Nonlactating clients

      a) Avoid nipple stimulation

      b) Cold compress

      c) Pain medication

      d) Supportive bra

   4) Lactating clients

      a) Manually express some milk to facilitate latch

      b) Frequent feeding or pumping

      c) Warm shower

      d) Breast massage

      e) Supportive bra

      f) Maternal medications immediately after to minimize cross-over to breast milk

NOTE: For engorgement, breastfeed every 2 to 3 hr. Encourage a warm shower immediately prior to breastfeeding. Immediately after and between feedings, apply cold compresses or ice-cold green cabbage leaves to breasts.

NOTE: Know the differences between mastitis and engorgement.

4. Uterus

a. Involution

   1) Firm

   2) Fundus near umbilicus after delivery

   3) Descends approximately 1 cm/day

   4) Breastfeeding enhances

   5) Full bladder impedes involution

b. Subinvolution

   1) Massage

   2) Frequent voiding

   3) Oxytocin

c. Lochia: Note color, amount (scant to moderate), presence of clots and odor (fleshy).

   1) Color

      a) Rubra—bright red, can contain small clots, transient flow increases during breastfeeding and upon rising. Lasts 1 to 3 days.

      b) Serosa—brownish red or pink. Lasts from day 4 to day 10.

      c) Alba—yellowish, white creamy color. Lasts from day 11 up to and beyond 6 weeks postpartum.

d. Teach about return of menses.

   1) Ovulation can occur prior to first menses.

   2) Nonlactating client: 6 to 8 weeks.

   3) Breastfeeding exclusively: can be up to 6 months.

   4) Need for birth control.

5. Perineum

a. Evaluate perineum using **REEDA**:

   1) **R** – Redness

   2) **E** – Edema

   3) **E** – Ecchymosis

   4) **D** – Drainage

   5) **A** – Approximation

b. Comfort and healing

   1) Cold compress first 24 hr

   2) Sitz bath

   3) Positioning

   4) Perineal hygiene

   5) Kegel exercises

   6) Medication

NOTE: Saturation of one perineal pad in 15 min or less, numerous large clots, or pooling of blood under the buttocks are indicators of excessive blood loss.

6. Bladder

a. Potential problem due to effects of anesthesia and hormones.

   1) Distended bladder increases potential for uterine atony and bleeding. Fundus will deviate to the side and above umbilicus.

   2) Assist with frequent urination.

   3) Provide noninvasive measures to promote urination.

   4) Perform bladder scan.

   5) Catheterize if retention persists.

7. Bowel

a. Bowel movement in 1 to 2 days.

b. Observe for hemorrhoids.

   1) Promote fiber, activity, fluids.

   2) Administer stool softener.

   3) Provide sitz bath.

   4) Apply topical anesthetic.

8. Edema and DTRs
   a. Monitor for pitting edema.
   b. Excessive use of oxytocin increases risk for edema.
   c. 2+ DTRs normal.
9. Deep-vein thrombosis
   a. Prevention is key: early ambulation.
   b. Monitor for pain, redness, or swelling of lower extremities.
10. Infection
    a. Temperature normally elevated to 38° C (100.4° F) first 24 hr after delivery.
    b. WBCs may be elevated to 20,000 to 25,000/mm^3 the first 10 to 14 days.
    c. Do not assume "normal."
    d. Collaborate with health care team to consider possible sources of infection.

G. **Psychologic Adaptations**
   1. Support systems
   2. Self-concept
   3. Bonding
      a. Initial contact within 30 to 60 min after birth
      b. Client exploration of infant
         1) Fingertips, then palms
         2) Extremities, then trunk
         3) En face
      c. Collaborative Care
         1) Minimize pain, fatigue, hunger to enhance bonding.
         2) Describe newborn behaviors.
   4. Maternal Role Adaptation

PHASES OF MATERNAL ADJUSTMENT

	CHARACTERISTICS	COLLABORATIVE CARE
Taking in	24 to 48 hr after birth: dependent, passive; focuses on own needs; excited, talkative	Assist with care. Provide comfort, nutrition, and hygiene. Listen; review labor and delivery.
Taking hold	Second to tenth day postpartum, or up to several weeks: focuses on maternal role and care of newborn; eager to learn; may develop blues	Provide teaching, written material, follow-up appointments, community resources. Monitor emotional status; discuss blues.
Letting go	Focuses on family and individual roles	Monitor progress. Discuss community resources.

5. Postpartum blues and depression

POSTPARTUM BLUES AND DEPRESSION

	POSTPARTUM BLUES	POSTPARTUM DEPRESSION
Contributing Factors	Fatigue, hormonal changes, role change, family tension, finances	History of depression*; poverty; unwanted pregnancy; lack support systems; newborn health problems
Occurrence	50% to 60% of postpartum clients	10% to 15% of postpartum clients
Onset	1 to 10 days postpartum	Up to 1 year or more after delivery; may persist for years
Signs/ Symptoms	Emotionally labile	Persistent depression; overwhelmed; anxious; hopeless; unable to care for self and/or infant; thoughts of suicide
Collaborative Care	Teaching; need for sleep, exercise, adequate nutrition; seek support and assistance with newborn care; community resources.	Use depression screening tools, teaching. Recognize signs and symptoms. Seek assistance. Needs rapid intervention.

*Note: Medications used to treat depression, such as SSRIs, are frequently Category C or D drugs and may be discontinued during pregnancy. A nurse ensures that the medications are resumed as needed after delivery.

H. **Provide focused assessment: BUBBLE HERV**
   1. **B** – Breasts
   2. **U** – Uterus (fundal height, uterine placement, and consistency)
   3. **B** – Bowel and GI function
   4. **B** – Bladder function
   5. **L** – Lochia (color, odor, consistency, and amount [COCA])
   6. **E** – Episiotomy (redness, edema, ecchymosis, drainage, approximation [REEDA])
   7. **H** – Hemorrhoids
   8. **E** – Emotions
   9. **R** – Rubella (prevent pregnancy at least one month after receiving), Rhogam
   10. **V** – Vaccines (influenza, pneumonia, Tdap [needed only once as adult, to prevent pertussis, not given if received tetanus-diphtheria vaccine within 2 years])

Complications During Postpartum

A. **Hemorrhage:** Blood loss of greater than 500 mL with vaginal delivery or greater than 1,000 mL with cesarean birth

1. Contributing Factors

   a. Uterine atony

   b. Lacerations and hematomas.

   c. Complications during pregnancy (e.g., placenta previa, abruptio placenta)

   d. Complications during labor (e.g., prolonged labor, rapid labor, administration of magnesium sulfate, use of forceps, retained placenta)

   e. Overdistended uterus (e.g., macrosomia, multiple fetuses)

   f. Coagulopathies (DIC)

2. Manifestations

   a. Saturation of one pad or more in 15 min

   b. Large clots (uterine atony) or spurting of bright red blood (cervical or vaginal laceration)

   c. Formation of hematomas

   d. Boggy uterus (uterine atony)

   e. Persistent lochia rubra beyond day 3 (retained placental fragments)

   f. Change in level of consciousness

   g. Manifestations of shock

3. **Nursing Interventions**

   a. Collaborate with health care team to determine source of bleeding.

      1) Fundus (massage if boggy)

      2) Perineum (laceration, episiotomy site, or hematomas: notify provider)

   b. Monitor vital signs and oxygen saturation.

   c. Monitor bladder.

   d. Maintain or initiate isotonic IV fluids.

   e. Medications to treat hemorrhage

      1) Oxytocin

      2) Methergine, Cytotec, Hemabate

B. **Rh Incompatibility**

RHOGAM

MOTHER	BABY	MATERNAL COOMBS	RHOGAM GIVEN?
Rh⁺	Rh⁺	Not checked	No
Rh⁺	Rh⁻	Not checked	No
Rh⁻	Rh⁺	Negative	Yes
Rh⁻	Rh⁺	Positive	No
Rh⁻	Rh⁻	Not checked	No

1. **Nursing Interventions**

   a. Observe newborn for hyperbilirubinemia.

   b. Reinforce teaching with mother about Rh, Rhogam.

      1) Prevents, does not reverse, formation of antibodies

      2) Given prenatally with any invasive procedure, at 28 weeks, and after delivery

      3) Given IM within 72 hr after delivery

C. **Thromboembolic Disorder**

1. Contributing Factors

   a. Increased clotting factors postpartum

   b. Immobility

   c. Pelvic pressure during labor/delivery

   d. History of thrombosis, varicosities, heart disease

2. Manifestations

   a. Pain, heat, redness, swelling in lower leg or extremity

3. **Nursing Interventions**

   a. Monitor extremities including peripheral pulses, measuring and comparing circumferences of both legs.

   b. Homan's sign is not recommended.

   c. Venous Doppler to rule out DVTs. If DVT is suspected:

      1) Bed rest

      2) Elevation of affected extremity

      3) Anti-thrombolytic stocking to unaffected leg

      4) Anticoagulant

D. **Puerperal Infections** (Endometritis, Mastitis, and Wound Infections)

1. Elevated temperature of at least 38° C (100.4° F) for 2 or more consecutive days excluding the first 24 hr.

2. Endometritis usually begins on the second to 5th day postpartum.

   a. More common after cesarean birth

   b. Pelvic pain, uterine tenderness, foul smelling or profuse lochia plus; fever, tachycardia, elevated WBC and RBC sedimentation rate.

3. Mastitis usually unilateral occurring 2 to 4 weeks after delivery.

   a. Symptoms include chills, fever, malaise, and local breast tenderness and erythema.

POSTPARTUM NURSING CARE WORKSHEET

Prioritize which of the following patients the nurse should see first. Each of the following clients had a vaginal delivery 8 hr ago.

A. A client who has not voided

B. A client who refuses to ambulate

C. A client who requires Rhogam injection before discharge.

D. A client who had an estimated blood loss of 250 mL during delivery

Answer: The nurse should first see the client who has not voided since delivery. A full bladder will impede involution, which could lead to life-threatening hemorrhage. The nurse should determine fullness of the bladder, tone and location of the fundus, and color and amount of lochia. Interventions to promote elimination will be needed based on data collected. Rhogam may be given up to 72 hr after delivery and should be administered by the RN. A client who refuses to ambulate can be exhibiting signs of "taking in," fatigue, or pain. The nurse should encourage early ambulation to prevent potential complications (thrombus, respiratory compromise, constipation, urinary stasis). The average estimated blood loss during a vaginal delivery is 500 mL. The nurse should provide planned care and promote early ambulation.

Newborn

Neonatal Period: From Birth Through 28 Days

A. **Initial Care: Immediately after birth**

1. Airway, breathing, circulation (ABCs)
2. Thermoregulation
3. Umbilical cord
   a. Inspect for two arteries and one vein. Observe for any bleeding from the cord, and ensure that the cord is clamped securely to prevent hemorrhage.
4. Apgar
   a. Determine

APGAR: FIVE CATEGORIES

	0	1	2
Heart rate	Absent	Slow less than 100	Greater than 100
Respiratory effort	Absent	Slow weak cry	Good cry
Muscle tone	Flaccid	Some flexion of extremities	Well flexed extremities
Reflex irritability	No response	Grimace	Cry
Color	Blue, pale	Centrally pink with blue extremities	Completely pink

   b. Ratings
      1) 7 to 10 is within normal limits
      2) 4 to 6 is moderately distressed
      3) 0 to 3 is severely distressed
5. Vital signs

VITAL SIGN ASSESSMENTS

Heart Rate

NORMAL FINDINGS	100 to 160/min
NORMAL VARIATIONS	100/min when sleeping 180/min when crying
DEVIATIONS FROM NORMAL	Persistent tachycardia 160/min or greater Persistent bradycardia 100/min or lower
NURSING INTERVENTIONS	Monitor all pulses bilaterally; they should be equal and strong. Monitor apical pulse for 1 min. Auscultate for murmurs.

Respirations

NORMAL FINDINGS	40 to 60/min
DEVIATIONS FROM NORMAL	Bradypnea: less than 25/min Tachypnea: greater than 60/min
NURSING INTERVENTIONS	Monitor rate, rhythm, and adventitious breath sounds. Respirations will often be shallow and irregular in the newborn. Note any signs of distress. Nasal flaring grunting, intercostal retractions or see-saw breathing.

VITAL SIGN ASSESSMENTS (CONTINUED)

Temperature

NORMAL FINDINGS	Axillary 37° C
NORMAL VARIATIONS	36.5 to 37.2° C (97.7 to 98.9° F) axillary
DEVIATIONS FROM NORMAL	Temperature not stabilized after 10 hr
NURSING INTERVENTIONS	Prevent heat loss: dry infant thoroughly; cover head; place on warm, dry environment; skin to skin contact with mother is encouraged.

Blood Pressure

NORMAL FINDINGS	60 to 80 systolic; 40 to 50 diastolic
NORMAL VARIATIONS	Variations occur with crying or sleeping
DEVIATIONS FROM NORMAL	**Hypotension** = potential sepsis or hypovolemic **Hypertension** in upper extremities = potential coarctation of aorta
NURSING INTERVENTIONS	Monitor all four extremities on admission to nursery then if problem suspected. Check arms and legs for significant differences between the lower and upper extremities; can be an indication of coarctation of the aorta.

> NOTE: Rectal temperatures are contraindicated.

6. Safety
   a. Footprints and identification bands are applied in presence of parents and before infant leaves delivery room. Security system explained and initiated.

B. **Ongoing Newborn Care: Admission to Discharge**
1. Physical Assessment

PHYSICAL ASSESSMENT

	FINDINGS
Posture	General flexion Spontaneous movement
Head	Circumference 2 to 3 cm greater than chest circumference Fontanels › Posterior: Triangle shape, closes at 8 to 12 weeks › Anterior: Diamond shape, closes at 18 months, pulse visible › Observe for bulge or depression Shape › Molding › Caput succedaneum › Cephalhematoma
Eyes	Vision best within 12 inches Strabismus; pseudo strabismus Subconjunctival hemorrhage Congenital cataracts
Ears	Responds to voice and other sounds Check for low-set ears
Nose	Patent nares Preferential nose breather

PHYSICAL ASSESSMENT (CONTINUED)

	FINDINGS
Skin	Pink Acrocyanosis Erythema Jaundice Hyperpigmentations Milia Café au lait spots; giraffe spots Nevus flammeus (port wine stains) Telangiectasia nevi (stork bites) Vernix Lanugo
Mouth	Symmetry of lip movement Soft/hard palate intact Epstein pearls
Chest	Symmetrical chest movement Nipples prominent, well formed Nipple buds are sign of maturity
Abdomen	Umbilical cord Liver can be palpable
Musculoskeletal	Evaluate joints for full range of motion Note presence of asymmetrical gluteal folds Spine straight and easily flexed Clavicles intact
Genitalia	Female: prominent labia, pseudomenstruation Male: scrotum large, palpable testes on each side, meatus at tip of penis, foreskin
GI/GU	Voiding within 24 hr. Void 6 to 10 times a day after 4 days of life. Meconium passed 24 to 48 hr after birth Breastfed babies have more frequent stools that appear yellow and seedy.

REFLEXES

	EXPECTED FINDING	EXPECTED AGE
Sucking and rooting	Elicited by stroking the newborn's cheek or edge of his mouth. Normal response: newborn turns head toward the side that is touched and starts to suck.	Birth to 4 months
Palmar grasp	Elicited by placing an object in the newborn's palm. Normal response: Newborn grasps the object.	Present at birth and until 3 to 6 months
Plantar grasp	Elicited by touching the sole of the newborn's foot. Normal response: Newborn curls toes downward.	Birth to 8 months
Moro reflex (startle)	Elicited by striking a flat surface that the newborn is lying on, or allowing the head and trunk of the newborn in a semisitting position to fall backward to an angle of at least 30°. Normal response: Newborn's arms and legs extend and abduct symmetrically; fingers form a "C."	Birth to 4 months

REFLEXES (CONTINUED)

	EXPECTED FINDING	EXPECTED AGE
Tonic neck reflex (fencer position)	The newborn will extend the arm and leg on the side when the head is turned to that side with flexion of the arm and leg of the opposite side.	Birth to 3 to 4 months
Babinski	Elicited by stroking outer edge of sole of foot toward toes. Normal response: Toes fan upward and out.	Birth to 1 year

2. Reactivity

   a. Observe for periods of reactivity in the newborn.

     1) **First period of reactivity**: The newborn is alert and exhibits exploring activity, makes sucking sounds, and has a rapid heartbeat and respiratory rate, lasts 15 to 30 min after birth.

     2) **Period of relative inactivity**: Sleep. Heart rate and respirations decrease, lasts from 30 min to 2 hr after birth.

     3) **Second period of reactivity**: Reawakens, often gags and chokes on mucus that has accumulated in his mouth. This period usually occurs 2 to 8 hr after birth and can last 10 min to several hours.

C. **Gestational Age Assessment: New Ballard Score**

  1. Provides maturity rating. Performed within 48 hr after birth.

  2. Components of Gestational Age Assessment

   a. Physical Components

     1) Skin

     2) Lanugo

     3) Plantar surfaces

     4) Breast

     5) Eye/ear

     6) Genitals

   b. Neuromuscular

     1) Posture

     2) Square window

     3) Arm recoil

     4) Popliteal angle

     5) Scarf sign

     6) Heel to ear

  3. Medications

   a. Eye prophylaxis

     1) Erythromycin or tetracycline administered within 1 hr after birth.

   b. Vitamin K (Aqua-Mephyton) IM administered within 1 hr of birth.

   c. Hepatitis vaccine administered within 12 hr of birth

4. Diagnostic and Therapeutic Procedures
   a. Cord blood: ABO blood type and Rh-status if the mother's blood type is "O" or she is Rh-negative.
   b. CBC (anemia, polycythemia, infection, or clotting problems)
   c. Glucose level
   d. Serum bilirubin
   e. Newborn metabolic screen
   f. PKU
   g. Newborn hearing screen
   h. Pulse oximetry

5. Collaborative Care

   a. **Nursing Interventions**
      1) Monitor for manifestations of respiratory distress.
      2) Promote patent airway.
         a) Perform oral and nasal suction only if needed.

NOTE: When using bulb syringe, remember M before N.

NOTE: Newborns delivered by cesarean birth are more susceptible to fluid remaining in the lungs than newborns who were delivered vaginally.

      3) Promote thermoregulation.
         a) Maintain body temperature of 36.5°C (97.7°F) axillary.
         b) Prevent heat loss.
      4) Monitor glucose levels.

NOTE: Identify potential risks and prevent heat loss by evaporation, conduction, convection, and radiant.

   b. Monitor nutrition.
      1) Initiate feedings immediately after birth (breast or formula).
         a) Maintain a fluid intake of 100 to 140 mL/kg/24 hr.
         b) Monitor for normal weight gain (both breast milk and formula provide 20 kcal/oz).
   c. **Nursing Interventions** to promote successful breastfeeding
      1) Explain breastfeeding techniques to the mother. Have the mother wash her hands, get comfortable, and have fluids to drink during breastfeeding.
      2) Offer the newborn the breast immediately after birth and feed every 2 to 3 hr.
      3) Explain the let-down reflex (stimulation of maternal nipple releases oxytocin that causes the letdown of milk).
      4) Reassure the mother that uterine cramps are normal during breastfeeding, resulting from oxytocin.
      5) Express a few drops of colostrum or milk and spread it over the nipple to lubricate the nipple and entice the newborn.
      6) Show the mother the proper latch-on position.

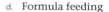

   d. Formula feeding
      1) Feed every 3 to 4 hr.
      2) **Nursing Interventions** to promote successful formula feeding
         a) Always hold the bottle and never prop it.
         b) Avoid supine position during feeding (danger of aspiration).
         c) Hold newborn close and at 45° angle during feeding.
         d) Teach how to prepare formula, bottles, and nipples.
         e) Check the flow of formula from the bottle to ensure it is not coming out too slowly or quickly.
         f) Place the nipple on top of the newborn's tongue.
         g) Keep the nipple filled with formula to prevent the newborn from swallowing air.
         h) Burp several times during a feeding, usually after each ½ to 1 oz of formula.
         i) Discard unused formula and after opened for 1 hr. Increased possibility of bacterial contamination.
         j) Discard any unused formula when the newborn is finished feeding due to the possibility of bacterial contamination.
   e. Monitor elimination.
      1) Document number of voidings and stools.
      2) Keep the perineal area clean and dry. Should have first void and stool within 24 hr.
   f. Provide skin care.
      1) Cord care: Cleanse with neutral pH cleanser and sterile water. The cord should be kept clean and dry to prevent infection.

NOTE: Cleansing of the umbilical cord with a neutral pH cleanser and sterile water is the most current EBP according to AWHONN.

      2) First bath after temperature stabilizes

NOTE: When handling the newborn, gloves should be worn by providers until after the first bath.

   g. Promote bonding.
      1) Encourage mothers and family to hold the newborn.
   h. Promote safety and security for the newborn and family
      1) Verify that identification bands are correctly placed according to facility protocol.
      2) Identity verification protocol should be followed each time the newborn is taken to the parent.
      3) All facility staff who assist in caring for the newborn are required to wear identification badges.

i. Provide circumcision care.

   1) Before procedure, check for family history of bleeding tendencies; hypospadias or epispadias; ambiguous genitalia; illness or infection.

   2) Obtain informed consent.

   3) Monitor for complications: bleeding or swelling with urine retention.

   4) Reinforce teaching with parents to:

      a) Change diaper at least every 4 hr.

      b) Clean penis with warm water.

      c) With clamp procedures, apply petroleum jelly with each diaper change for at least 24 hr.

      d) Expect a yellowish mucus over the glans by day 2 and do not wash it off.

      e) Avoid premoistened towelettes (contain alcohol) to clean the penis, which heals within 2 weeks.

6. Client Education

   a. Safety

      1) Position on back to sleep

      2) Thermoregulation

      3) Nutrition and weight gain (healthy newborn needs 100 to 140 mL/kg/24 hr, no water supplement; loss of 5% to 10% immediately after birth normal: regain in 10 to 14 days)

      4) Elimination (voiding 6 to 8 diapers a day)

      5) Avoid submerging in water until cord falls off—around 10 to 14 days after birth

      6) CPR

      7) Newborn behaviors

      8) Car seat regulations

      9) Oral and nasal suctioning

      10) Sudden infant death syndrome (no exposure to secondhand smoke)

      11) Signs of illness to report

      12) Newborn follow-up care and immunization schedule

      13) Crib safety: Space between mattress and sides of crib should be less than 2 fingerbreadths; slats on crib should be no more than 2.5 inches apart.

Q&A

1. Discuss topics for teaching about bathing a newborn that should be reinforced prior to discharge.

2. Identify priority nursing interventions postcircumcision.

Answer Key: 1. Should be performed before feeding. Use mild soap without hexachlorophene. No lotions, oils, or powders No tub bath until cord falls off and is healed. 2. Observe the newborn for bleeding. Check site every 15 min for 1 hr and then every hour for at least 12 hr. Also check for voiding and swelling.

Complications of the Newborn

It is essential for a nurse to immediately identify and report complications.

A. **Maternal Substance Abuse**

   1. General Information

      a. Intrauterine alcohol and drug exposure can cause anomalies, neurobehavioral changes, and signs of withdrawal in the neonate.

      b. Response is dependent on specific drug, dosage, metabolism, and excretion by the mother and fetus, timing of exposure, and length of exposure.

   2. Fetal alcohol syndrome (FAS)

      a. Contributing Factors

         1) Amount and duration of consumption (chronic or periodic intake)

         2) Daily intake increases the risk of FAS

      b. Manifestations—will have signs in three categories

         1) Growth restriction

         2) CNS alterations such as intelligence deficit, attention deficit disorder, diminished fine motor skills, poor speech

         3) Craniofacial features such as microcephaly, small eyes or short palpebral fissures, thin upper lip, flat midface.

         4) Other signs

            a) Feeding problems

            b) Increased wakefulness

            c) Hearing loss

   3. Tobacco use during pregnancy

      a. Manifestations

         1) Prematurity, low birth weight

         2) Increased risk for sudden infant death syndrome

         3) Increased risk for bronchitis, pneumonia

         4) Developmental delays

   4. Drug and Alcohol Withdrawal Syndrome in the Newborn

      a. Objective data: Use a neonatal abstinence scoring system.

         1) CNS

            a) Increased wakefulness

            b) High-pitched, shrill cry, incessant crying

            c) Irritability, tremors

            d) Hyperactive with an increased Moro reflex. Heroin withdrawal will see decreased Moro reflexes, and hypothermia or hyperthermia.

            e) Increased deep-tendon reflexes, increased muscle tone

            f) Seizures

         2) Skin

            a) Abrasions and/or excoriations on the face and knees

3) Metabolic, vasomotor, and respiratory findings
   a) Nasal congestion with flaring
   b) Frequent yawning, skin mottling
   c) Tachypnea greater than 60/min
   d) Sweating and a temperature greater than 37.2°C (99°F)
4) Gastrointestinal
   a) Poor feeding, regurgitation (projectile vomiting)
   b) Diarrhea, and excessive, uncoordinated, and constant sucking
5) Vital organ anomalies
   a) Heart defects, including atrial and ventricular septal defects, tetralogy of Fallot, and patent ductus arteriosus

b. Medications
   1) Phenobarbital (Solfoton): anticonvulsant
      a) It is prescribed to decrease CNS irritability and control seizures for neonates who have alcohol or opioid addiction.

c. Diagnostic Procedures
   1) Laboratory tests: Blood tests should be done to differentiate between neonatal drug withdrawal and central nervous system irritability.
      a) CBC
      b) Blood glucose
      c) Calcium and magnesium
      d) TSH, T_4, T_3
      e) Drug screen of urine or meconium to reveal the agent abused
      f) Hair analysis
   2) Diagnostic Procedures
      a) Chest x-ray to rule out congenital heart defects

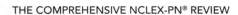

d. Collaborative Care
   1) **Nursing Interventions** will include normal newborn care plus the following.
      a) Perform a neonatal abstinence scoring system assessment.
      b) Monitor newborn reflexes.
      c) Monitor ability to feed and digest intake.
      d) Monitor fluid and electrolytes, skin turgor, fontanelles, and I&O.
      e) Observe behavior including crying, sleep patterns, and tremors.
      f) Maintain IV.
      g) Reduce external stimuli: swaddle, do not place next to nurses' desk.
      h) Small, frequent feedings with high-calorie formula—can need gavage feedings.
      i) If sucking is a problem, use preterm nipples and nipples with larger holes.
      j) Have suction immediately available (risk for aspiration).
      k) For newborns who are addicted to cocaine, avoid eye contact and use vertical rocking and a pacifier.
      l) Initiate a consult with child protective services.
      m) Consult lactation services to evaluate if breastfeeding is desired and not contraindicated.

B. **Hypoglycemia:** A serum glucose level of less than 40 mg/dL.
1. Contributing Factors
   a. Maternal diabetes mellitus
   b. Preterm infant
   c. LGA or SGA
   d. Stress at birth, such as cold stress and asphyxia
2. Manifestations
   a. Objective data: physical assessment findings
      1) Poor feeding
      2) Jitteriness/tremors
      3) Hypothermia
      4) Diaphoresis
      5) Weak cry
      6) Lethargy
      7) Flaccid muscle tone
      8) Seizures/coma
3. Diagnostic Laboratory Tests and Procedures
   a. Two consecutive plasma glucose levels less than 40 mg/dL in a newborn who is term, and less than 25 mg/dL in a newborn who is preterm
4. Collaborative Care
   a. **Nursing Interventions**
      1) Perform heel stick for blood glucose within 2 hr of birth.
      2) Provide frequent oral and/or gavage feedings.
      3) Monitor the neonate's blood glucose level closely per facility protocol.
      4) Monitor IV if the neonate is unable to orally feed.

C. **Respiratory Distress Syndrome (RDS)**
1. RDS occurs as a result of surfactant deficiency in the lungs and is characterized by poor gas exchange and ventilatory failure.
2. Surfactant is a phospholipid that assists in alveoli expansion.
3. Surfactant keeps alveoli from collapsing and allows gas exchange to occur.
4. Contributing Factors
   a. Preterm gestation
   b. Perinatal asphyxia (meconium staining, cord prolapse, and nuchal cord)
   c. Stress/asphyxia during labor (maternal hypotension, UPI)
5. Manifestations: Physical Assessment
   a. Objective data
      1) Tachypnea (respiratory rate greater than 60/min)
      2) Nasal flaring
      3) Expiratory grunting
      4) Intercostal and substernal retractions
      5) Labored breathing
      6) Fine rales on auscultation
      7) Cyanosis
      8) Unresponsiveness, flaccidity, and apnea with decreased breath sounds (manifestations of worsened RDS)

6. Diagnostic Procedures and Laboratory Tests

   a. Culture and sensitivity of the blood, urine, and cerebrospinal fluid (rule out sepsis)

   b. Blood glucose and serum calcium

   c. ABGs reveal hypercapnia (excess of carbon dioxide in the blood) and respiratory or mixed acidosis.

   d. Chest x-ray

7. Nursing Interventions

   a. Infant will receive lung surfactant—beractant (Survanta).

   b. Avoid suctioning ET tube for 1 hr after administration of medication.

D. **Preterm Newborn:** Birth occurs after 20 weeks of gestation and before 38 weeks gestation.

1. Contributing Factors

   a. Maternal gestational hypertension

   b. Multiple pregnancies

   c. Adolescent pregnancy

   d. Lack of prenatal care

   e. Substance abuse

   f. Smoking

   g. Previous history of preterm delivery

   h. Abnormalities of the uterus or cervix

   i. Premature rupture of the membranes

2. Manifestations: Physical Assessment

   a. Objective data

      1) New Ballard assessment shows a physical and neurological assessment totaling less than 37 weeks of gestation.

      2) Episodes of apnea (pause in respirations longer than 15 seconds)

      3) Signs of increased respiratory effort and/or respiratory distress.

      4) Physical characteristics: Typically has low birth weight, minimal subcutaneous fat, head large in comparison to body, wrinkled features, weak grasp reflex, before 34 weeks has inability to coordinate suck and swallow, and weak or absent gag, suck, and cough reflex.

3. **Nursing Interventions**

   a. Perform rapid initial assessment.

   b. Transfer to high-risk nursery.

   c. Maintain thermoregulation.

   d. Administer respiratory support.

   e. Administer parenteral or enteral nutrition and fluids (less than 34 weeks).

   f. Provide nonnutritive sucking.

   g. Minimize stimulation (cluster care, smooth and light touch, dim lighting, and noise reduction).

E. **Post-Term Infant**

1. Contributing Factors

   a. Gestational age more than 42 weeks

2. Manifestations: Physical Assessment

   a. Dry, parchment-like skin

   b. Longer, harder nails

   c. Profuse scalp hair

   d. Absent vernix

   e. Hypoglycemia

3. Complications

   a. Progressive aging of placenta

   b. Difficult delivery

   c. High perinatal mortality

   d. Jaundice (hyperbilirubinemia)

4. Nursing Interventions

   a. Early and frequent heel sticks (glucose testing)

   b. Initiate early feeding

   c. Observe for birth injuries (from shoulder dystocia—fractured clavicle, brachial plexus injury, facial paralysis)

F. **Hyperbilirubinemia**

1. Physiologic Jaundice (benign)

   a. Caused by breakdown of fetal RBCs, excessive bruising, and liver immaturity.

   b. Jaundice appears after 24 hr of age.

2. Pathologic Jaundice (underlying disease; increased RBC production or breakdown)

   a. Appears before 24 hr of age or is persistent after day 7.

   b. Usually caused by blood group incompatibility (Rh or ABO incompatibility) or an infection.

   c. Kernicterus (bilirubin encephalopathy) bilirubin levels at or higher than 25 mg/dL. Can lead to anemia and brain damage.

3. Manifestations

   a. Yellowish tint to skin, sclera, and mucous membranes.

   b. Jaundice assessed best by blanching skin on the cheek or sternum.

   c. Note time of onset to distinguish between physiologic and pathologic jaundice.

   d. Determine the underlying cause by reviewing the maternal prenatal, family, and newborn history.

4. Diagnostic and Laboratory Procedures

   a. Monitor the infant's bilirubin levels every 4 hr until the level returns to normal.

   b. Check maternal and newborn blood type to determine if there is a presence of ABO-incapability. This occurs if the newborn has blood type A, B, or AB, and the mother is type O.

   c. Review Hgb and Hct.

   d. A direct Coombs' test reveals the presence of antibody-coated (sensitized) Rh-positive RBCs in the newborn.

   e. Monitor electrolyte levels for indications of dehydration during phototherapy.

   f. Transcutaneous level is a noninvasive method to measure an infant's bilirubin.

5. **Nursing Interventions**

a. Phototherapy, sunlight, and/or exchange transfusion is administered to the newborn.

b. Monitor vital signs.

c. Maintain an eye mask over the newborn's eyes for protection of corneas and retinas.

d. Keep newborn undressed. Cover male genitals to prevent possible testicular damage from heat and light waves.

e. Avoid applying lotions or ointments to the infant because they absorb heat and can cause burns.

f. Remove the newborn from phototherapy every 4 hr and unmask the newborn's eyes, checking for signs of inflammation or injury.

g. Reposition the newborn every 2 hr to expose all of the body surfaces to the phototherapy lights and prevent pressure sores. Check the lamp energy with a photometer per unit protocol.

h. Turn off the phototherapy lights before drawing blood for testing.

i. Observe the newborn for side effects of phototherapy.
   1) Bronze discoloration: not a serious complication
   2) Maculopapular skin rash: not a serious complication
   3) Development of pressure areas
   4) Dehydration (poor skin turgor, dry mucous membranes, decreased urinary output)
   5) Elevated temperature

j. Monitor elimination and daily weights, watching for signs of dehydration.

k. Monitor newborn's axillary temperature every 4 hr during phototherapy because temperature can become elevated.

l. Feed the newborn early and frequently—every 3 to 4 hr to promote bilirubin excretion in the stools.

m. Continue to breastfeed the newborn. Supplementing with formula may be prescribed.

n. Maintain adequate fluid intake to prevent dehydration.

o. Reassure the parents that most newborns experience some degree of jaundice.

p. Explain hyperbilirubinemia, its causes, diagnostic tests, and treatment to parents.

q. Explain that the newborn's stool contains some bile that will be loose and green.

r. Administer an exchange transfusion for infants who are at risk for kernicterus.

ADAPTING NURSING CARE FOR GESTATIONAL AGE WORKSHEET

1. A nurse observes the following characteristics for a newborn: weak muscle tone, ample vernix caseosa, abundant lanugo, weak suck reflex, absent swallow reflex, and undescended testicles. The gestational age is likely to be: _____ (preterm, full term, postterm).

2. Based on the gestational age, what are three priority actions the nurse should include when providing care?

Answers: 1. The newborn is likely to be preterm. Weak muscle tone and diminished reflexes might be caused by maternal medications or birth trauma. However, the presence of large amounts of vernix caseosa and lanugo, as well as undescended testicles, indicate the infant is likely to be preterm. 2. Priority nursing care for preterm newborns: Airway/respirations (Preterm infants are likely to have immature lungs.); Temperature control (Preterm infants have poorly developed thermoregulation and often lack adequate adipose tissue, including brown fat.); Nutrition (Preterm infants are fed with caution related to diminished suck/swallow/gag reflexes. Tube feeding may be required.)

SECTION 10

Women's Health

A. **Contraception:** Methods of contraception include natural family planning, barrier, hormonal, and intrauterine methods, as well as surgical procedures.

1. A nurse should evaluate a client's need/desire for contraception.

2. A thorough discussion of benefits, risks, and alternatives of each method should be discussed.

3. Nurses should support clients in making the decision that is best for their individualized situations.

4. Refer to table in Unit Four: Pharmacology in Nursing – Contraceptives.

B. **Infertility:** An inability to conceive despite engaging in unprotected sexual intercourse for a period of at least 12 months

1. Contributing Factors

   a. Structural or hormonal disorders (e.g., tubal occlusion, endometriosis, obesity)

   b. Decreased or abnormal sperm

   c. STIs (see the "Sexually Transmitted Infections" table on page 215)

   d. Exposure to radiation or toxic substances

2. Diagnostic Procedures

   a. Infertility procedures
      1) Semen collection
      2) Pelvic examination
      3) Ultrasonography
      4) Hysterosalpingography
      5) Hysteroscopy
      6) Laparoscopy

3. Collaborative Care

   a. Perform infertility assessment.

   b. **Nursing Interventions**

      1) Encourage couples to express and discuss their feelings.

      2) Monitor for side effects associated with medications to treat female and male infertility.

      3) Advise that the use of medications to treat female infertility can increase the risk of multiple births by more than 25%.

      4) Provide information regarding assisted reproductive therapies.

   c. Referrals to support groups

      1) Genetic counseling

C. **Vaginal Infections**

   1. Normal vaginal secretions are clear to cloudy, nonirritating, nonoffensive odor, with pH of 4 to 5.

   2. Most common vaginal infections: bacterial vaginosis (BV), candidiasis, and trichomoniasis.

   3. Most common causes: irritations (bath salts or bubble bath), tight-fitting clothing (especially jeans), or anything that disrupts the normal vaginal flora, such as douching, sexual activity, contamination by feces.

   4. Teach preventive measures: genital hygiene, avoid douching, use condoms, void before and after intercourse, decrease dietary sugar, drink yeast-active milk, and eat yogurt with lactobacilli.

      a. If at risk for STIs, should not use IUD or diaphragm for contraception.

   5. Bacterial vaginosis: Etiology unknown. Associated with preterm labor and birth.

      a. Manifestations

         1) Increased thin vaginal discharge and fishy odor.

      b. Collaborative Care and Nursing Interventions

         1) Administer metronidazole (Flagyl).

         2) Treatment of partner is not routinely recommended.

   6. *Vulvovaginal candidiasis*, or yeast infection: most common organism is *Candida albicans*.

      a. Contributing Factors

         1) Use of oral contraceptives, frequent use of antibiotics, and frequent douching; diabetes mellitus and immunosuppression.

         2) Ensure that both partners are treated.

      b. Manifestations

         1) Yellow, green, or gray discharge

         2) Discomfort with urination and intercourse

         3) Irritation and itching

   7. Sexually transmitted infections (see the "Sexually Transmitted Infections" table on page 215)

D. **Cancer**

   1. **Cervical Cancer:** Forms in the tissue of the cervix

      a. Contributing Factors

         1) Human papillomavirus is responsible for most cervical cancer

         2) Multiple partners with initial sex before age 18

         3) History of STIs

         4) Immunosuppression

         5) Cigarette smoking

      b. Manifestations

         1) Abnormal bleeding

         2) Pelvic pain or pain during intercourse

      c. Diagnostic Screening

         1) Annual Pap smear

         2) HPV, DNA test

      d. Collaborative Care/Treatment

         1) Conization, laser surgery, loop electrocautery excision procedure, cryosurgery, hysterectomy, radiation, and/or chemotherapy

         2) Prevention

            a) Delay initial intercourse.

            b) Avoid smoking.

            c) Practice safe sex.

            d) Gardasil (human papillomavirus quadrivalent) is a vaccine that is given as three injections over a 6-month period. Initiate as early as age 11 or up to 26 years.

   2. Endometrial Cancer: Is often detected at an early stage, as it produces early vaginal bleeding between menstrual cycles or after menopause.

      a. Contributing Factors

         1) Obesity: increases risk three-fold for women who are 21 to 50 lb overweight

         2) Nulliparity

         3) Late menopause

      b. Manifestations

         1) Postmenopausal bleeding

         2) Abnormal bleeding

      c. Diagnostic Screening

         1) There is no specific diagnostic test.

         2) At the time of menopause, all women should be informed about the risks and symptoms of endometrial cancer.

         3) Report any unusual bleeding to the provider.

      d. Collaborative Care

         1) Radium

         2) X-ray therapy

         3) Hysterectomy

e. **Nursing Interventions**
   1) Monitor for grieving.
   2) Provide preoperative teaching.
   3) Provide postoperative care.
   4) Monitor psychosexual needs.

3. Ovarian Cancer: Cancerous growth originating from different parts of the ovary.
   a. Contributing Factors
      1) Over 40 years of age
      2) Nulliparity or first pregnancy after 30 years of age
      3) Family history of ovarian, breast, or colon cancer
      4) History of dysmenorrhea or heavy bleeding
      5) Hormone replacement therapy
      6) Use of infertility medications
   b. Manifestations
      1) Early symptoms are not obvious.
      2) Later symptoms can include:
         a) Pressure or pain in the abdomen, pelvis, back, or legs.
         b) Swollen or bloated abdomen, nausea and indigestion, constipation or diarrhea, fatigue, shortness of breath, frequent urination, and/or vaginal bleeding.
   c. Diagnostic Screening
      1) CA 125 blood test: more than 35 u/mL is considered abnormal
      2) Intravaginal ultrasound
      3) Pelvic exam
   d. Collaborative Treatment
      1) Chemotherapy
      2) Radiation, surgery

4. **Breast Cancer:** Abnormal growth of breast tissue
   a. Contributing Factors
      1) Family history (first-degree relative)
      2) Early menarche (before 12 years) and late menopause (after age 51 years)
      3) Nulligravida or first pregnancy after age 30
      4) Early or prolonged use of oral contraceptives
      5) Long-term use of HRT
      6) Lifestyle: overweight, sedentary, excessive alcohol intake.
   b. Manifestations
      1) Lump in breast or axilla region
      2) Thickening, dimpling, redness, pain, or asymmetry in breasts
      3) Pulling, discharge, or pain in nipple area

   c. Diagnostic Screening
      1) Mammogram: Women 40 and older should get a mammogram every 1 to 2 years.
      2) Clinical breast exam: Women should receive this exam annually.
      3) Breast self-exam: Women should perform this monthly, 1 week after menses.
      4) BRCA1 and BRCA2 gene test (cannot be done within 3 months of a blood transfusion).
   d. Treatment
      1) Surgery (mastectomy) postoperative care
         a) Head of the bed elevated 30° when awake and arm supported on pillow.
         b) Position on unaffected side.
         c) Sling on affected side while ambulating.
         d) No injections, blood pressures or blood draws from affected side. Place sign above bed regarding these precautions.
         e) Monitor incision and drainage tubes. (Drains are usually left in for 1 to 3 weeks.)
      2) Chemotherapy (combination therapy)
         a) Cyclophosphamide, doxorubicin, fluorouracil
      3) Radiation
      4) Hormone therapy
         a) Gonadotropin-releasing hormone (GnRH): leuprolide (Lupron)
         b) Selective estrogen receptor modulators (SERMs): tamoxifen (Nolvadex) and raloxifene (Evista).
            (1) SERMs are used in women who are at high risk for breast cancer or who have advanced breast cancer.
            (2) Tamoxifen increases risk of endometrial cancer, DVT, and pulmonary embolism. Raloxifene does not have these side effects.
   e. Preventative Teaching
      1) Encourage screenings.
      2) Diet should include five servings of fruits and vegetables daily.
      3) Maintain healthy weight, and exercise regularly.
      4) Limit alcohol intake and avoid or cease smoking.

E. **Uterine Disorders**
   1. **Myomas (uterine fibroids):** Benign fibroid tumors of the uterine muscle
      a. Contributing Factors
         1) African Americans older than age 30 who have never been pregnant
      b. Manifestations
         1) Pelvic pain or pressure
         2) Hypermenorrhea
      c. Collaborative Treatment
         1) Medication
         2) Surgery

2. **Endometriosis:** Endometrial tissue located outside of the uterus

   a. Contributing Factors

     1) Can involve retrograde menstruation

     2) Hereditary factors

     3) Impaired immune function

   b. Manifestations

     1) Severe dysmenorrhea

     2) Lower abdominal pain, pain during intercourse, back and rectal pain

     3) Abnormal bleeding

   c. Collaborative Treatment

     1) Oral contraceptives (hormone therapy), surgery, or pregnancy

F. **Menopause:** Complete cessation of menstruation for 1 year

  1. Manifestations

   a. Vasomotor symptoms: hot flashes

   b. Genitourinary: atrophic vaginitis, vaginal dryness, and incontinence

   c. Psychologic: mood swings, changes in sleep patterns, and decreased REM sleep

   d. Skeletal: decreased bone density

   e. Cardiovascular: decreased HDL and increased LDL

   f. Dermatologic: decreased skin elasticity and loss of hair on head and in the pubic area

   g. Reproductive—breast tissue changes, irregular menses

2. Collaborative Care and **Nursing Interventions**

   a. Monitor the client's psychosocial response.

   b. Discuss hormone replacement therapy (HRT): advantages and disadvantages, administration, and safety measures.

     1) Instruct in self-administration of HRT.

     2) Advise to immediately quit smoking if applicable.

     3) Reinforce teaching to prevent and monitor for development of venous thrombosis.

   c. Reinforce education about alternative hormone therapies: dong quai, black cohosh, vitamin E. They decrease hot flashes in some women.

   d. Older adult clients may decrease risk of osteoporosis by performing regular weight-bearing exercises; increasing intake of high-protein and high-calcium foods; avoiding alcohol, caffeine, and tobacco; and taking calcium with vitamin D supplements.

   e. Reinforce education on health promotion

     1) Schedule annual exams including physical, pelvic, and mammogram.

     2) Schedule bone density test.

     3) Instruct on atypical manifestations of MI.

     4) Discuss diet, exercise, and alternative therapies.

SEXUALLY TRANSMITTED INFECTIONS

SYMPTOMS IN WOMEN	SYMPTOMS IN MEN	COMPLICATIONS	TREATMENTS

Chlamydia
If symptoms appear usually not until several weeks after infected.

Vaginal discharge	Small amounts of clear or cloudy penile discharge	Can pass to sexual partners and to neonate during childbirth (conjunctivitis, pneumonia)	Oral antibiotics, usually azithromycin (Zithromax) or doxycycline.
Vaginal bleeding			
Painful/frequent urination	Painful/frequent urination	PID	Preventive treatment in newborn: erythromycin (Ilotycin) ointment in eyes within 1 hr of birth.
Abdominal pain	Swollen/tender testicles	Can lead to infertility in women and sterility in men	
Fever/nausea			
Usually asymptomatic			

Genital herpes
Transmission most commonly occurs from infected partner who has no visible lesion.

Most are asymptomatic	Some have no symptoms	No cure; symptoms are treated	Caused by a virus
Initial outbreak: painful blisters and possible systemic symptoms (fever, body aches, enlarged lymph nodes)	Blisters on mouth or genital region	Can pass to sexual partners and to neonate during childbirth	The antiviral medications acyclovir (Zovirax), famciclovir, and valacyclovir can shorten and prevent outbreaks.
Recurrences: mild tingling or shooting pains hours to days before herpetic eruption.	Blisters last 7 to 21 days		Cesarean birth indicated if active lesions present during the last 2 weeks before delivery.
Blisters last 7 to 21 days	Blisters can reoccur		Antiviral medication (acyclovir) started at 36 weeks gestation to prevent outbreak before delivery.

Gonorrhea
Symptoms may appear 2 to 21 days after infection.

Yellow/gray vaginal discharge	Yellow/green penile discharge	Transmitted to sexual partner and to the neonate in uterus/during childbirth (opthalemia neonatorum)	First-line treatment is single intramuscular injection of ceftriaxone, 250 mg.
Vaginal bleeding between periods	Painful urination/bowel movement	Can lead to infertility in women and sterility in men	Ceftriaxone routinely accompanied by azithromycin or doxycycline to address the likelihood of coinfection with chlamydia
Symptoms mild and nonspecific	Frequent urination	Untreated GC can cause urogenital, anorectal, conjunctival, and pharyngeal infections. Can also spread to the blood and cause disseminated gonococcal infection (DGI). DGI is usually characterized by arthritis, tenosynovitis, and/or dermatitis.	Because of high reinfection rates, patients should be retested in three to six months.
Dysuria	Swollen/tender testicles (epididymitis)		Preventive treatment of newborn: erythromycin (Ilotycin) ointment in eyes.

HIV
Symptoms can appear months to several years after infection.

Acute retroviral syndrome is characterized by non-specific symptoms, including fever, malaise, lymphadenopathy, and skin rash. Frequently occurs in the first few weeks after HIV infection, before antibody test results become positive.

Can be infected for several years without symptoms	Can be infected for several years without symptoms	There is no cure for HIV, but treatment is available.	HIV is a virus that progressively depletes CD4 lymphocytes.
Weight loss/fatigue	Weight loss/fatigue	Can be passed by sex, sharing needles, during childbirth, or during breastfeeding	Prevention counseling is key. Screening with early detection is critical.
Recurring vaginal yeast infections	Diarrhea/flu-like symptoms		Medication includes: Antiretroviral therapy (HAART)
Diarrhea/flulike symptoms	Oral thrush		Management for obstetrical clients include: Antiretroviral regimens and obstetrical interventions, such as zidovudine or nevirapine (Viramune) and elective Cesarean birth at 38 weeks of pregnancy, and education to avoid breastfeeding.
Oral thrush			

SYMPTOMS IN WOMEN	SYMPTOMS IN MEN	COMPLICATIONS	TREATMENTS

Human papillomavirus (HPV)
There are multiple strains. Some may cause genital warts and others have been linked to cervical cancer. Symptom appearance time varies.

SYMPTOMS IN WOMEN	SYMPTOMS IN MEN	COMPLICATIONS	TREATMENTS
Genital warts, also referred to as condylomas. Appear as small, flesh-colored or gray swelling in the genital area. They can clump together and form a cauliflower shape. Itching/burning around the genitalia Abnormal pap smear	Genital warts Warts can recur Itching/burning around the genitalia	Can pass to sexual partners and neonate during childbirth Warts can spread. Certain strains may lead to cancer. A rare complication includes recurrent respiratory papillomatosis (RRP).	HPV vaccines (Gardasil or Cervarix) recommended for 11- or 12-year-old boys and girls. May be given to girls beginning at age 9. Medications to treat genital warts include imiquimod (Aldara) and podophyllin (Condylox)

Pelvic inflammatory disease (PID)
Several different bacteria can cause PID, and many cases have been related to chlamydia and gonorrhea.

SYMPTOMS IN WOMEN	SYMPTOMS IN MEN	COMPLICATIONS	TREATMENTS
Lower abdominal pain Vaginal discharge May have unpleasant odor Painful intercourse/urination Abnormal vaginal discharge; yellow or green Fever, chills and nausea and vomiting	PID does not occur in males	Can cause ectopic pregnancy Can lead to infertility May cause chronic pain in abdominal area	Depending on the severity of PID, the following may be used for treatment › Antibiotics › Hospitalization/bed rest › Outpatient intensive treatment

Syphilis
There are three stages of syphilis. Stage 1 symptoms can appear 1 week to 3 months after infection.

SYMPTOMS IN WOMEN	SYMPTOMS IN MEN	COMPLICATIONS	TREATMENTS
Stage 1 › Sore(s) on genitalia or mouth › The sore(s) can last 2 to 6 weeks Stage 2 › Rash on body › Flu-like symptoms Tertiary (last) Stage › Neurological/ cardiovascular complications	Stage 1 › Sore(s) on genitalia or mouth › The sore(s) can last 2 to 6 weeks Stage 2 › Rash on body › Flu-like symptoms Tertiary (last) Stage › Neurological/ cardiovascular complications	Can pass to sexual partners and to the neonate during pregnancy May cause miscarriage in women May cause heart disease, blindness, and/or brain damage Can lead to death	Caused by bacteria Penicillin is drug of choice

Trichomoniasis (Trich)
Symptoms can appear 3 days to 2 weeks after infection.

SYMPTOMS IN WOMEN	SYMPTOMS IN MEN	COMPLICATIONS	TREATMENTS
May be asymptomatic Common symptom: yellowish to greenish, frothy, mucopurulent, copious, malodorous discharge. Dysuria and dyspareunia Vaginal irritation and pruritus	Often no symptoms White, watery penile discharge Painful/frequent urination	Can pass to sexual partners Can lead to prostate infection in men	Recommended treatment is metronidazole (Flagyl) or tinidazole unless client in first trimester of pregnancy. Partner(s) should also be treated

Nursing Care of Children

Foundations of Nursing Care of Children

Family

A. Identify legal guardian.

B. Build relationship with family and child.

C. Monitor family dynamics.

D. Collaborative Care

   1. Nursing Interventions

      a. Respect family diversity.

   2. Observe parent-child interactions.

      a. Assist families to understand growth and development needs.

      b. Assist families to adapt to the needs of child with a health problem.

      c. Assist families to participate in care as appropriate.

      d. Use community resources for family adaptation.

SECTION 2

Growth and Development

Expected Growth and Development of the Infant (1st Year of Life)

A. **Physical Development**

   1. Fontanelles

      a. Posterior closes by 2 to 3 months of age

      b. Anterior closes by 12 to 18 months of age

   2. Dentition

      a. First tooth appears at 6 or 7 months of age

      b. Additional 1 tooth per month

      c. Pain relief

         1) Acetaminophen (Tylenol)

         2) Cold

            a) Refrigerated pacifier

            b) Frozen cloth

      d. Tooth care

         1) Clean teeth with wet cloth.

         2) Do not prop bottles.

         3) Give only formula or breast milk in bottle; juices should be avoided.

3. Vision

      a. Infant vision is undeveloped

      b. Best able to focus on objects 10 to 12 inches from face

      c. Best able to discern shapes with contrast such as black/white and primary colors.

4. Measurements of growth

      a. Height, weight, and head circumference plotted on graph

         1) Height usually measured lying supine until age 2

         2) If weighed with diaper, assess weight of diaper

         3) Head circumference measured at widest point

      b. Identify issues

         1) Weight/height ratio

         2) Weight below 5th percentile or above 95th percentile

         3) Failure to thrive

         4) Parental educational needs

      c. Rules of thumb

         1) 5% to 7% weight loss immediately after birth is common.

         2) Birth weight is reattained by 2 weeks of age.

         3) Birth weight doubles by 6 months of age.

         4) Birth weight triples by 12 months of age.

MOTOR SKILL DEVELOPMENT OF THE INFANT

AGE	GROSS MOTOR SKILLS	FINE MOTOR SKILLS
1 month	Demonstrates head lag	Strong palmar grasp reflex
2 months	Lifts head off mattress	Holds hands
3 months	Raises head and shoulders off mattress	Palmar grasp reflex begins to diminish Voluntary grasp present
4 months	Rolls from back to side	Places objects in mouth
5 months	Rolls from front to back	Strong palmar grasp (Do not confuse with palmar grasp reflex.)
6 months	Rolls from back to front	Holds bottle
7 months	Bears full weight on feet	Moves objects from hand to hand
8 months	Sits unsupported	Begins using pincer grasp
9 months	Pulls to a standing position	Pincer grasp is more precise
10 months	Changes from a prone to a sitting position	Grasps rattle by its handle Picks up finger foods
11 months	Walks while holding onto something	Places objects into a container
12 months	Sits down from a standing position without assistance	Tries to build a two-block tower without success

INFANT DEVELOPMENT MILESTONES

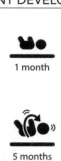

| 1 month | 2 months | 3 months | 4 months |

| 5 months | 6 months | 7 months | 8 months |

| 9 months | 10 months | 11 months | 12 months |

GETTY IMAGES/ISTOCKPHOTO

B. **Cognitive Development**

1. Piaget: Sensorimotor stage (birth to 24 months)

   a. Separation: Infant learns that other people and objects are separate from himself.

   b. Object permanence: Around 9 months of age the infant learns objects exist when hidden from view.

   c. Mental representation: Infant recognizes some symbols.

2. Language

   a. Vocalizes with cooing noises

   b. Responds to noises

   c. Turns head to the sound of a rattle

   d. Laughs and squeals

   e. Pronounces single-syllable words

   f. Begins speaking two-word phrases and progresses to speaking three-word phrases

C. **Psychosocial Development**

1. Erikson: Trust vs. Mistrust

   a. Trust develops as needs are met

2. Attachment and bonding occur

3. Separation anxiety begins 4 to 8 months of age. Peaks in toddler.

D. **Age-Appropriate Activities**

1. Infants enjoy watching faces and listening to voices.

2. Infants have a short attention span.

3. Infants engage in solitary play.

4. Appropriate toys include:

   a. Rattles

   b. Mobiles

   c. Teething toys

   d. Nesting toys

   e. Playing pat-a-cake

   f. Playing with balls

   g. Listening to someone read

E. **Health Promotion for Infants**

1. Immunizations

> NOTE: Always refer to the CDC website (www.cdc.gov) for the latest immunization requirements and schedules.

2. Nutrition

   a. First 6 months

      1) Breastfeeding or iron-fortified formula provides a complete diet for the first 6 months of life.

   b. 4 to 6 months

      1) Introduce solids.

      2) Introduce no more than one food at a time to evaluate allergy and tolerance.

      3) Start with iron-fortified rice cereal.

      4) Later, introduce yellow/orange vegetables and fruits.

      5) Around 9 months of age, infant will have pincer grasp and be able to self-feed some foods.

      6) Foods to avoid in first year

         a) Milk

         b) Eggs

         c) Wheat

         d) Peanuts (any form)

         e) Honey

         f) Citrus fruits

   c. Weaning from a bottle: Around 6 months, begin introducing a "baby cup."

   d. At 12 months, whole cow's milk is introduced. Reduced-fat (2%) cow's milk may be used for infants who have or are at risk for obesity and elevated cholesterol.

II Safety – Infant

A. **Aspiration and Suffocation**

1. Toys must be age-appropriate.

2. Chop food in fine pieces.

3. Check clothing and household objects for hazards such as loose buttons or draw strings.

4. Plastic bags and balloons should not be near infants. Latex balloons are the leading cause of pediatric choking deaths. Substitute mylar or paper balloons for latex.

5. Cribs should follow standards: firm mattress, nothing in crib with baby, slats no more than 6 cm (2.4 in) apart, mobiles removed before child pulls to sitting. Position cribs away from window coverings and large furniture.

B. **Bodily Harm**

1. Keep sharp objects out of reach.

2. Keep infants away from heavy objects that they can pull down onto themselves.

3. Do not leave infants unattended with any animals present.

4. Monitor infants for shaken baby syndrome.

C. **Burns**

1. The temperature of bath water should be checked.

2. Thermostats on hot water heaters should be turned down to a safe temperature of 49° C (120° F)

3. Working smoke detectors should be kept in the home.

4. Handles of pots and pans should be kept turned to the back of stoves.

5. Sunscreen should be used when infants will be exposed to the sun.

6. Electrical outlets should be covered.

7. Microwave ovens: Stir food and check temperature before feeding.

8. Infant clothing should be flame retardant.

D. **Drowning**

1. Infants must always be supervised near water such as tubs, toilets, and swimming areas.

E. **Falls**

1. Never leave an infant unattended.

2. Place safety gates on stairs.

F. **Poisoning**

1. All potentially toxic substances should be locked or removed.

2. Medications should be stored in safety bottles in a locked cupboard. Never refer to medicine as candy.

3. Carbon monoxide detectors should be working.

4. Poison control number should be readily available.

G. **Motor Vehicle Injuries**

1. Infants should be placed in approved rear-facing car seats in the backseat, preferably in the middle (away from air bags and side impact). Infants should be in rear-facing car seats until 2 years of age and they exceed the manufacturer's recommended weight.

2. A five-point harness or T-shield should be part of a convertible restraint.

   a. According to the National Highway Traffic Safety Administration, infants should remain rear-facing until they outgrow the height or weight limit of the seat.

   b. The American Academy of Pediatrics (AAP) recommends rear-facing until age 2—longer if the child has not yet reached the weight/height limits of the seat. This change was made in April 2011.

   c. The safest location is the center of the rear seat.

   d. If air bags are near the infant, the air bags should be inactivated.

H. **Sudden Infant Death Syndrome (SIDS)**

1. Risks

   a. Males

   b. Age 2 to 4 months

   c. Preterm infants with apnea problems

   d. Cigarette smoke

   e. Multiple births

   f. Sleeping in any position other than supine

   g. Soft mattress or added pillows, blankets, etc.

   h. Co-sleeping

2. Prevention

   a. Place babies on their backs to sleep.

   b. Breast feeding may provide some protection.

   c. AAP recommends use of a pacifier when sleeping.

III Expected Growth and Development of the Toddler (Ages 1 to 3 Years)

A. **Physical Development**

1. Anterior fontanelles close by 18 months of age.

2. Weight: At 30 months of age, toddlers should weigh about four times their birth weights.

MOTOR SKILL DEVELOPMENT OF THE TODDLER

AGE	GROSS MOTOR SKILLS	FINE MOTOR SKILLS
15 months	Walks without help Uses a cup well	Creeps up stairs Builds a tower of two blocks
18 months	Assumes a standing position	Manages a spoon without rotation Turns pages in a book, two or three at a time
2 years	Walks up and down stairs	Builds a tower of six or seven blocks
2.5 years	Jumps in place with both feet Stands on one foot momentarily	Draws circles Has good hand-finger coordination

TODDLER DEVELOPMENT MILESTONES

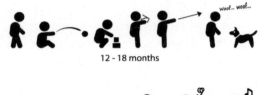

12 - 18 months

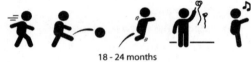

18 - 24 months

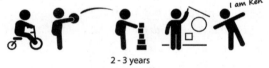

2 - 3 years

GETTY IMAGES/ISTOCKPHOTO

B. **Cognitive Development**

1. Piaget: The sensorimotor stage transitions to the preoperational stage

   a. Object permanence is developed

   b. Memory develops

   c. Preoperational thought allows the toddler to use symbols to represent objects

2. Language development

   a. Language increases to about 400 words, with toddlers speaking in two- to three-word phrases.

C. **Psychosocial Development**

1. Erikson

    a. Autonomy vs. Shame and Doubt

    b. Toddlers want to make choices; parents should offer healthy, age-appropriate options.

    c. Temper tantrums should be ignored after ascertaining child is safe.

    d. Separation anxiety peaks.

    e. Rituals are important.

2. Moral Development

    a. Toddlers are egocentric.

    b. Toddlers understand that good behavior is rewarded and bad is punished.

3. Body Image Changes

    a. Toddlers appreciate the usefulness of various body parts.

    b. Toddlers will develop gender identity by 3 years of age.

D. **Age-Appropriate Activities**

1. Solitary play evolves to parallel play.

2. Activities

    a. Filling and emptying containers

    b. Blocks

    c. Looking at books

    d. Push-pull toys

    e. Ball toss

3. Toilet training

    a. Begins when toddler is able to recognize the urge to urinate or defecate.

    b. Parents should allow the child to set the pace.

    c. Nighttime continence usually occurs last.

E. **Health Promotion for Toddlers**

1. Immunizations

2. Nutrition

    a. Offer nutritious choices for meals and snacks.

    b. Serving size is about 1 tbsp per year of age.

    c. Whole cow's milk (3%) is recommended for ages 12 to 24 months. Reduced-fat cow's milk (2%) may be used for children who have or are at risk for obesity and elevated cholesterol.

    d. Low-fat milk (1%) is recommended for all children after 24 months of age.

    e. By 12 months, bottles should be avoided to decrease ear infections and tooth decay.

    f. Finger foods may increase autonomy.

3. Dental Care

    a. Dental checks

    b. Parents and child brush teeth

IV Safety – Toddler

A. **Aspiration and Suffocation**

1. Small toys and objects should be kept out of reach.

2. Avoid common causes of choking: hot dogs, nuts, grapes, peanut butter, raw carrots, tough meat, popcorn.

3. No balloons or plastic bags.

4. Crib mattresses should fit tightly.

5. Crib slats should be no farther apart than 6 cm (2.4 in).

6. Pillows should be kept out of cribs.

7. Drawstrings should be removed from jackets and other clothing.

B. **Bodily Harm**

1. Sharp objects should be kept out of reach.

2. Firearms should be kept in locked boxes or cabinets.

3. Toddlers should not be left unattended with any animals present.

4. Toddlers should be taught stranger safety.

C. **Burns**

1. The temperature of bath water should be checked.

2. Thermostats on hot water heaters should be turned down to a safe temperature of 49° C (120° F).

3. Working smoke detectors should be kept in the home.

4. Pot handles should be turned toward the back of the stove.

5. Electrical outlets should be covered.

6. Toddler should wear sunscreen when outside.

D. **Drowning**

1. Toddlers should not be left unattended in bathtubs.

2. Toilet lids should be kept closed.

3. Toddlers should be closely supervised when near pools or any other body of water.

4. Toddlers should be taught to swim.

E. **Falls**

1. Doors and windows should be kept locked.

2. Crib mattresses should be kept in the lowest position with the rails all the way up.

3. Safety gates should be used across stairs both at the top and bottom of stairs.

F. **Motor Vehicle Injuries**

1. According to the National Highway Traffic Safety Administration, children should remain in the forward-facing car seat until they exceed the height/weight limit of the seat.

2. After children have exceeded the height/weight limits of the forward-facing car seat, they may sit in a booster seat. The safest place is the back seat.

3. Any air bags by the child should be inactivated.

G. **Poisoning**

1. Exposure to lead paint should be avoided.

2. Safety locks should be placed on cabinets that contain cleaners and other chemicals.

3. The phone number for a poison control center should be kept near the phone.

4. Medications should be kept in childproof containers, away from the reach of toddlers.

5. A working carbon monoxide detector should be placed in the home.

v Expected Growth and Development of the Preschooler (3 to 6 Years of Age)

A. **Physical Development**

1. The preschooler gains greater control of fine and gross motor skills.

2. The preschooler dresses independently.

MOTOR SKILLS OF THE PRESCHOOLER

AGE	GROSS MOTOR SKILLS
3 years	Rides a tricycle Jumps off bottom step Stands on one foot for a few seconds
4 years	Skips and hops on one foot Throws a ball overhead
5 years	Jumps rope Walks backward with heel to toe Moves up and down stairs easily

B. **Cognitive and Language Development**

1. Piaget

    a. Preconceptional thought: 2 to 4 years

        1) Judgments made by appearance

        2) Animation—inanimate objects are alive

    b. Intuitive thought: 4 to 7 years

        1) Become aware of cause and effect

    c. Time—understand past, present, future and begin to understand days of the week

2. Language Development

    a. Speaks with sentences

C. **Psychosocial Development**

1. Erikson—Initiative vs. Guilt

    a. Guilt may occur if unable to successfully complete a task or if they are "punished" for an unsuccessful try

    b. Adults can try to guide preschoolers to tasks that are appropriate

2. Moral Development

    a. Begin to understand behaviors that are socially acceptable

3. Social Development

    a. Separation anxiety tapers.

    b. Pretend play; may develop imaginary friends.

    c. Sleep disturbances are common; night lights may be useful.

    d. Preschoolers need about 12 hr of sleep per day. Bedtime routines are important.

D. **Age-Appropriate Activities**

1. Associative play with some cooperation

2. Appropriate activities

    a. Playing ball

    b. Puzzles

    c. Tricycles

    d. Playing pretend and "dress-up"

    e. Painting

    f. Reading books

E. **Health Promotion for Preschoolers**

1. Immunizations: Follow CDC guidelines.

2. Health screening

    a. Vision screening

    b. Dental care

3. Nutrition

    a. May be selective with food choices.

    b. Require about 50% of adult calories.

    c. All nutrients are important.

vi Safety for Preschoolers

A. **Bodily Harm**

1. Place all firearms and ammunition in locked safes.

2. Teach stranger safety.

3. Encourage protective equipment (e.g., helmet).

B. **Burns**

1. Thermostats should be turned down on hot water heaters.

2. Working smoke detectors should be kept in the home.

3. Preschoolers should have sunscreen applied when outside.

C. **Drowning**

1. Preschoolers should not be left unattended in bathtubs.

2. Preschoolers should be closely supervised when near the pool or any other body of water.

3. Preschoolers should be taught to swim.

D. **Motor Vehicle Injuries**

1. According to the National Highway Traffic Safety Administration, children should remain rear-facing until they outgrow the height or weight limit of the seat.

2. The American Academy of Pediatrics recommends rear-facing until age 2—longer if the child has not yet reached the weight/height limits of the seat. This change was made in April 2011.

3. After the child exceeds the weight/height limits of the rear-facing car seat, the child should be placed in a front-facing car seat but remain in the back seat.

4. Any air bags by the child should be inactivated.

E. **Poisoning**

1. Keep the phone number for a poison control center near the phone.

2. Avoid exposure to lead paint.

3. Keep plants out of reach.

4. Place safety locks on cabinets with cleaners and other chemicals.

5. Keep medications in childproof containers, out of reach of preschoolers.

6. Place a working carbon monoxide detector in the home.

VII Expected Growth and Development of the School-Age Child (6 to 12 Years)

A. **Physical Development**

1. Puberty

   a. Females

      1) Onset around 10 to 14 years of age

      2) Onset of menarche increases iron needs

   b. Males

      1) Onset around 12 to 16 years of age

2. Permanent teeth erupt.

3. Visual acuity improves to 20/20.

4. Auditory acuity and sense of touch is fully developed.

5. Fine and gross motor development continue to improve.

B. **Cognitive and Language Development**

1. Piaget: Concrete Operations

   a. Understands time

   b. Understands analogies

   c. Understands some emotions

   d. Able to solve problems

2. Language

   a. Defines many words and understands rules of grammar

   b. Understands that a word may have multiple meanings

C. **Psychosocial Development**

1. Erikson—Industry vs. Inferiority

   a. A sense of industry is achieved through advancements in learning.

   b. Fears of ridicule are common.

2. Moral development

   a. Early on, may not understand the reasoning behind many rules and may try to find ways around them. Instrumental exchange ("I'll help you if you help me") is in place. Children want to make the best deal, and they do not really consider elements of loyalty, gratitude, or justice as they make decisions.

   b. In the latter part of the school-age years, children move into a law-and-order orientation with more emphasis placed on justice being administered.

3. Self-concept development

   a. Strive to develop a healthy self-respect by finding out in what areas they excel.

   b. Need parents to encourage them regarding educational or extracurricular successes.

4. Body image changes

   a. Solidification of body image occurs.

   b. Curiosity about sexuality should be addressed with education regarding sexual development and the reproductive process.

   c. More modest than preschoolers and place more emphasis on privacy issues.

5. Social development

   a. Peer groups play an important part in social development. Peer pressure begins to take effect.

   b. Friendships begin to form between same-gender peers. Clubs and best friends are popular.

   c. Children prefer the company of same-gender companions.

   d. Most relationships come from school associations.

   e. Children may rival same-gender parents.

   f. Conformity becomes evident.

D. **Age-Appropriate Activities**

1. Play is competitive and cooperative

2. Common activities

   a. Board games

   b. Jump rope

   c. Collecting

   d. Bicycles

   e. Sports

   f. Crafts

E. **Health Promotion for School-Age Children**

1. Immunizations: Follow current CDC guidelines.

2. Nutrition

   a. Nutritious choices, regular meals, and avoiding fast-food is important.

   b. Obesity is an increasing problem.

   c. The CDC provides BMI charts to use in assessment of appropriate BMI based upon the child's age, height, weight, and sex.

3. Health screenings

   a. Scoliosis

      1) May appear during growth spurts

      2) Scoliosis screening

   b. Dental health

      1) Brush and floss daily.

      2) Have regular checkups.

      3) Have regular fluoride treatments.

VIII Safety for School-Age Children

A. **Bodily Harm**

1. Firearms should be kept in locked cabinets or boxes.

2. Children should not be allowed to use trampolines.

3. Safe play areas should be identified.

4. Stranger safety should be taught.

5. Children should be taught to wear helmets and/or pads when skating, skateboarding, bicycling, riding scooters, skiing, and snowboarding.

B. **Burns**

1. Teach children fire safety and potential burn hazards.

2. Keep working smoke detectors in the home.

3. Children should use sunscreen when outside

C. **Drowning**

1. Supervise children when swimming or when near a body of water.

2. Teach children to swim.

D. **Motor Vehicle Injuries**

1. A child whose weight or height is above the forward-facing limit for the car seat should use a belt-positioning booster seat until the seat belt in the vehicle fits the child properly. AAP states this occurs when the child has reached a height of 4 feet 9 inches, generally between the ages of 8 and 12 years.

2. Children should not use a seat belt until the lap belt fits snugly across the upper thighs (not abdomen) and the shoulder restraint lies snugly across the shoulder and chest (not neck or head). The child should remain in the back seat.

3. Any child younger than 13 years should be restrained in the rear seats of vehicles for optimal protection.

4. Air bags should be inactivated.

E. **Substance Abuse**

1. Community resources

2. Family involvement

3. Commonly abused substances change rapidly and may include:

   a. Alcohol

   b. Cannabinoids (e.g., marijuana, hashish)

   c. Prescription drugs (may abuse family members' or their own prescription, or obtain illegally)

   d. Inhalants (e.g., adhesives, aerosols, paint thinner)

   e. Stimulant street drugs (e.g., cocaine, amphetamines)

IX Expected Growth and Development of the Adolescent (12 to 20 Years)

A. **Physical Development**

1. Puberty is completed and adult height attained.

2. Acne is common.

3. Sleep needs may increase related to increased metabolism and rapid growth.

B. **Cognitive and Language Development**

1. Piaget—Formal Operations

   a. Able to think abstractly

   b. Idealistic

   c. Logical thinking

   d. Capable of deductive thinking

2. Language

   a. Adolescents develop jargon within their peer groups. They are able to communicate one way with peer groups and another way with adults or teachers.

   b. Development of communication skills is essential for adolescents.

C. **Psychosocial Development**

1. Erikson—Identity vs. Role Confusion

   a. Families strongly influence personal identity

   b. Peer groups greatly influence behavior

   c. Career planning

   d. Interest in opposite sex

   e. May see themselves as invincible

2. Moral development

   a. Conventional law and order: Rules are not seen as absolutes. Each situation needs to be looked at, and perhaps the rules will need to be adjusted. Not all adolescents attain this level of moral development during these years.

3. Self-concept development

   a. A healthy self-concept is developed by having healthy relationships with peers, family, and teachers. Identifying a skill or talent helps maintain a healthy self-concept. Participation in sports, hobbies, or the community can have a positive outcome.

4. Body image

   a. May be concerned with image related to peers, parents, and media

   b. May lead to depression or eating disorders

5. Body image changes

   a. Adolescents seem particularly concerned with body images portrayed by the media. Changes that occur during puberty result in comparisons between individual adolescents and their surrounding peer groups. Parents also give their input as to hair styles, dress, and activities. Adolescents may require help if depression or eating disorders result due to poor body image.

D. **Age-Appropriate Activities**

1. Nonviolent video games

2. Nonviolent music

3. Sports

4. Caring for a pet

5. Career training programs

6. Reading

7. Social events (going to movies, school dances)

E. **Health Promotion for Adolescents**

1. Immunizations

2. Screenings

   a. Scoliosis

   b. Pap and pelvic exam if female is sexually active

   c. STI screening if sexually active

   d. Education about birth control and "safer" sex

   e. Testicular self exam—testicular cancer is the most common solid tumor in males 15 to 34 years old.

3. Nutrition

    a. Rapid growth and high metabolism require increases in quality nutrients. Nutrients that tend to be deficient during this stage of life are iron, calcium, and vitamins A and C.

    b. Eating disorders (see "Body Image" above)

F. **Dental health**

  1. Brush and floss daily.

  2. Have regular checkups.

  3. Have regular fluoride treatments.

x Safety for the Adolescent

A. **Three leading causes of death in adolescents** are homicide, suicide, and motor vehicle accidents.

B. **Additional common safety issues:** Burns, drowning, and substance abuse.

C. **Car restraints:** When the child's weight and height are adequate, the child may use the seat belt provided in the vehicle. However, the seat belt should always be a lap/shoulder combination.

xı Child Neglect and Abuse

While evaluating growth and development, the nurse may find indications of neglect and/or abuse.

A. **Types**

  1. Physical neglect: failure to provide necessities of life

  2. Physical abuse: deliberate infliction of injury

  3. Emotional neglect: failure to provide emotional nurturing, deliberate or unintentional

  4. Sexual abuse: use of child to meet adult's sexual needs

  5. Munchausen syndrome by proxy (MSBP): a disorder in which a caregiver (usually parent) falsely reports or intentionally causes symptoms in his or her own child to seek attention

B. **Contributing Factors**

  1. Parental

    a. Poor self-esteem

    b. Abused as a child

    c. Lack of knowledge

    d. Lack of support system

    e. Poor coping skills

    f. Unwanted pregnancy or sex

  2. Child

    a. Difficult temperament or behaviors

  3. Environment

    a. Chronic stress

    b. Socioeconomic factors

C. **Manifestations of Abuse and Neglect**

  1. Physical neglect

    a. Failure to thrive: disruption in maternal-infant bonding; poor feeding behaviors; mother does not respond to infant's cues; weight less than 5th percentile; developmental delay

    b. Poor health care, lack of immunizations

    c. Failure to meet basic needs: malnutrition, poor hygiene

  2. Physical abuse

    a. Bruises: not on bony prominences, in varying degrees of healing, with patterns

    b. Burns: with immersion lines, in patterns

    c. Fractures: spiral, twisting

    d. Shaken baby: unconscious infant with retinal hemorrhage and no external signs of trauma

    e. Conflicting stories given by parents, child, or others

    f. History incompatible with physical findings or developmentally improbable

    g. Delay in seeking medical attention

  3. Emotional neglect and abuse

    a. Extremes of behavior

    b. Poor self-esteem

  4. Sexual abuse

    a. Bruising of the genitalia

    b. STI

    c. Sudden change in behavior, regressive behavior

  5. Munchausen syndrome by proxy

    a. Victims usually under age 6 years

    b. May have lasting emotional impact

    c. Increased risk for child to develop Munchausen syndrome as adult

    d. Parent well versed in medical knowledge

D. **Collaborative Care**

  1. Nursing Interventions

    a. Do not leave child unattended.

    b. Establish trust with child.

    c. Follow agency policy to notify social services.

    d. Arrange needed referrals.

    e. Document findings objectively.

Adapting Nursing Care for the Child

EXPECTED VITAL SIGNS

AGE	BLOOD PRESSURE	TEMPERATURE	HEART RATE	RESPIRATORY RATE
1 year	95/65 mm Hg	37.7° C (99.7° F)	80 to 150/min	30/min
6 years	105/65 mm Hg	37° C (98.6° F)	70 to 110/min	21/min
13 years	110/65 mm Hg	36.6° C (97.8° F)	55 to 90/min	18/min
17 years	120/75 mm Hg	37° C (98.6° F)	55 to 90/min	16 to 18/min

AGE-RELATED NURSING INTERVENTIONS

AGE	INTERVENTIONS
Infant	Place infants whose parents are not in attendance close to nursing stations so that their needs may be quickly met.
Toddler	Provide consistency in assigning caregivers. Encourage parents to provide routine care, such as changing diapers and feeding. Encourage the child's autonomy by giving appropriate choices. Provide consistency in assigning caregivers.
Preschooler	Explain all procedures using simple, clear language. Avoid medical jargon and terms that can be misinterpreted by the child. Encourage independence by letting the child provide self-care. Encourage the child to express feelings. Validate fears and concerns. Provide toys that allow for emotional expression, such as a pounding board to release feelings of protest. Provide consistency in assigning caregivers. Give choices when possible, such as "Do you want your medicine in a cup or a spoon?" Allow younger children to handle equipment if it is safe.
School-age	Provide factual information. Encourage the child to express feelings. Try to maintain a normal routine for long hospitalizations, including time for school work. Encourage contact with peer group.
Adolescent	Provide factual information. Include the adolescent in the planning of care to relieve feelings of powerlessness and lack of control. Encourage contact with peer group.

Stress of Hospitalization

A. **Separation Anxiety**
   1. Protest (e.g., screaming)
   2. Despair (regression, e.g., bed wetting)
   3. Detachment (e.g., lack of interaction)

B. **Nursing Interventions**
   1. Reinforce teaching with the child and family what to expect during hospitalization.
   2. Encourage parents or family members to stay with the child during the hospital experience to reduce the stress.
   3. Attempt to maintain routine as much as possible.

II Therapeutic Play

A. **Uses**

1. Play may allow for expression of feelings.
2. Play facilitates development physically, cognitively, and socially.
3. Play may be used for education.
4. Play should be age-appropriate.

B. **Purpose**

1. Acting out feelings
2. Coping with environment
3. Teaching

C. **Appropriate Activity for Age and Health Status**

1. **Nursing Interventions**

    a. Select activity to enhance physical needs (such as blowing bubbles for deep breathing).
    b. Select activity to enhance coping (such as drawing pictures).
    c. Use toys from home as appropriate.

        1) Avoid toys that are difficult to disinfect if contagious process is involved.
        2) Avoid toys that might spark if oxygen is in use.

    d. Provide adequate rest periods.
    e. Monitor response to activity.

D. **Collaborative Care**

1. Consult child life specialist.
2. Consult social services if needed.
3. Consult resource management as needed.

EFFECT OF HOSPITALIZATION ON CHILDREN

LEVEL OF UNDERSTANDING	EFFECT OF HOSPITALIZATION
Infant	
Inability to describe symptoms and follow directions	Experiences stranger anxiety between 6 to 18 months of age
Lack of understanding for the need of therapeutic procedures	Displays physical behaviors as expressions of discomfort due to inability to verbalize
	May experience sleep deprivation due to strange noises, monitoring devices, and procedures
Toddler	
Limited ability to describe symptoms	Experiences separation anxiety
Poorly developed sense of body image and boundaries	May exhibit an intense reaction to any type of procedure due to the intrusion of boundaries
Limited understanding for the need for therapeutic procedures	
Limited ability to follow directions	
Preschooler	
Limited understanding of the cause of illness but knows what illness feels like	May experience separation anxiety
Limited ability to describe symptoms	May harbor fears of bodily harm
Fears related to magical thinking	May believe illness and hospitalization are a punishment
Ability to understand cause and effect inhibited by concrete thinking	
School-age child	
Beginning awareness of body functioning	Fears loss of control
Ability to describe pain symptoms	Seeks information as a way to maintain a sense of control
Increasing ability to understand cause and effect	May sense when not being told the truth
	May experience stress related to separation from peers and regular routine
Adolescent	
Increasing ability to understand cause and effect	Develops body image disturbance
Perceptions of illness severity are based on the degree of body image changes	Attempts to maintain composure but is embarrassed about losing control
	Experiences feelings of isolation from peers
	Worries about outcome and impact on school/activities
	May not adhere to treatments/medication regimen due to peer influence

III Pain Management

TOOLS USED IN PAIN ASSESSMENT

FORM OF EVALUATION	AGE OF CHILD
CRIES Neonatal Postoperative Scale	
Pain rated on a scale of 0 to 10 Behavior indicators › Crying › Changes in vital signs › Changes in expression › Altered sleeping patterns	32 weeks of gestation to 20 weeks of life
Faces, Legs, Activity, Cry, and Consolability (FLACC) Postoperative Pain Tool	
Behavior indicators › Facial expressions › Position of legs › Activity › Crying › Ability to be consoled	2 months to 7 years
FACES Pain Rating Scale	
Rating scale uses drawings of happy and sad faces to depict levels of pain.	3 years and older
Visual Analog Scale (VAS)	
Pain is rated on a scale of 0 to 10. Child points to the number that best describes the pain he is experiencing	7 years and older (may be effective with children as young as 4.5 years)
Noncommunicating Children's Pain Checklist	
Pain is rated on a scale of 0 to 10. Behavior indicators › Vocalization › Socialization › Facial expressions › Activity level › Movement of extremities › Physiologic changes	3 to 18 years of age (for children with or without cognitive impairments)

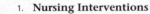

A. **Collaborative Care**

1. **Nursing Interventions**

   a. Interventions should be determined in conjunction with the family and child. Severity of the pain will also guide the choice of treatment.

   b. Medications

      1) Administer medications routinely vs. PRN (as needed) to manage pain that is expected to last for an extended period of time.

      2) Use caution when administering medications to newborns less than 2 to 3 months of age because of immature liver function.

c. Nonpharmacologic Measures

   1) Positioning

   2) Reinforcing breathing and relaxation techniques

   3) Splinting

   4) Maintaining a calm environment (low noise, reduced lighting)

   5) Providing ice to swollen or injured area

   6) Offering warm blankets

   7) Assisting with guided imagery

   8) Offering distractions (video games, cartoons, movies)

   9) Providing comfort with physical contact (holding, rocking)

   10) Administering sucrose pacifiers for infants during procedures

ANALGESIA FOR CHILDREN

ROUTE	NURSING IMPLICATIONS
Oral	Oral medications take 1 to 2 hr to reach peak analgesic effects. These medications are not suited for children experiencing pain that requires rapid relief or pain that is fluctuating in nature.
Topical/ transdermal	Eutectic mixture of local anesthetics (EMLA) contains equal quantities of lidocaine and prilocaine in the form of a cream or disk. › Use for any procedure in which the skin will be punctured (IV insertion, biopsy) 60 min prior to a superficial puncture and 2 hr prior to a deep puncture. › Place an occlusive dressing over the cream after application. › Prior to the procedure, remove the dressing or disk and clean the skin. An indication of an adequate response is reddened or blanched skin. › Demonstrate to the child that the skin is not sensitive by tapping or scratching lightly. › Instruct parents to apply at home prior to coming to a health care facility for a procedure. Fentanyl › Use for children older than 12 years of age. › Use to provide continuous pain control. It has an onset of 12 to 24 hr and a duration of 72 hr. › Use an immediate-release opioid for breakthrough pain. › Treat respiratory depression with naloxone (Narcan).
Continuous intravenous (IV)	Use provide stable blood levels.
Patient-controlled analgesia (PCA)	Use to control pain from injury and chronic conditions. Administer morphine, fentanyl, and hydromorphone (Dilaudid). Allow child to control if appropriate. Designate one family member or one nurse to control.

IV Safe Medication Administration

A. Overview

1. Organ system immaturity affects drug sensitivity in infants and children.

   a. Newborns and young infants may have intense and prolonged responses to medications.

   b. In comparison to adults, medications administered by IM injection are absorbed more slowly in newborns, but faster in infants.

B. Pediatric-Specific Considerations of Safe Medication Administration

1. **Right client:** Verify the client's identification each time a medication is administered.

   a. Infants and young children cannot be relied upon to identify themselves.

   b. Young children may answer to any name that is called. A parent or guardian should be asked to identify an infant or young child.

2. **Right dose:** Calculate the correct medication dose; many pediatric medication doses will be weight-based. Check medication reference to ensure the dose is within the safe and therapeutic range. Have a second nurse check if unsure or if facility policy requires it.

3. **Right route:** If administering an oral medication, the nurse should use a pediatric-approved medication administration device. The nurse should also educate parents not to use household measuring devices for medication administration.

C. Collaborative Care

1. **Nursing Interventions**

   a. Adaptations for Oral Medication Administration to Children

      1) The oral route is preferred for children.

      2) Strategies

         a) When administering the medication, hold the child in a semi-reclining position to prevent aspiration.

         b) A needleless syringe provides the most accurate measurement of dose. Droppers vary in size and should not be used to measure the medication unless the dropper has been provided with the medication.

         c) Administer the medication with the needleless syringe if the dose is less than a teaspoon and/or the medication is thick. Place the syringe along the side of the infant/child's tongue. Administer in small amounts to allow the infant/child time to swallow between amounts.

         d) Do not provide medication in a bottle.

         e) Avoid using a cup because medication may stick to the cup and could spill.

         f) Do not mix a medication with formula or breast milk.

         g) Avoid mixing a medication with any food because child may not eat all of food.

   b. Other Adaptations for Administering Medications to Children

      1) Otic administration

         a) Pull the auricle down and back when instilling otic solutions for children up to 3 years of age. Pull the auricle up and back for older children.

         b) Warm otic solutions to room temperature before instilling.

      2) Subcutaneous and Intradermal Medication Administration

         a) Apply a eutectic mixture of local anesthetics (EMLA) in the form of a cream or disk 60 min prior to injection.

         b) Ensure the amount of medication injected is appropriate for the child's amount of subcutaneous tissue (approximately 0.5 mL for infants and up to 2 mL in the adolescent).

         c) Subcutaneous injection sites are the same for all ages.

         d) Select the smallest syringe possible for the dose.

         e) Use a 26- to 30-gauge needle.

      3) Intramuscular (IM) Medication Administration

         a) Apply EMLA in the form of a cream or disk a minimum of 60 min, preferably 2 to 2.5 hr, prior to injection.

         b) Ensure the amount of medication injected is appropriate for the child's muscle size (approximately 0.5 mL for infants and up to 2 mL in the adolescent).

         c) The preferred IM injection site for infants and small children is the vastus lateralis. The ventrogluteal may also be used. The dorsogluteal is not a safe site until sufficiently developed.

         d) Use the smallest syringe that will accommodate the dose.

         e) Use a 0.5- to 2-inch needle, depending upon the child's body size.

      4) Intravenous (IV) Medication Administration

         a) Short-term use may decrease pain/fear from injections.

         b) Long-term use may require home administration and family education.

         c) Restraints used only if needed; allow maximum safe ROM.

V Adapting Care for the Child Experiencing Surgery

A. **Assess parents' and child's understanding.**

B. **Involve parents as appropriate.**

C. **Teach at the developmental level of the child.**

   1. Dolls

   2. Books

   3. Tours

D. **Document findings, including behaviors, to compare postoperatively.**

VI Nursing Care of Children: Death and Dying

A. Overview

1. The death of a child may be traumatic and devastating for a family.

2. Children, regardless of age, will experience grief and loss, which is expressed sporadically through behavior and play and is present for a long period of time.

CHILDREN'S RESPONSE TO DEATH/DYING

AGE	RELEVANT FACTORS
Infants/toddlers (birth to 3 years)	Have little to no concept of death
	Have egocentric thinking that prevents them from understanding death (toddlers)
	Mirror parental emotions (sadness, anger, depression, anxiety)
	React in response to the changes brought about by being in the hospital (change of routine, painful procedures, immobilization, less independence, separation from family)
	May regress to an earlier stage of behavior
Preschool children (3 to 6 years)	Have egocentric thinking
	Have magical thinking that allows them to believe that their thoughts can cause an event such as death (may feel guilty and shameful)
	Interpret separation from parents as punishment for bad behavior
	Because the preschooler does not have a concept of time, the permanence of death is not understood. The preschooler will not understand that death is "forever."
School-age children (6 to 12 years)	Start to respond to logical or factual explanations
	Begin to have an adult concept of death (inevitable, irreversible, universal). This generally applies to school-age children who are older (9 to 12 years)
	Experience fear of the disease process, the death process, the unknown , and loss of control
	› Fear is often displayed through uncooperative behavior.
	May be curious about funeral services and what happens to the body after death
Adolescents (12 to 20 years)	May have an adultlike concept of death
	May have difficulty accepting death because they are discovering who they are, establishing an identity, and dealing with issues of puberty
	Rely more on their peers rather than the influence of their parents, which may cause the reality of a serious illness to cause adolescents to feel isolated
	May be unable to relate to peers and communicate with their parents
	May become more stressed by changes in physical appearance from the medications or illness than the prospect of death
	May experience guilt and shame

B. Collaborative Care

1. **Nursing Interventions:** Terminally Ill Children

CARE FOR TERMINALLY ILL CHILDREN

CARE	FOCUS
Hospital care	The child cannot be managed at home (the family does not want or is not able to provide necessary care, the child requires intensive nursing care).
Home care	A home care agency nurse provides assessments, treatments, medications, supplies, and equipment under the direction of the health care provider.
Hospice care	The psychological, spiritual, physical, and social needs of the child and family will be managed.
	Family members providing most of the care with support from the hospice team.
	Priority is given to pain and symptom control.
	Support to the family will continue post-death. Family needs will be addressed after death occurs.

a. Allow an opportunity for anticipatory grieving, which affects the way a family will cope with the death of a child.

b. Offer primary nursing.

c. Offer strategies specific to developmental level.

STRATEGIES FOR CARING FOR TERMINALLY ILL CHILDREN

AGE GROUP	DEVELOPMENTAL APPROACH
Infants and toddlers	Encourage parents to stay with the child.
	Attempt to maintain a normal environment.
Preschoolers	Encourage parents to stay with the child.
	Communicate with the child in honest, simple terms.
	Be aware of medical jargon that may frighten the child.
School-age children	Encourage parents to stay with the child.
	Use language that is clear regarding the disease, medications, procedures, and expectations.
	Encourage self-care to promote independence and self-esteem.
	Allow participation in plans for funeral services.
Adolescents	Be honest and respectful when communicating.
	Encourage self-care to promote independence and self-esteem.
	Allow participation in plans for funeral services.
	Encourage parents or other family members to stay with the adolescent.

d. Provide information to the child and family about the disease, medications, procedures, and expected events.

e. Encourage and support parents to participate in caring for the child.

f. Encourage parents to remain near the child as much as possible.

g. Encourage the child's independence and control as developmentally and physically appropriate.

h. Allow for visitation of family and friends as desired.

i. Emphasize open, honest communication among the child, family, and health care team.

j. Provide support to the child and family with decision making.

k. Provide opportunities for the child and family to ask questions.

l. Assist the child with completion of unfinished tasks.

m. Assist parents to cope with their feelings and help them to understand the child's behaviors.

n. Use books, movies, art, music, and play therapy to stimulate discussions and provide an outlet for emotions.

o. Provide and encourage professional support and guidance from a trusted member of the health care team.

p. Remain neutral and accepting.

q. Give reassurance that the child is not in pain and that all efforts are being made to maintain comfort and support of the child's life.

r. Recognize and support the individual differences of grieving. Advise families that each member may react differently on any given day.

s. Give families privacy, unlimited time, and opportunities for any cultural or religious rituals. Respect the family's decisions regarding care of the child.

t. Encourage discussion of special memories and people, reading of favorite books, providing favorite toys/objects, physical contact, sibling visits, and continued verbal communication, even if the child seems unconscious.

u. After death, validate the loss.

v. Issues and decisions to be addressed when appropriate include the following:

1) Organ and/or tissue donation if applicable

2) Autopsy

3) Viewing of the body

4) Sibling's attendance at the funeral

SECTION 4

Nursing Care of the Child with a Congenital Anomaly

A. **Congenital Heart Disease**

1. Contributing Factors

   a. Maternal factors

      1) Rubella in early pregnancy

      2) Alcohol and/or other substance abuse during pregnancy

      3) Diabetes mellitus

   b. Genetic factors

      1) History of congenital heart disease in other family members

      2) Trisomy 21 (Down syndrome)

      3) Presence of other congenital anomalies or syndromes

CONGENITAL HEART ANOMALIES

ANOMALY	HEMODYNAMICS	MANIFESTATIONS	TREATMENT
Defects with Increased Pulmonary Blood Flow			
Patent ductus arteriosus A vascular channel between the left main pulmonary artery and the descending aorta, as a result of failure of the fetal ductus arteriosus to close	Shunt of oxygenated blood from the aorta into the pulmonary artery Increased left ventricular output and work load	Usually asymptomatic, but frequent impairment of growth or heart failure "Machinery murmur" Wide pulse pressure	Medical: administration of indomethacin (Indocin) (prostaglandin inhibitor) is effective in some newborns and premature newborns Surgical: ligation of patent ductus (in infancy)
Ventricular septal defect In membranous muscular portion of the ventricular septum; may vary from small to large defect	Shunt of oxygenated blood from left to right ventricle Leads to right ventricular hypertrophy Needs surgical repair Bidirectional shunting may occur with very large defect (Eisenmenger's complex)	May be asymptomatic Heart murmur is heard in first week of life (systolic) Growth failure, feeding problems during the first year of life; failure to thrive; frequent respiratory infections Heart failure	Some small defects may close spontaneously Open heart: direct closure suturing with plastic prosthesis (usually preschooler; may be done earlier in infancy for large defects)
Atrial septal defect Malfunctioning foramen ovale, or abnormal opening between the atria	Shunting of oxygenated blood from the left to right atrium Increased right ventricular output and work load May develop pulmonary hypertension in adulthood (if not surgically treated in childhood)	Acyanotic; asymptomatic Soft blowing, systolic murmur Thin and asthenic Frequent episodes of pulmonary inflammatory diseases Poor exercise intolerance	Open heart with direct closure or suturing with plastic prosthesis (usually preschooler)

ANOMALY	HEMODYNAMICS	MANIFESTATIONS	TREATMENT

Defects with Decreased Pulmonary Blood Flow

Tetralogy of Fallot Combination of four defects › Pulmonary stenosis › Ventricular septal defect (VSD) › Overriding aorta › Hypertrophy of right ventricle	Obstruction to outflow of blood from the right ventricle into pulmonary circuit and increased pressure in the right ventricle leads to right to left shunting of oxygenated blood through the VSD directly into the aorta Severity of defect depends on degree of pulmonary stenosis and size of VSD	Acute cyanosis at birth Cyanosis developing during early months that increases with physical exertion Clubbing of fingers and toes Systolic murmur Acute episodes of cyanosis and hypoxia called "tet spells" or hypercyanotic episodes occur if oxygen supply cannot meet demand (crying, exertion, exercise, feeding) Squatting Growth retardation	Surgical—Blalock-Taussig procedures; provides blood flow to pulmonary arteries from the left to right subclavian artery Repair—open heart closure of VSD and resection of stenosis; usually performed in the first 2 years of life.

Defects with Mixed Blood Flow

Transposition of great vessels (TGV) The aorta originates from the right ventricle and the pulmonary artery from the left ventricle	Two separate circulations without mixture of oxygenated and unoxygenated blood except through shunts Mixture of blood may occur through one or more septal defects › Ventricular septal defect (VSD) › Atrial septal defect (ASD) › Patent ductus arteriosus (PDA)	Usually deep cyanosis shortly after birth or after closing of ductus Early clubbing of toes and fingers Poor growth and development, failure to thrive Rapid respirations; fatigue Heart failure	Prostaglandin medications are given to keep ductus arteriosus open until surgery. Prostaglandin inhibitors are given to close duct. Repair—arterial switch treatment of choice; must be done within the first few days of life; great vessels reimplanted under complete circulatory arrest Several other types of repair are all multiple stage approaches

Defects with Obstructive Blood Flow

Coarctation of aorta Preductal constriction of the aorta between subclavian artery and ductus arteriosus Postductal constriction of aorta directly beyond the ductus	Obstructions of the flow of blood through the constricted segments Increased left ventricular pressure and work load Extensive collateral circulation bypasses coarctated area to supply lower extremities with blood	Hypertension in upper extremities with decreased blood pressure in lower extremities Weak or absent pulsations in lower extremities Heart failure May be asymptomatic; occasionally fatigue, headaches, leg cramps, epistaxis	Surgical resection of coarctated area with direct anastomosis or use of a graft Correction usually done by 2 years of age to prevent permanent hypertension

B. **Heart failure (HF):** Impaired myocardial function

1. Contributing factors

    a. Structural anomalies such as septal defects

    b. Increased blood volume and pressure within the heart

    c. Decreased contractility of the heart

    d. Excessive demands on the cardiac muscle such as sepsis, and severe anemia

    e. Pulmonary congestion

2. Collaborative Care

    a. **Nursing Interventions**

        1) Conserve the child's energy by providing frequent rest periods; clustering care; providing small, frequent meals; bathing PRN; and keeping crying to a minimum in cyanotic children.

        2) Allow the child to sleep with several pillows.

        3) Allow the infant to rest during feedings, taking approximately 30 min to complete the feeding.

        4) Gavage feed the infant if he is unable to consume enough formula or breast milk.

        5) Closely monitor fluid balance with weight and I&O.

        6) Closely monitor for infections especially pulmonary.

        7) Assist family with adaptation.

    b. Medications

        1) Digoxin (Lanoxin): improves myocardial contractility

            a) The earliest sign of toxicity in infants and children is bradycardia. Hold if apical pulse is less than 90/min for infants; less than 70/min for children.

            b) Observe for other early signs of toxicity such as vomiting or poor feeding.

            c) If given as a PO liquid, provide oral care if teeth are present to prevent tooth decay.

        2) Captopril (Capoten) or enalapril (Vasotec)

        3) Furosemide (Lasix) or chlorothiazide (Diuril)

    c. Client Education and Referrals

        1) Dietitians should be consulted to assist the family with appropriate food choices.

C. **Down Syndrome**

1. Manifestations at birth (vary by client)

  a. Head

    1) Small, abnormally shaped

    2) Eyes round or upward slanting; Brushfield spots

    3) Small low-set ears

    4) Flattened nose

  b. Heart murmur usually caused by AVSD

  c. Hands

    1) Single palm crease

    2) Short fingers

2. Manifestations in childhood (vary from client to client)

  a. Cognitive

    1) Slow learning

    2) Short attention span

    3) Poor judgement

  b. Visual problems

  c. Leukemia

  d. Hearing loss

  e. Frustration with inabilities

D. **Collaborative Care**

1. **Nursing Interventions**

  a. Assist with highest level of functioning through collaboration with health team: physician, physical therapy, occupational therapy, speech therapy, audiology, and educational system.

  b. Assist with genetic counseling and prenatal screening.

  c. Provide emotional support to family and client.

  d. Modify activity with health status.

E. **Club Foot**

1. Contributing Factors

  a. Positional (intrauterine crowding)

  b. Syndromic (associated with other deformities).

  c. Congenital anomalies

2. Manifestations

MANIFESTATIONS OF CLUBFOOT

DEFORMITY NAME	MANIFESTATION
Talipes equinovarus (most common)	Plantar flexion with feet bending inward
Talipes calcaneus	Dorsiflexion of feet with toes higher than heels
Talipes equinus	Plantar flexion of feet with toes lower than heels
Talipes varus	Inversion of feet (toes pointing toward midline)
Talipes valgus	Eversion of feet (toes pointing laterally)

3. Diagnostic Procedures

  a. Prenatal ultrasound: used to identify the deformity

  b. Radiograph: used to determine bone placement and tissue involvement for clubfoot

4. Collaborative Care

  a. **Nursing Interventions**

    1) Encourage parents to hold and cuddle the child.

    2) Encourage parents to meet the developmental needs of the child.

    3) If cast or harness is used, monitor skin, circulation, and neuromuscular function.

  b. Therapeutic Measures

    1) Management of clubfoot will depend upon the severity of the deformity.

    2) Passive exercise may be performed for a minor deformity.

    3) Serial casting is begun after birth before the newborn is discharged home. Weekly casting to stretch the skin and other structures of the foot is done until maximum correction is accomplished.

    4) Surgical intervention should occur if maximum correction is not achieved by 3 months of age.

  c. Client Education

    1) Reinforce teaching with the family about how to perform gentle stretching of the foot as prescribed.

    2) Reinforce teaching with the family about the importance of serial casting, cast care, and follow-up appointments.

F. **Developmental Dysplasia of the Hip (DDH):** A variety of disorders resulting in abnormal development of the hip structures; may be identified during prenatal or postnatal periods or early in childhood.

1. Contributing Factors

  a. Family history, gender, birth order, intrauterine position, and/or laxity of a joint.

  b. Intrauterine placement, mechanical situations (e.g., size of infant, multiple births, breech presentation), and genetic factors.

2. Manifestations

  a. Asymmetrical gluteal and thigh folds

  b. Limited abduction of hips; one knee that appears shorter when the infant is supine with thighs flexed at 90° toward the abdomen (Allis sign)

  c. For infants from birth to 3 months of age, the provider performs the Barlow and Ortolani tests

    1) Barlow test: The hips are taken through adduction (the thighs are brought toward the midline) and abduction, and an audible click or clunk is heard from the head of the femur on the affected hip, which can be moved from the socket.

    2) Ortolani test: The affected hip is then reduced back into the socket by manipulation of the joint.

  d. For children able to walk, observe postural gait

    1) Trendelenburg sign: Abnormal downward tilting of pelvis on the unaffected side when bearing weight on the affected side

    2) Waddling gait or abnormal lordosis of spine if bilateral dislocation

3. Diagnostic Procedures

   a. Ultrasound: Should be performed at 2 weeks of age to determine the cartilaginous head of the femur.

   b. X-ray: Can diagnose DDH in infants older than 4 months.

4. Collaborative Care

   a. **Nursing Interventions**

     1) Perform circulatory, neurovascular, and skin integrity assessments after cast and/or harness placement. Ensure proper positioning of Pavlik harness at all times.

     2) Assess and maintain the hip spica cast.

     3) Perform range of motion with the unaffected extremities.

     4) Use appropriate pain tool in planning care.

     5) Evaluate hydration status frequently.

     6) Assess elimination status daily.

   b. Therapeutic Measures

     1) A Pavlik harness can be used from birth up to 5 or 6 months of age, until the hip is determined, by radiograph, to be stable. Frequent follow-up will be needed for strap adjustment.

     2) Hip spica cast can be used for infants older than 6 months of age. It can also be used in children whose hips were not stabilized by use of the Pavlik harness. A short course of traction is sometimes used prior to the application of a hip spica cast.

   c. Client Education and Referrals

     1) Keep the Pavlik harness on continuously, except during bathing, if prescribed.

     2) Return for follow-up visits weekly at the start of therapy and then as needed.

     3) Reinforce teaching about skin care.

     4) Use a cotton shirt and cotton socks under the Pavlik harness to prevent irritation. Avoid powders and lotions.

     5) Position casts on pillows.

     6) Reinforce to parents the importance of monitoring color and temperature of toes on casted extremity.

     7) Encourage parents to hold and cuddle the child.

     8) Encourage parents to meet the developmental needs of the child.

     9) Reinforce teaching for discharge with emphasis on using appropriate equipment (stroller, wagon, car seat) for maintaining mobility.

G. **Hydrocephalus:** An imbalance in either absorption or production of cerebrospinal fluid within the intracranial cavity. Classification is either congenital or acquired. Usually diagnosed at birth or within 2 to 4 months of life. Often associated with other neural tube defect (myelomeningocele).

1. Contributing Factors

   a. Impaired absorption of cerebrospinal fluid (CSF) within the subarachnoid space

   b. Obstruction to the flow of CSF through the ventricular system

   c. Developmental malformations: neoplasm, infection, and trauma

2. Manifestations (categorized by age)

   a. Infant: increased head circumference, tense bulging anterior fontanel, distended scalp veins, high-pitched cry, irritability, feeding problems, discomfort when held

   b. Older child: headache, vomiting (especially in the morning), diplopia, blurred vision, behavioral changes, decreased motor function, decreased level of consciousness, seizures

3. Diagnostic Procedure

   a. May be detected on prenatal sonogram

   b. Clinical signs

     1) Increased intracranial pressure

     2) Increased head circumference

   c. Computed tomography or magnetic resonance imaging scan confirms diagnosis by showing excessive fluid in ventricles

4. Collaborative Care

   a. **Nursing Interventions**

     1) **Preoperatively**

       a) Institute seizure precautions.

       b) Provide frequent neurological checks.

       c) Measure head circumference by obtaining occipitofrontal measurement.

     2) **Postoperatively**

       a) Institute seizure precautions.

       b) Perform frequent neurological checks including lethargy, vomiting, and irritability.

       c) Measure head circumference daily.

       d) Position on nonoperative side; check anterior fontanel to determine positioning of the head; do not pump shunt without order.

       e) Decrease shunt infection.

         (1) Monitor for elevated vital signs, decreased level of consciousness, vomiting, and feeding problems.

         (2) Monitor the incision site frequently for manifestations of inflammation or leakage.

         (3) Implement care to meet physiologic and developmental needs.

b. Medications

   1) Administer IV antibiotics.

   2) Assist provider with intraventricular instillation of antibiotics.

c. Therapeutic Measures

   1) Surgical placement of a ventriculoperitoneal (VP) shunt

   2) Endoscopic third ventriculostomy-only used for children with a noncommunicating hydrocephalus.

d. Client Education and Referrals

   1) Reinforce teaching with caregivers to recognize signs and symptoms of shunt malfunction.

   2) Reinforce teaching with caregivers to recognize signs and symptoms of infection as well as how to prevent infection.

   3) Reinforce teaching with caregivers of safe transportation and positioning of child.

   4) Reinforce teaching with caregivers how to pump shunt when necessary.

   5) Collaborate with home health when indicated.

   6) Collaborate with the National Hydrocephalus Foundation and the Hydrocephalus Foundation.

NOTE: Arbitrary pumping of the VP shunt can cause obstruction and should be avoided unless ordered by the physician.

NOTE: Shunts will need to be routinely replaced as the child grows.

H. **Neural Tube Defects**

1. Types

a. Myelomeningocele (Spina Bifida): A spinal defect, in which a fissure in spinal column is open, leaving meninges and spinal cord exposed; the sac also includes spinal fluid and nerves. The level of impairment depends on the level of the neural tube defect on the spine.

b. Meningocele: A spinal defect and saclike protrusion are present, but only spinal fluid and meninges are present in the sac. After the sac is repaired, no further symptoms are usually seen because spinal nerves are not damaged.

2. Contributing Factors (etiology unknown)

a. Failure of posterior laminae to fuse with herniation of saclike cyst of meninges, cerebrospinal fluid, spinal nerves

b. Usually associated with other neurological defects (hydrocephalus)

c. May be prevented by folic acid supplementation for women of childbearing age prior to conception and through first trimester

d. Collect data for family history of neural tube defects

3. Manifestations

a. Partial to complete paralysis determined by location of defect (usually lumbosacral)

b. Musculoskeletal problems such as clubfoot, scoliosis, congenital hip dysplasia

c. Varying degrees of sensory disturbances

d. Parallel motor dysfunction

e. Bowel and bladder problems including constipation, incontinence, and neurogenic bladder

4. Diagnostic Procedure

a. An elevated maternal serum alpha-fetoprotein is a screening tool for neural tube defects.

b. Amniocentesis: 98% accurate; elevated amniotic alpha-fetoprotein, confirmed by prenatal sonogram.

c. Apparent at birth: visible sac.

d. MRI, ultrasound, and CT are used to determine the degree and causative factors of NTDs.

e. Early closure of myelomeningocele when possible.

5. Collaborative Care

a. **Nursing Interventions**

   1) **Preoperatively**

     a) Priority of care is to preserve integrity of sac.

       (1) Keep infant in prone position.

       (2) Cover sac with 4 × 4 gauze moistened with sterile saline.

       (3) Check sac frequently for tears or cracks.

       (4) Do not cover sac with clothing or diapers.

     b) Prevent infection.

       (1) Perform perineal care to prevent contamination of sac.

       (2) Monitor for manifestations of meningitis such as irritability, anorexia, fever, and seizures.

   2) **Postoperatively**

     a) Preserve neurological integrity.

       (1) Place the infant in a prone position with head slightly lower than body.

       (2) Monitor for manifestations of increased intracranial pressure.

       (3) Perform neurological checks by measuring head circumference daily.

       (4) Promote effective parental and familial coping strategies.

     b) Prevent infection.

       (1) Place a protective barrier across the incision to prevent contamination.

       (2) Monitor for signs of infection.

b. Therapeutic Measures

   1) Pressure is relieved by surgically inserting a VP shunting device for associated hydrocephalus.

   2) Early treatment is necessary to prevent progressive mental retardation.

   3) Decision to correct the defect or not is difficult as well as controversial.

   4) Early surgical closure is advocated to preserve neural function, reduce risk of infection, and control hydrocephalus.

c. Client Education and Referrals

   1) Reinforce teaching with parents about how to use the Credé maneuver.

   2) Encourage independent intermittent self-catheterization, which can be performed as early as 5 to 6 years of age.

   3) Stress hydration and early recognition of urinary tract infections.

   4) Explain to parents that urinary diversion procedures are often required.

   5) Refer to appropriate disciplines for optimal outcomes

     a) Orthopedics

     b) Physical therapy

     c) Neurosurgery

     d) Pediatrics

     e) Urology

     f) Physical therapy

     g) Rehabilitation services

     h) Social services

NOTE: Children who have neural tube defects are at increased risk for latex allergy to common medical (or other) products containing latex. Avoid latex gloves and balloons.

I. **Cerebral Palsy**

1. Contributing Factors

  a. Causes undetermined; may be related to prenatal, perinatal, or postnatal factors

  b. Birth asphyxia

  c. Prenatal brain abnormalities

2. Manifestations (Early): Parents should be instructed to report any of these symptoms immediately.

  a. Persistent primitive reflexes

  b. Hyper- or hypotonicity (stiff or floppy arms and legs)

  c. Poor hand control and body control

  d. Feeding difficulties

  e. Irritability

  f. Delayed attainment of developmental milestones

3. Diagnostic Procedures

  a. Classified by nature and distribution of neuromuscular dysfunction

  b. May not be diagnosed until child is several months old

  c. Confirmed by physical evaluation or supplemental tests (electroencephalogram test, tomography, or metabolic screening)

4. Collaborative Care

  a. **Nursing Interventions**

    1) Institute seizure precautions if appropriate.

    2) Encourage physical safety techniques such as aspiration precautions and adequate rest.

    3) Encourage self-care activities to foster independence and confidence.

    4) Modify the environment and introduce devices to enhance development, enhance safety, and increase functional abilities.

  b. Medications

    1) Administer anticonvulsants and antispasmodics if ordered.

    2) Administer antibiotics and analgesics as ordered pre- and postoperatively

  c. Therapeutic Measures

    1) Treatment (based on degree of disability)

    2) Physical therapy (active and passive)

    3) Occupational therapy

    4) Potentially speech therapy

    5) Modified toys or equipment to enhance development

    6) Modify the environment to enhance safety

    7) Surgery to correct contractures or spastic deformities

  d. Client Education and Referrals

    1) Refer to occupational and speech therapy for evaluation and development of verbal and nonverbal communication skills.

    2) Encourage alternative communication methods to facilitate positive adjustments of child and family.

J. **Gastrointestinal Structural Disorders—see following chart.**

CONGENITAL GASTROINTESTINAL DISORDERS

Hypertrophic pyloric stenosis

DESCRIPTION AND CONTRIBUTING FACTORS	A thickening of the pyloric sphincter. There is a genetic component.	
MANIFESTATIONS	**Vomiting** that often occurs 30 to 60 min after a meal and becomes projectile as obstruction worsens **Constant hunger** **Olive-shaped mass** in the right upper quadrant of the abdomen and possible peristaltic wave that moves from left to right when lying supine	**Failure to gain weight and signs of dehydration**, such as skin that is dry and/or pale, cool lips, dry mucous membranes, decreased skin turgor, diminished urinary output, concentrated urine, thirst, rapid pulse, sunken eyes, and decreased blood pressure
DIAGNOSTIC PROCEDURES	Ultrasound of the abdomen. An ultrasound will reveal an elongated, sausage-shaped mass and an elongated pyloric area.	
NURSING INTERVENTIONS	Position the child on her side or with her head elevated when vomiting to prevent aspiration. Document the amount and characteristics of vomitus, and describe vomiting behavior to aid in diagnosis of etiology. Monitor fluid and electrolyte balance to assess for deficits. Daily weight and I&O	Monitor IV fluid replacement Nothing by mouth Monitor NG tube Preoperative teaching Postoperative care including NG tube and NPO until bowel sounds return
MEDICATIONS	Analgesics	
THERAPEUTIC MEASURES	Surgical incision into the pyloric sphincter (pylorotomy)	
CLIENT EDUCATION AND REFERRALS	Parents will need to know signs and symptoms of dehydration Parents will need to know to observe the incision and identify signs of infection	Demonstrate proper hand hygiene techniques. Encourage the parents to be active in the care of the child.

Hirschsprung's disease (congenital aganglionic megacolon)

DESCRIPTION AND CONTRIBUTING FACTORS	Occurs when a section of the colon is aganglionic. Stool accumulates in this aganglionic section.	
MANIFESTATIONS	**Newborn** – Failure to pass meconium within 24 to 48 hr, refusal to eat, episodes of vomiting bile, and abdominal distention **Infant** – Failure to thrive, constipation, abdominal distention, episodes of vomiting and diarrhea **Older child** – Constipation, abdominal distention, visible peristalsis, ribbon-like stool, palpable fecal mass, and a malnourished appearance	
DIAGNOSTIC PROCEDURES	Rectal biopsy Full-thickness biopsies to reveal the absence of ganglion cells	
NURSING INTERVENTIONS	Position the child on her side or with her head elevated when vomiting to prevent aspiration. Document the amount and characteristics of vomitus, and describe vomiting behavior to aid in diagnosis of etiology. Monitor fluid and electrolyte balance to assess for deficits.	Provide oral care after the child vomits to prevent damage to teeth from hydrochloric acid contact. Preoperative teaching Postoperative care including NG tube and NPO until bowel sounds return
MEDICATIONS	Analgesics PRN Antibiotics per prescription	
THERAPEUTIC MEASURES	Surgical removal of the aganglionic section (colostomy may be temporary). Serial rectal irrigation may be used to decompress the bowel prior to surgery.	
CLIENT EDUCATION AND REFERRALS	Parents will need to know signs and symptoms of dehydration Parents will need to know to observe the incision and identify signs of infection Demonstrate proper hand hygiene techniques.	Encourage the parents to be active in the care of the child. Reinforce teaching with parents about feeding/nutrition information. If present, reinforce teaching with parents about colostomy care.

CONGENITAL GASTROINTESTINAL DISORDERS (CONTINUED)

Intussusception

DESCRIPTION AND CONTRIBUTING FACTORS	The telescoping of the intestine upon itself. Intussusception is not a congenital condition but often occurs with congenital conditions such as cystic fibrosis.
MANIFESTATIONS	Normal comfort interrupted by periods of sudden and acute pain Palpable, sausage-shaped mass in the right upper quadrant of the abdomen and/or a tender, distended abdomen Stools that are mixed with blood and mucus that resemble the consistency of red currant jelly
DIAGNOSTIC PROCEDURES	Ultrasound, barium enema
NURSING INTERVENTIONS	Position the child on her side or with her head elevated when vomiting to prevent aspiration. Document the amount and characteristics of vomitus, and describe vomiting behavior to aid in diagnosis of etiology. Monitor fluid and electrolyte balance to assess for deficits. Provide oral care after the child vomits to prevent damage to teeth from hydrochloric acid contact. Assess for current jelly stools. Preoperative teaching Postoperative care related to procedure
MEDICATIONS	Proton pump inhibitors (Prilosec) H_2 receptor antagonist (Zantac) Antibiotics per prescription
THERAPEUTIC MEASURES	Surgical reduction if inflating the bowel with air or administering a barium enema is not successful
CLIENT EDUCATION AND REFERRALS	Reinforce teaching with parents about signs and symptoms to report if recurrence occurs, especially in the first 72 hr after enema or postoperative. Reinforce teaching with parents that prognosis is excellent if treated early. Parents will need to monitor the incision and monitor for signs of infection. Demonstrate proper hand hygiene techniques. Encourage the parents to be active in the care of the child.

Cleft lip (CL) and cleft palate (CP)

DESCRIPTION AND CONTRIBUTING FACTORS	**Multifactorial**, but there are strong indicators of genetic or environmental factors **Cleft palate** is more common in males **Cleft lip** is more common in females and may or may not be accompanied by cleft palate **Heredity** (as the incidence of cleft palate is higher in relatives of people with the defect) **Teratogens** (especially maternal intake of phenytoin [Dilantin]), maternal smoking, and family tendency)
MANIFESTATIONS	Cleft lip is visible. Cleft palate alone may only be visible when examining the mouth. Individuals are prone to ear, nose, and throat infection. Long-term problems include speech, hearing, and dentition problems.
DIAGNOSTIC PROCEDURES	Cleft lip visible Cleft palate palpated during the newborn assessment.
NURSING INTERVENTIONS	**Preoperative nursing care** Monitor respiratory status and ease of respiratory effort. Keep suction equipment and bulb syringe at bedside. Encourage the parents to express feelings. Monitor ability to suck and swallow. Follow precautions during feedings. Modify feeding techniques utilizing obturators, special nipples, and feeders. Feed in upright position in frequent, small amounts; burp frequently. Monitor I&O. Weigh daily. **Postoperative nursing care** Monitor for respiratory distress. Maintain suture integrity. Provide age-appropriate activities. Preserve suture line. Restrain elbows. Avoid sucking. Cleanse suture after each feeding. Maintain airway and prevent aspiration. Provide support to the parents.
MEDICATIONS	Antibiotics and pain medications as ordered
THERAPEUTIC MEASURES	Repair usually completed by 12 to 18 months of age to prevent speech problems. Surgery may be performed in stages.
CLIENT EDUCATION AND REFERRALS	Reinforce teaching with parents about appropriate feeding and prevention interventions prior to discharge. Encourage the parents to verbalize feelings, and offer emotional support.

Nursing Care of the Child with an Acute Condition

A. **Fever:** Temperature in excess of 38°C (100.4°F)

1. Contributing Factors

   a. Not always related to severity of illness; varies by child

   b. Age of the child (below 6 months is a more serious concern)

   c. Child who is immunosuppressed or receiving chemotherapy

   d. Most fevers in children are viral and self-limiting; may play a role in recovery from infection

2. Manifestations

   a. May vary secondary to the source of fever

3. Diagnostic Procedures

   a. Feeling a child's skin for warmth is not an accurate indicator.

   b. Always investigate family epidemiology and take a careful history for exposure to communicable diseases.

   c. Diet, activity level, and behavioral changes are subtle diagnostic clues.

   d. Laboratory tests may include CBC, urinalysis, chest film, and blood cultures.

      1) A "septic workup" includes all of the above with the addition of a lumbar puncture and urine culture.

4. Collaborative Care

   a. **Nursing Interventions**

      1) Maintain fluid and electrolyte balance.

      2) Monitor for signs of dehydration.

      3) Provide IV fluids.

      4) Monitor renal function.

      5) Frequently assess temperature.

      6) Encourage clear liquids.

      7) Expose skin and avoid excessive clothing.

      8) Provide safe care during febrile seizure.

         a) Maintain airway.

         b) Prevent aspiration and injury.

         c) Observe the seizure.

   b. Medications

      1) Fever management is questionable because fever is considered a part of the body's defense mechanism.

      2) Antipyretics, such as acetaminophen (Tylenol) or ibuprofen (Motrin), should be given in weight-appropriate dose.

      3) No aspirin is allowed due to the risk of Reye syndrome.

   c. Client Education

      1) Reinforce teaching with parents about

         a) seizure precautions.

         b) fever control.

         c) preventing dehydration.

         d) how to correctly measure temperature (age appropriate).

         e) how to manage febrile seizures (ensure safety and call 911).

B. **Vomiting**

1. Contributing Factors: Vomiting causes a loss of hydrochloric acid, which leads to metabolic alkalosis.

   a. Short-term illness such as a virus

   b. Children with GERD

   c. Related to medications or treatments such as chemotherapy

   d. Postoperative nausea

2. Manifestations

   a. Emaciation

   b. Dry skin and mucous membranes

   c. Sunken fontanels or lack of tears in infants

   d. Lethargic

   e. Potential metabolic alkalosis

   f. Poorly perfused

   g. Hyperventilating

3. Diagnostic Procedures: The following may be done for prolonged or unusual emesis.

   a. Upper GI series

   b. CT of abdomen

   c. pH probe

   d. Esophagoscopy

4. Collaborative Care

   a. **Nursing Interventions**

      1) Monitor and document:

         a) Amount, color, and consistency of emesis.

         b) Time and frequency of emesis.

         c) Relationship to meals or medication.

      2) Monitor for signs of dehydration.

      3) Maintain fluid and electrolytes.

      4) Adhere to strict I&O and daily weights.

      5) Maintain NPO status until asymptomatic.

      6) Introduce clear liquids slowly and frequently.

      7) Monitor for metabolic alkalosis.

   b. Medications

      1) OTC and prescription medications to treat nausea and vomiting are usually not recommended for infants and young children.

      2) IV fluids if indicated

C. **Gastroenteritis (Diarrhea):** Expelled forcefully; Na⁺, K⁺, and bicarbonate are lost via the stool. Diarrhea is serious in young children because dehydration can occur very rapidly.

1. Contributing Factors
   a. Bacteria (salmonella or shigella)
   b. Viral (rotavirus), allergies
   c. Emotional disturbances
   d. Dietary and malabsorption problems
   e. Chronic nonspecific diarrhea

2. Manifestations
   a. An increase in fluid, frequency and volume of stool
   b. Usually results from increased rate of peristalsis
   c. Stools that are watery, acidic, green in color
   d. Weight is a critical indicator of fluid loss in young children.
      1) 1 g of weight equals 1 mL of body fluid; a weight loss or gain of 1 kg in a 24-hr period represents a fluid shift of 1,000 mL.
   e. The loss of fluid and electrolytes in the diarrhea stool results in dehydration and electrolyte depletion.

3. Diagnostic Procedures
   a. Serum electrolytes
   b. CBC
   c. Blood cultures
   d. Antibiotic therapy is a common cause of diarrhea; obtain a thorough history including dietary habits, family history, recent travel, or exposures to contagious illness.

4. Collaborative Care

   a. **Nursing Interventions**
      1) Monitor for signs of dehydration or poor skin turgor.
      2) Maintain fluid and electrolyte balance.
      3) Monitor daily weights and strict I&O.
      4) Apply skin barrier (zinc products).
      5) Monitor for metabolic acidosis.
      6) Maintain NPO status until asymptomatic.
      7) Introduce clear liquids slowly and frequently. Oral rehydration solutions are recommended. Avoid apple juice.
      8) Administer antidiarrheal as prescribed.
   b. Therapeutic Measures
      1) Mild dehydration (2% to 9%) without hypernatremia; generally treated with oral rehydrating solutions; critical behaviors that demand immediate attention are persistent diarrhea, weight loss, bloody stools, or physiological changes such as deep breathing, listlessness, or reduced urinary output.
      2) Secondary lactose intolerance may occur following gastroenteritis; child may be maintained temporarily on a lactose-free diet.
      3) Stool cultures may be indicated.

D. **Infections**

1. **Acute otitis media** (most prevalent childhood disease)
   a. Contributing Factors
      1) Middle ear infections are common in children under age 5; breastfed infants have decreased incidence.
      2) Eustachian tube is shorter, wider, and straighter.

   b. Manifestations: Fever; irritability; pulling, tugging or rubbing the affected ear; anorexia; signs of a upper respiratory infection; older children may report earache or pain when chewing or sucking; purulent discharge may be present.

   c. Diagnostic Procedure
      1) Otitis media: otoscopy reveals an intact tympanic membrane that appears inflamed, bulging, and without a light reflex.
      2) Chronic otitis media: otoscopy reveals dull, gray membrane with visible fluid behind eardrum.

   d. Collaborative Care
      1) **Nursing Interventions**
         a) Administer analgesics such as acetaminophen and ibuprofen as needed. Topical pain ear drops such as benzocaine may be used. Warm compresses may be soothing. Avoid foods that require chewing.
         b) Monitor for nonverbal signs of discomfort; changes in behavior can be an early indicator of pain.
      2) Medications
         a) Oral antibiotics are not always required. If they are used, parents should know to continue use until entire dose is given.
         b) Amoxicillin (Amoxil) is commonly administered. If child is sensitive to penicillin or has a resistant infection, another antibiotic may be used, such as the cephalosporin ceftriaxone (Rocephin).
         c) Oral decongestants such as sympathomimetics (vasoconstriction) or antihistamines (reduce congestion) may be used with caution in children over 2 years of age. They should not be used for children 2 or younger. Analgesics such as acetaminophen may be used for pain.
         d) Following completion of the antibiotic regimen, treatment effectiveness should be evaluated.
      3) Therapeutic Measures
         a) Children with recurrent otitis media should be tested for hearing loss.
         b) Myringotomy (surgical incision of the ear drum) and insertion of pressure-equalizing (PE) tubes may be ordered in cases of recurrent chronic otitis media
      4) Client Education and Referral
         a) Reinforce teaching with parents regarding the importance of antibiotic compliance; medication should be taken for 10 to 14 days (even after manifestations have gone away).
         b) Reinforce teaching with parents in feeding techniques to reduce the incidence of ear infection (upright when feeding; breast-feeding offers protection against pathogens).
         c) Eliminate tobacco smoke and known or potential allergens from environment.
         d) Following myringotomy and PE tubes insertion, some drainage from the ears is expected; report obvious bleeding and an abrupt rise in temperature; the ear should be kept dry; avoid activities that require submerging the head in water (use earplugs for bathing).

COMMUNICABLE DISEASES GUIDE

TRANSMISSION	INCUBATION	MANIFESTATIONS	TREATMENT AND NURSING INTERVENTIONS	PREVENTION
Bacterial epiglottitis (*H. influenza* – ages 2 to 8 years)				
Direct contact or droplet	Probably less than 1 week	Sudden onset of sore throat and dysphagia. Child often sits up, leaning forward (tripod position) and drools. There is usually a high fever.	Do NOT place anything in the mouth or throat. Monitor for respiratory distress; have emergency cart in room. Administer humidified oxygen; maintain NPO; administer antibiotics, steroids, bronchodilators, antipyretics.	HIB vaccine
Conjunctivitis – viral or bacterial				
Direct transmission from fingers or other objects. In newborn may be transmitted via vaginal canal.	Days to weeks (varies with contaminate)	Bacterial: purulent discharge, swollen lids, conjunctivitis (pink eye), itching Viral: as with bacterial, but discharge may be serous.	Isolate from cause and prevent spread to opposite eye and others; antibiotics for bacterial; warm moist compress to remove discharge and crusting.	Best prevention is good hand washing and avoid contact with eyes. Newborns: erythromycin at birth.
Epstein-Barr infectious mononucleosis (EBV – common in adolescence)				
Direct contact with saliva	10 days to 6 weeks	May be mild: headache, fatigue, anorexia, mild fever. If progresses, liver and spleen enlargement may occur.	Symptomatic relief; bed rest; no contact sports if hepatomegaly or splenomegaly occur.	Avoid contact with saliva (straws, sharing utensils, kissing). Stay healthy—diet and exercise.
Erythema infectiosum (fifth disease/human parvovirus [HPV] B19)				
Droplet and blood	4 to 21 days	"Slapped face"; maculopapular rash appears on extremities proximal to distal. Fever, malaise, vomiting may occur.	Symptomatic relief; bed rest; acetaminophen for pain or fever; antihistamines for itching with children over 2 years. Immunoglobulins may be used if the child has other health problems.	Hand washing, standard precautions.
Impetigo contagiosa (*Streptococcus* or *Staphylococcus*, including MRSA common in toddler and preschooler)				
Intact skin provides a barrier to these common bacteria. Infection may occur when skin is broken by bites, scratches, or other trauma. May occur as a secondary infection when a child has pruritus. May occur with intact skin. Contact transmission.	1 to 3 days	Begins as macular rash, changing to papular then vesicular. Vesicles rupture leaving a moist ulcerated lesion which will form a honey-colored crust. Itching. Generally heal without scarring.	May clean with mild soap and water or a solution such as Burrows. Topical antibiotic. If severe may use systemic antibiotics.	Do not share towels or other linens. Clients with impetigo should use a clean towel with each hand washing. Wash hands thoroughly after touching lesions.
Laryngotracheobronchitis (Croup – commonly Parainfluenza virus)				
Droplet and contact	2 to 3 days	Fever, hoarseness, sore throat, and cough often described as a "barking seal." Respiratory distress sometimes occurs.	Keep child hydrated. Provide humidified air. Bed rest. If child requires hospitalization, suction and emergency intubation equipment should be kept at the bedside. Monitor respiratory status frequently. Medications may include acetaminophen, bronchodilators, corticosteroids, and epinephrine.	Good hand hygiene. Avoid contact with sick people. Keep children well-hydrated and healthy. Avoid respiratory irritants such as secondhand smoke.

TRANSMISSION	INCUBATION	MANIFESTATIONS	TREATMENT AND NURSING INTERVENTIONS	PREVENTION
Meningitis – viral or bacterial (*H. influenza* – 3 months to 3 years; meningococcal meningitis)				
Direct invasion via otitis media, upper respiratory infection, head injury	2 to 10 days	Onset abrupt with fever, headache, irritability, altered level of consciousness, nuchal rigidity, increased intracranial pressure; must do lumbar puncture to isolate organism.	Isolate; reduce environmental stimuli; monitor hydration; seizure precautions; IV antibiotics	Rifampin given to contacts of client with meningococcal meningitis as prophylaxis
Mumps – viral (paramyxovirus)				
Saliva, direct contact or droplet	14 to 21 days	Prodromal stage—headache, malaise, anorexia, followed by earache; parotitis 3 days later with pain/tenderness	Symptomatic and supportive; analgesics; antipyretics; hydration	MMR
Pediculosis capitis (head lice) – Pediculus humanus capitis				
Sharing of personal items (hair ornaments, caps, hats)	Eggs hatch in 7 to 10 days	Intense itching; can visually see nits attached to base of hair shafts; differentiate from dandruff.	Do not share personal items. Shampoo with anti-lice products; wash linens and clothing in hot water Caution: medicated shampoos may be neurotoxic.	Caution children about sharing hair items.
Pertussis (whooping cough) – _Bordetella pertussis_				
Respiratory droplets and direct contact	7 to 21 days	Initially "cold" manifestations; progresses to spasms or paroxysmal coughing (whooping cough)	Antibiotics; corticosteroids; supportive care; isolation; stay with child during coughing spells	DTaP
Rabies – viral				
Contact with saliva of infected animal	10 days to 3 months	Prodromal—malaise, sore throat followed by hypersensitivity, excitation, convulsions, paralysis; high mortality	Irrigate wound; psychological follow-up	Avoid contact with wild animals; rabies shot (given after exposure).
Respiratory syncytial virus (RSV) – common under 1 year				
Direct and droplet	5 to 8 days	Early: symptoms of URI. If progresses, may develop bronchiolitis and respiratory distress.	Usually managed at home with hydration, rest, and symptomatic relief. Medications may include steroids, bronchodilators, and Virazole (antiviral aerosol).	Avoid tobacco smoke. Promote hand hygiene. Palivizumab (Synagis) may be given for at-risk children or children with recurrent RSV infections.
Reye syndrome				
Reye syndrome is not an infection or a communicable disease. It is a possible response to a viral infection.	Usually occurs after recovery from a viral infection but may occur earlier.	Prodromal—malaise, cough, upper respiratory infection. 1 to 3 days after fever—decreased level of consciousness, hepatic and cerebral dysfunction; high mortality	Monitor live function; peak age 4 to 11 years; neurological assessments; intracranial pressure monitoring	Avoid the use of aspirin in adolescents and children.
Rheumatic fever – Group A beta-hemolytic strep				
Nasopharyngeal secretions; direct contact with infected person or droplet spread	1 to 3 weeks after acute infection, develops inflammatory disease	Carditis, arthritis, chorea (involuntary ataxic movements), subcutaneous nodules, erythema marginatum (rash)	Bed rest in acute phase to decrease cardiac workload; full course of antibiotics (penicillin/erythromycin); high dose of aspirin therapy (monitor for toxicity tinnitus)	Adequate, prompt treatment of strep infection (must finish entire course of therapy)

TRANSMISSION	INCUBATION	MANIFESTATIONS	TREATMENT AND NURSING INTERVENTIONS	PREVENTION
Roseola (exanthem subitum) – viral (human herpes virus type 6)				
Unknown (limited to children 6 months to 2 years of age)	Unknown	Persistent high fever for 3 to 4 days; precipitous drop in fever with appearance of rash (rose-pink maculopapule on trunk, then spreading to neck, face, and extremities); lasts 1 to 2 days	Antipyretics to control temperature and prevent febrile seizures; hydrate	None
Rubella (German measles) – viral (rubella virus)				
Nasopharyngeal secretions—direct contact, indirect via freshly contaminated nasopharyngeal secretions or urine	14 to 21 days	Prodromal phase; absent in children, present in adults; rash; first face and rapidly spreads downward to neck, arms, trunk, and legs; teratogenic to fetus	No treatment necessary; isolate child from pregnant women; women of childbearing years should have rubella titer done	MMR
Rubeola (measles) – viral				
Respiratory—airborne	10 to 21 days	Prodromal stage—fever and malaise, coryza, conjunctivitis, Koplik's spots (spots with blue/white center on buccal mucosa opposite molars); rash that starts on the face, spreads downward, may desquamate (peel)	Antipyretics to control temperature and prevent seizures; dim lights if photophobia; respiratory precautions	MMR
Scabies – *Sarcoptes scabiei*				
Direct contact with the person or objects the infected person has touched.	Mites will begin laying eggs shortly after contact.	Streaking (burrows), itching	Medications may be neurotoxic. Follow directions closely. All clothes and bedding should be washed in hot water and dried in a hot dryer.	Do not share personal clothing or bedding.
Scarlet fever – Group A beta-hemolytic strep				
Nasopharyngeal secretions, direct contact with infected person or droplet spread	2 to 4 days	Prodromal stage—abrupt high fever, pulse increased, vomiting, chills, malaise, abdominal pain; enanthema—tonsils enlarged, edematous reddened, covered with patches of exudate; strawberry tongue; exanthema—rash appears 12 hr after prodromal signs	Full course of antibiotics (penicillin/erythromycin); isolate; monitor for rheumatic fever; glomerulonephritis hydrate	Adequate, prompt treatment of strep infection (must finish entire course of therapy)
Tetanus – *Clostridium tetani*				
Deep puncture, not contagious, "anaerobic"	7 to 14 days	Gradual stiffening of voluntary muscles until rigid (lockjaw, rigid abdomen); sensitive to stimuli; clear sensorium	Eliminate stimuli; monitor respirations, blood gases; muscle relaxants; monitor hydration	DTaP, Td
Varicella (chickenpox – varicella zoster virus)				
Direct, contact with contaminated objects, airborne	2 to 3 weeks	Malaise and low fever followed by a rash progressing from macular to papular to vesicular lesions. Spreads from face to proximal extremities. Itching.	At-risk child may receive immunoglobulins and antiviral. Symptomatic relief. Contagious until all lesions have scabbed. Pregnant women should not be in contact. Shingles may occur later in life.	Immunization. Isolation of infected clients.

NURSING CARE FOR COMMON CHILDHOOD INFECTIONS

Fill in the blanks.

A nurse is assigned to provide care for each of the following clients. Which client should the nurse see first? Which prioritizing guideline is used? Complete the table below.

Client	LIKELY CAUSE OF INFECTION	PRECAUTIONS REQUIRED IN ADDITION TO STANDARD	PRIORITY NURSING CARE AND PREVENTION
1. Child A, a 6-month-old who has a maculopapular red rash and slight excoriation on the buttocks.			
2. Child B, a 2-year-old who is drooling while sitting with arms propped against the bed table.			
3. Child C, a 4-year-old who has crusty drainage from the left eye.			
4. Child D, a 6-year-old who has liquid brown stools for 2 days.			

Answers

Prioritization: Child B who has symptoms of epiglottis should be seen first (ABCs). The airway could become obstructed. Immediate referral/reporting is required. Child D who has diarrhea for 2 days is the second priority (Maslow). Children are at high risk for dehydration and fluid and electrolyte imbalances. Child C might have a localized infection requiring precautions and treatment (Maslow). Child A has signs of diaper dermatitis requiring topical treatment, frequent diaper changes, and consoling.

1. Child A. Likely cause of infection: Candida albicans. Precautions: Standard. Priority Nursing Care: Decrease irritation to the area and prevent future infection. Keep diapers dry. If using cloth diapers, launder in mild soap. Clean area with water. Avoid soap and disposable wipes. Do not rub area. Leave area open to air to dry thoroughly prior to re-diapering. To relieve itch, bathe in oatmeal bath. Zinc oxide or petroleum jelly may be applied to protect and lubricate the area and to make future cleaning easier. Antifungal ointment such as nystatin (Micostatin) can be needed. Steroid creams can reduce inflammation but will not rid the infection. Prevention: Continue the diaper care as outlined. There is no vaccine.

2. Child B. Likely cause of infection: Bacterial epiglottitis, possibly Haemophilus influenzae type B. Precautions: Droplet. Priority Nursing Care: Maintain patent airway. Do not place anything in mouth/throat. NPO. Provide humidity, IV fluids, and antibiotics. Signs and symptoms: Dysphagia, drooling, sitting in tripod position. Agitation and change in LOC can occur if O_2 levels are affected. There is usually no coughing. Prevention: HIB vaccine.

3. Child C. Likely cause of infection: Bacterial or viral conjunctivitis. Precautions: Standard unless there is copious drainage, then use contact. Priority Nursing Care: This child is 4 and might understand the need to prevent spreading the infection to the other eye and others. Reinforce hand hygiene. Warm compresses and "milking" the tear duct can help decrease the drainage. If drops or ointment is prescribed, reinforce proper administration. Prevention: Reinforce to the child to avoid touching eyes.

4. Child D. Likely cause of infection: Rotovirus (likely). Precautions: Contact. Priority Nursing Care: Monitor for dehydration, electrolyte imbalances, and metabolic acidosis. Monitor fever and other symptoms. Typically, fluids will be replaced with clear liquids. If severe, electrolyte solutions and IV fluids will be used. Prevention: Three-step oral vaccine.

E. **Tonsillectomy and Adenoidectomy (T&A)**

1. Tonsils help protect body from infections; typically enlarged in children

2. Contributing Factors

   a. Chronic tonsillitis (controversial)

   b. Massive hypertrophy that interferes with breathing (obstructive apnea)

3. Collaborative Care

   a. **Nursing Interventions**

      1) **Preoperative**

         a) Monitor bleeding and coagulation time.

         b) Confirm child is free from current infection.

         c) Prepare the child.

   2) **Postoperative**

      a) Hemorrhage risk is greatest in the first 48 hr and then at 7 days after procedure.

         (1) Manifestations include frequent swallowing, clearing the throat, bright red emesis, change in level of consciousness, and shock.

         (2) Prevention: Avoid coughing, sneezing, blowing the nose, or placing any object in the mouth other than clear liquids. Avoid suctioning. If nausea is present, use an antiemetic to prevent vomiting.

      b) Offer cool fluids to decrease edema and to relieve pain.

b. Medications

   1) Administer analgesics regularly first 24 hr—acetaminophen (Tylenol); may require rectal or parenteral route due to throat pain

c. Client Education and Referrals

   1) Child may return to school in 1 to 2 weeks.

   2) Child should avoid: Avoid red-colored foods. Avoid pretzels, crackers, chips, and dairy products.

F. Appendicitis

1. Manifestations

  a. Periumbilical pain radiating to right-lower quadrant; rebound tenderness; positive McBurney's sign; abdominal guarding

  b. Fever, may be low-grade

  c. Nausea and vomiting

  d. Elevated WBC count

  e. May perforate and lead to peritonitis; sudden relief of pain followed by increased pain and rigid abdomen; high fever

> **NOTE:** If appendicitis is suspected, avoid laxatives or applying heat to the area.

2. Collaborative Care

  a. **Nursing Interventions**

    1) **Preoperative nursing care**

      a) Provide pain relief.

      b) Perform abdominal assessment frequently.

      c) Maintain NPO status.

      d) Provide fluid and electrolyte balance.

      e) Provide patient and family education for diagnostic tests such as CT scan and blood work.

    2) **Postoperative nursing care**

      a) Monitor vital signs and perform abdominal assessment frequently.

      b) Monitor for signs of infection.

      c) Promote mobility.

      d) Promote respiratory toileting.

  b. Medications

    1) Provide analgesics as ordered.

G. Accidental Ingestion of Toxic Substances

1. Provide emergency care—ABCs.

2. Identify substance; save evidence of poison.

3. Call poison control center for treatment advice.

4. Remove substance.

  a. Activated charcoal

  b. Gastric lavage

  c. Specific antidote

5. Provide supportive therapy.

6. Reinforce teaching with parents to childproof environment.

7. Evaluate event to rule out intentional abuse or a suicide attempt.

8. Provide anticipatory guidance.

  a. Infants and toddlers: at risk because everything goes into the mouth

  b. Adolescents: at risk for intentional ingestion

9. Types of ingestions—see following chart.

OVERVIEW OF COMMON ACCIDENTAL INGESTION

MANIFESTATIONS	TREATMENT	NURSING INTERVENTIONS
Salicylate (Aspirin)		
Tinnitus	Emesis	Anticipatory guidance
Hyperpyrexia	Hydration	
Seizures	Vitamin K	Bleeding precautions
Bleeding	Activated charcoal	
Hyperventilation		
Acetaminophen (Tylenol)		
Liver necrosis in 2 to 5 days	Emesis	Liver assessment
Nausea	Mucomyst (antidote)	
Vomiting		
Pain in right upper quadrant		
Jaundice		
Coagulation abnormalities		
Hepatotoxic		
Lead (paint, soil near heavily traveled roads, household dust)		
Developmental regression	Chelation therapy—to remove heavy metals	Neurological assessment
Impaired growth (encephalopathy)		Diet high in calcium, iron
Irritability	Promote hydration	Educate the parents to wash the child's hands and toys, and to frequently remove lead dust
Increased clumsiness		
		Lead abatement
Hydrocarbons (kerosene, turpentine, gasoline)		
Burning in the mouth	Do not induce emesis	If vomiting, reduce aspiration
Choking and gagging	Activated charcoal	
CNS depression	Gastric lavage	
Corrosives (drain or oven cleaner, chlorine bleach, battery acid)		
Burning in the mouth	Do not induce emesis	Keep warm and inactive
White, swollen mucous membranes	Dilute toxin with water	
Violent vomiting	Activated charcoal	

H. **Burns**

1. Manifestations

   a. Due to the difference in proportions of head, trunk, and limbs, burn percentages are rated differently for children.

   b. Manifestations vary based on the TBSA, type and depth of burn.

   c. Due to the high percentage of extracellular fluids in the child, fluid loss can quickly lead to hypovolemic shock.

2. Collaborative Care

   a. **Nursing Interventions**

      1) Similar to adult with modifications in the fluid replacement formulas.

      2) Monitor for signs of infection.

      3) Monitor I&O.

      4) Perform dressing changes using sterile technique.

   b. Medications

      1) Administer IV fluids.

      2) Administer analgesics.

      3) Administer antibiotics.

      4) Administer nutritional supplements as ordered. Children are likely to resist eating enough calories to sustain healing and growth needs Parenteral or enteral feedings are usually necessary.

   c. Client Education and Referrals

      1) Reinforce teaching with parents how to recognize signs and symptoms of infection.

      2) Incorporate play into the physical or occupational therapy regimens for improved success.

      3) Consider psychosocial needs of the child.

      4) Adjustment and transition back to school may be very difficult for the child who has sustained a disfiguring burn.

      5) Ensure parents understand all instructions and have necessary follow-up appointments.

I. **Fractures**

1. Manifestations

   a. Due to immaturity of bones and incomplete ossification, greenstick (incomplete) fractures are commonly seen.

   b. Fractures to the epiphysis (growth plate) are of greater concern, as growth in limb can be stunted depending on the amount of injury.

2. Collaborative Care

   a. Therapeutic Measures

      1) Similar to adult, although pediatric fractures often have shorter healing times and may need to be replaced if the infant or child outgrows the cast

      2) May use cast (plaster or, more commonly, fiberglass), soft splint, traction, or bracing

Nursing Care of the Child with a Chronic Condition

A. **Immune Disorders**

1. Eczema

   a. Contributing Factors

      1) Etiology: May be hereditary and related to allergies.

      2) Family history is common.

   b. Manifestations

      1) Rash

      2) Pruritus

      3) Dry skin

      4) Secondary infection from scratching—often staph aureus

   c. Collaborative Care

      1) **Nursing Interventions**

         a) Hydrate skin.

            (1) Tepid baths daily with mild soap or oil followed by an emollient

         b) Relieve pruritus.

            (1) Wash cloths in mild detergent and rinse well.

            (2) Apply cool compresses.

            (3) Topical steroids, diphenhydramine, or hydroxyzine (Atarax) may reduce itching.

         c) Reduce flare-ups.

            (1) Encourage soft cotton clothing.

            (2) Encourage hypoallergenic diet (avoid dairy, eggs, chocolate, wheat).

         d) Prevent secondary infection.

            (1) Clip nails.

            (2) Keep hands clean and place cotton gloves or stockings on hands.

            (3) Monitor for honey-colored crust and other signs of infection over hands.

            (4) Administer antibiotics if infection occurs.

B. **Bronchial asthma**

1. Collaborative Care

   a. Nursing interventions as with an adult.

   b. Developmentally appropriate instructions for child; include family.

   c. Avoid triggers, including allergens and smoke.

   d. Plan activities and sports that require stop-and-start energy; teach use of medication related to activity.

   e. Reinforce teaching on use of a peak-flow meter to monitor airway status.

   f. Involve school staff, including coaches, in planning care.

C. **Rheumatic fever**

1. Manifestations

   a. Arthralgia; low-grade fever that spikes in the afternoon; hot, red, swollen joints (polyarthritis); tachycardia with precordial friction rub; subcutaneous nodules; truncal rash (erythema marginatum)

   b. Chorea

      1) Sudden, involuntary movements with involuntary facial grimaces

      2) Muscle weakness and speech disturbances

      3) Transitory; reassure parents that chorea will self-resolve

2. Diagnosis Procedure

   a. Elevated or rising antistreptolysin O (ASO) titer with elevated erythrocyte sedimentation rate (ESR)

   b. Jones criteria (presence of two major, or one major and two minor manifestations)

3. Collaborative Care

   a. **Nursing Interventions**

      1) Monitor vital signs.

      2) Control joint pain and inflammation with massage and alternating hot and cold applications.

      3) Provide bed rest in acute febrile phase.

      4) Initiate seizure precautions if child is experiencing chorea.

   b. Medications

      1) Provide prophylactic antibiotics with all dental work.

      2) Administer antibiotics and anti-inflammatory medications as prescribed.

   c. Client Education

      1) Reinforce teaching with parents about the importance of follow-up.

      2) Reinforce teaching with parents that prophylactic antibiotics may be required when the child is at increased risk of infection, such as dental work and other invasive procedures.

D. **Scoliosis**

1. Contributing Factors

   a. No apparent cause identified

2. Diagnostic Procedure

   a. Screening exam in school: child flexes at waist; one scapula more prominent

   b. Spinal x-ray

3. Collaborative Care

   a. **Nursing Interventions**

      1) Provide postoperative nursing care.

      2) Log roll for first 24 hr.

      3) Perform neurovascular assessments frequently.

      4) Promote pulmonary toileting.

      5) Provide pain management.

      6) Encourage age-appropriate activities.

   b. Therapeutic Measures

      1) Mild scoliosis (less than 20° curvature): observation, encourage physical exercise

      2) Moderate scoliosis (20° to 40° curvature): fitted Milwaukee brace

      3) Goal is to prevent worsening of curve

      4) Severe scoliosis (greater than 40° curvature): requires surgery

      5) Spinal fusion with instrumentation

      6) Requires prolonged immobilization in cast, brace, or body jacket

   c. Client Education and Referral

      1) Address developmental needs of client.

      2) Provide client teaching—skin care, commitment of therapy, and fashion concerns.

      3) Reinforce the importance of compliance with all follow-up appointments.

E. **Juvenile rheumatoid arthritis (JRA)**

1. Classification

   a. Systemic (fever, rash, and organomegaly in addition to joint involvement)

   b. Polyarticular (many joints)

   c. Pauciarticular (few joints)

2. Manifestations

   a. Swelling, thickening of joint

   b. Pain, stiffness, impaired range of motion

   c. Lethargy, weight loss

   d. Supportive treatment to maintain joint mobility

3. Collaborative Care

   a. **Nursing Interventions**

      1) Promote mobility and range of motion.

      2) Encourage nutritional intake.

      3) Provide pain relief (medication, heat, and cold).

      4) Monitor for exacerbation of symptoms.

   b. Medications

      1) NSAIDs

      2) Methotrexate

      3) Corticosteroids

F. **Type 1 diabetes mellitus**

1. Collaborative Care

   a. **Nursing Interventions**

      1) Monitor exercise patterns.

      2) Collect data about the child's, family's, and school's level of comfort with blood sugar monitoring as well as insulin administration.

         a) If using an insulin pump, assess that the catheter is changed at least every 3 days.

         b) Observe the child assess blood sugar and administer insulin.

      3) Collect data about psychosocial stresses.

4) Monitor the child's and family's ability to adapt care for sleepovers and meals away from home.

5) Provide information for glucagon administration. The child receiving glucagon may lose consciousness and vomit. The child should be placed side-lying to avoid aspiration.

6) Reinforce teaching about long-term complication avoidance and prevention.

7) Evaluate family and child's understanding of nutritional guidelines and reinforce education as needed.

   a) Plan meals to achieve appropriate timing of food intake, activity, onset, and peak of insulin. Calories and food composition should be similar each day.

   b) Eat at regular intervals and do not skip meals.

   c) Restrict calories and increase physical activity as appropriate to facilitate weight loss (for children who are obese or to prevent obesity).

   d) Include fiber in the diet to increase carbohydrate metabolism and to help control cholesterol levels.

8) Reinforce to the child about guidelines to follow when sick.

   a) Monitor blood glucose levels every 3 to 4 hr.

   b) Continue to take insulin or oral antidiabetic agents.

   c) Consume 4 oz sugar-free, noncaffeinated liquid every 0.5 hr to prevent dehydration.

   d) Meet carbohydrate needs by eating soft foods if possible. If not, consume liquids that are equal to the usual carbohydrate content.

   e) Test urine for ketones and report if abnormal (should be negative to small).

   f) Rest.

9) Call the provider if:

   a) Blood glucose remains above 240 mg/dL or if urinary ketones remain high.

   b) Fever higher than 38.9°C (102°F), fever does not respond to acetaminophen (Tylenol), or fever lasts more than 12 hr.

   c) Disorientation or confusion occurs.

   d) Rapid breathing is experienced.

   e) Vomiting occurs more than once.

   f) Diarrhea occurs more than five times or for longer than 24 hr.

   g) Liquids cannot be tolerated.

   h) Illness lasts longer than 2 days.

10) Teach the child measures to take in response to signs and symptoms of hypoglycemia.

G. **Hemophilia**

1. Contributing Factors

   a. Deficiency of clotting factors

   b. Sex-linked recessive trait more common in males

   c. Factor VIII and IX are most common deficiencies

   d. Hemarthrosis (bleeding into joint cavities), bruises easily

2. Manifestations

   a. Bleeding into subcutaneous and intramuscular tissue

   b. Hemarthrosis characterized by swelling, warmth, redness, pain, and loss of movement in joints

   c. Bruising

3. Collaborative Care

   a. **Nursing Interventions**

      1) Control bleeding.

      2) Provide supportive therapy.

      3) Immobilize joint.

      4) Provide ice packs.

   b. Medications

      1) Administer Cryoprecipitate (transfusion that replaces missing clotting factor)

      2) Risk for AIDS and/or hepatitis is decreased because of screening, but does still exist.

   c. Client Education

      1) Safety is directed toward developmental level to prevent injury, bleeding.

      2) Avoid contact sports (difficult for children).

      3) Childproof environment.

      4) Avoid aspirin.

      5) Provide parental education and support.

H. **Sickle cell anemia**

1. Contributing Factors

   a. Sickling occurs in response to

      1) Infection, stress

      2) Dehydration

      3) Decreased oxygen

      4) High altitude

2. Types of crisis

   a. Vaso-occlusive: "hand-foot syndrome" caused by stasis of blood in capillaries; schema and infarction

   b. Sequestration: pooling of large amounts of blood in liver, spleen; hypovolemia and shock

3. Manifestations

   a. Shortness of breath, fatigue

   b. Tachycardia, pallor, jaundice

   c. Lethargy, irritability, weakness

   d. Pain, nausea, vomiting, anorexia

   e. Swelling, fever

4. Collaborative Care
   a. **Nursing Interventions**
      1) Provide hydration.
      2) Provide oxygen as needed.
      3) Administer analgesics, antibiotics as prescribed.
      4) Reduce stress of hospitalization.
      5) Provide parental support.
   b. Medications
      1) Analgesics
   c. Therapeutic Measures
      1) Eliminate cause of crisis.
      2) Blood transfusions
         a) Monitor complications:
            (1) Anemia
            (2) Splenic sequestration
            (3) Cerebrovascular accidents

I. **Renal Disorders**—see following chart.

RENAL DISORDERS

	Nephrotic Syndrome	Acute Glomerulonephritis
OTHER NAMES	Childhood nephrosis	Poststreptococcal glomerulonephritis
CONTRIBUTING FACTORS	Cause unknown; likely autoimmune	Antigen–antibody reaction secondary to infection elsewhere in the body; usually a streptococcus ß-hemolytic, group A of the upper respiratory tract
INCIDENCE	Average age of onset about 2.5 years; more common in boys	Two-thirds of cases are in children who are under 4 to 7 years; more common in boys
PATHOLOGY	Increased permeability of the glomerular membrane to protein	Inflammation of the kidneys; damage to the glomeruli allows excretion of RBCs
MANIFESTATIONS	Edema—appears insidiously; usually first noticed in the eyes and can advance to the legs, arms, back, peritoneal cavity, and scrotum; massive proteinuria; anorexia; pallor	Periorbital edema—appears insidiously; tea-colored urine from hematuria; hypertension; oliguria
BLOOD PRESSURE	Usually normal; transient elevation may occur early	Varying degrees of hypertension may be present; when blood pressure is elevated, cerebral manifestations may occur as a result of vasospasm; these may include headache, drowsiness, diplopia, vomiting, convulsions
DIAGNOSTIC PROCEDURES	Urine shows heavy hematuria	Urine contains RBCs; has a high specific gravity
DIAGNOSTIC LAB	Involves reduction in protein (mainly albumin); gamma globulin is reduced; during the active stages of the disease, the sedimentation rate is greatly increased	BUN value is elevated; anemia (reduction in circulating RBCs, in Hgb, or both) tends to develop rapidly
MEDICATIONS AND TREATMENTS	Prednisone Furosemide (Lasix) Salt-poor albumin	Antibiotics for strep infection Diuretics and antihypertensives used to remove accumulated fluid and manage hypertension. **Nursing Interventions** › Monitor blood pressure. › Monitor I&O. › Monitor for electrolyte imbalances, such as hypokalemia. Observe for side effects of medications. › Corticosteroids

	Nephrotic Syndrome	Acute Glomerulonephritis
NURSING INTERVENTIONS	Control edema; provide skin care; prevent infection; monitor nutrition (low sodium, high protein, high potassium); monitor urine for proteinuria; monitor for side effects from steroid therapy. Provide rest. Monitor I&O. Monitor urine for specific gravity and protein. Monitor daily weights; weigh the child on the same scale with the same amount of clothing. Monitor edema and measure abdominal girth daily. Measure at the widest area, usually at or above the umbilicus. Assess degree of pitting, color, and texture of skin. Monitor and prevent infection. Assist the child to turn, cough, and deep breathe to prevent pulmonary involvement. Monitor vital signs, especially temperature, for changes secondary to infection. Maintain good hand hygiene. Administer antibiotic therapy as prescribed. Encourage nutritional intake within restriction guidelines. Salt and fluids may be restricted during the edematous phase. Increase protein in diet to replace protein losses. Cluster care to provide for rest periods. Monitor skin for breakdown areas. Prevent pressure sores. Avoid use of urinary collection bags in very young children. Pad bony prominences or use a specialty mattress to reduce breakdown of skin. Encourage frequent turning and repositioning of the child. Keep the child's skin dry. Elevate edematous body parts.	Monitor I&O. Monitor daily weights Weigh the child on the same scale with the same amount of clothing daily. Monitor vital signs. Monitor neurological status and observe for behavior changes, especially in children who have edema, hypertension, and gross hematuria. Implement seizure precautions if condition indicates. Encourage adequate nutritional intake within restriction guidelines. A regular diet with elimination of high-sodium foods will be appropriate for most. Restrict foods high in potassium during periods of oliguria. Provide small, frequent meals of favorite foods due to a decrease in appetite. Manage fluid restrictions as prescribed. Fluids may be restricted during periods of edema and hypertension. Monitor skin for breakdown areas and to prevent pressure sores. Encourage frequent turning and repositioning. Keep skin dry. Pad bony prominences and use a specialty mattress. Elevate edematous body parts. Monitor tolerance for activity. Provide for frequent rest periods. Monitor and prevent infection. Advise the child to turn, cough, and deep breathe to prevent pulmonary involvement. Monitor vital signs, especially temperature, for changes secondary to infection. Maintain good hand hygiene.
COLLABORATIVE CARE	Refer the child for dietary consultation if indicated. Provide for age-appropriate diversional activities. Consult child life specialist. Cluster care to facilitate rest and tolerance of activity. Provide emotional support.	Refer the child for dietary consultation if indicated. Provide for age-appropriate diversional activities. Consult child life specialist. Cluster care to facilitate rest and tolerance of activity. Provide emotional support.
CLIENT EDUCATION	Encourage the child to eat food high in potassium if potassium-sparing diuretics are not used. Inform the child and family that dizziness can occur with the use of antihypertensives. Encourage the child to verbalize feelings related to body image. Educate the child regarding appropriate dietary management. Educate the family about the need for follow-up care. The child should be seen by the provider weekly for several weeks and then monthly until the disease is fully resolved.	Encourage the child to eat food high in potassium if potassium-sparing diuretics are not used. Inform the child and family that dizziness can occur with the use of antihypertensives. Encourage the child to verbalize feelings related to body image. Reinforce education regarding appropriate dietary management. Reinforce education with the family about the need for follow-up care. The child should be seen by the provider weekly for several weeks and then monthly until the disease is fully resolved.

J. **Cystic fibrosis (CF)**

1. Contributing Factors

   a. Inherited disease

   b. Requires inheritance of two mutated CF genes, one from each parent

2. Manifestations

   a. Chronic respiratory infection

   b. Accumulation of sticky, thick mucus in the lungs, adventitious or decreased breath sounds, wheezing and chronic cough with blood streaking, changes in color and amount of sputum

   c. Stools pale or clay colored, foul smelling, float on surface of water

   d. Weight loss, failure to thrive in infants, abdominal swelling

   e. Excessive salt in sweat, dehydration

   f. Abdominal pain, flatulence

   g. Fatigue

   h. Clubbing of fingertips

3. Collaborative Care

   a. **Nursing Interventions**

      1) Monitor respiratory status; oxygenation, color, and amount of sputum.

      2) Provide consistent, scheduled chest physiotherapy and postural drainage with cough and deep breathing.

      3) Monitor daily weight and I&O.

      4) Provide small frequent feedings with pancreatic enzymes with each meal.

      5) Provide parental education and emotional support.

      6) Reinforce teaching with parents how to avoid exposing the child to infection, and to avoid environments containing smoke.

   b. Medications

      1) Hypoglycemic agents: Monitor blood glucose levels and administer hypoglycemic agents as prescribed.

      2) Bronchodilators (inhalers)

         a) Short-acting β_2-agonists, such as albuterol (Proventil), provide rapid relief.

         b) Cholinergic antagonists (anticholinergics), such as ipratropium (Atrovent), block the parasympathetic nervous system, providing relief of acute bronchospasms.

         c) Instruct the child and family in the proper use of an MDI, DPI, or nebulizer.

         d) Monitor the child for tremors and tachycardia when he is taking albuterol.

         e) Observe the child for dry mouth when taking ipratropium.

      3) Antibiotics

         a) Antibiotics are used to treat bacterial infections.

         b) The child should finish the full course of antibiotics.

      4) Dornase alfa (Pulmozyme)

         a) Decreases the viscosity of mucus and improves lung function.

         b) Monitor the child for improvement in PFTs.

         c) Reinforce teaching with the child about the use of a nebulizer.

         d) Reinforce teaching with the child to use once daily.

      5) Pancreatic enzymes: pancrelipase (Pancrease)

         a) Used to treat pancreatic insufficiency associated with cystic fibrosis.

         b) Capsules should be given with all meals.

         c) Capsules can be swallowed whole or sprinkled on food.

   c. Therapeutic Measures

      1) Encourage exercise.

      2) Pulmonary postural drainage, aerosol therapy, and treatment with antibiotics for infection.

      3) Pancreatic enzymes with meals and supplementation of fat-soluble vitamins—A, D, E, K (twice the normal daily age requirement). Give pancreatic enzymes in food.

      4) Free use of salt.

      5) Possible lung transplantation.

      6) Monitor for signs of pneumothorax in clients who have repeated infections.

   d. Client Education

      1) Ensure that the family has information regarding access to medical equipment.

      2) Provide teaching about equipment prior to discharge.

      3) Reinforce teaching with the family about ways to provide CPT and breathing exercises. For example, a child can stand on her head by using a large, cushioned chair placed against a wall.

      4) Promote regular primary care provider visits.

      5) Emphasize the need for up-to-date immunizations with the addition of an initial seasonal influenza vaccine at 6 months of age and then yearly.

      6) Promote regular physical activity.

      7) Encourage the family to participate in a support group and use community resources.

   e. Referrals

      1) Respiratory therapy, social services, and dietitians may be involved in the care of a child who has cystic fibrosis.

K. **Celiac disease**

1. Manifestations

   a. Diarrhea

   b. Large bulky stools

   c. Anemia

   d. Delayed growth and development

   e. Frequent infection

   f. Malabsorption of vitamin D

2. Diagnostic Procedure

   a. Bowel biopsy

3. Collaborative Care

   a. **Nursing Interventions**

      1) Monitor weight and dietary intake.

      2) Monitor I&O during acute episodes of diarrhea.

      3) Provide gluten-free diet.

   b. Medications

      1) Administer fat-soluble vitamins A, D, E, and K.

   c. Therapeutic Measures

      1) Provide emotional support.

      2) Collaborate with nutritionist.

   d. Client Education

      1) Instruct the parents to avoid giving the child foods made with gluten; also, avoid barley, rye, oats, wheat (BROW diet).

L. **Leukemia**

1. Manifestations

   a. Leukemic infiltrate

   b. Limb and joint pain

   c. Lymphadenopathy

   d. CNS involvement

   e. Hepatosplenomegaly/bleeding tendencies

   f. History of frequent infection and fever

   g. Decreased platelet and RBC count

   h. Increased immature WBCs

   i. Anemia, pallor, and fatigue from decreased RBCs, headache

   j. Low-grade fever

   k. Petechiae and epistaxis from decreased platelets

2. Diagnostic Procedure: Bone marrow aspiration reveals hypercellular marrow, abnormal cells.

3. Collaborative Care

   a. **Nursing Interventions**

      1) Take complete history and perform physical assessment.

      2) Monitor for anorexia, headache, and fatigue.

      3) Monitor vital signs and oxygenation.

      4) Monitor CBC, temperature fluctuations.

      5) Monitor for signs of infection.

      6) Weigh daily.

      7) Monitor I&O.

      8) Provide support care related to chemotherapy.

      9) Provide Age-Appropriate anticipatory guidance to the child and family.

         a) Teach family and child about therapeutic measures (below), infection prevention, and pain management.

      10) Provide emotional support and appropriate referrals.

      11) Complex home care management will be needed.

   b. Medications

      1) Chemotherapy

      2) Corticosteroids

      3) Hematopoietic growth factors

      4) Antimicrobials (prophylactically or for infection)

      5) Antifungals (prophylactically or for infection)

   c. Therapeutic Measures

      1) Lumbar puncture for analysis of CSF

      2) Ultrasound for liver and spleen infiltration

      3) Baseline liver and kidney function studies

      4) Radiation therapy for CNS involvement

M. **Nephroblastoma (Wilms' tumor):** Type of renal cancer with a peak age of 3 years

1. Contributing Factors

   a. Certain genetic conditions or birth defects can increase risk. Arises from embryonal tissue.

   b. Children at risk should be screened for Wilms' tumor every 3 months until age of 8 years.

2. Manifestations

   a. Most common clinical sign is swelling; mass within the abdomen

   b. Anemia, hypertension, hematuria

3. Diagnostic Procedure

   a. IV pyelogram

   b. Computerized tomography

   c. Bone marrow to rule out metastasis

4. Collaborative Care

  a. **Nursing Interventions**

    1) Preoperative care

      a) Support parents, and keep explanations simple.

      b) Monitor blood pressure due to excess renin production.

      c) Prevent rupture of encapsulated tumor.

      d) Post sign on bed: DO NOT PALPATE ABDOMEN.

      e) Bathe and handle child gently.

    2) Postoperative care

      a) Monitor vital signs, respiratory status, and oxygenation status.

      b) Monitor blood pressure.

      c) Monitor dressing for bleeding.

      d) Provide pain management.

      e) Monitor urinary output and kidney function; dipstick urine for protein or blood.

      f) Provide age-appropriate developmental support and emotional support to parents.

  b. Therapeutic Measures

    1) Nephrectomy and adrenalectomy

    2) Radiation and chemotherapy determined by staging

5. Manifestations

  a. Abdominal mass, urinary retention and frequency, lymphadenopathy, generalized weakness, and malaise

  b. Primary site is abdomen, most often in flank area

6. Diagnostic Procedures

  a. Computerized tomography

  b. Bone marrow to determine metastasis

  c. Excessive catecholamine production

7. Collaborative Care

  a. **Nursing Interventions**

    1) Monitor vital signs, height, and weight.

    2) Monitor I&O and nutritional status.

    3) Monitor for developmental delays related to illness.

    4) Provide education and support to child and family.

    5) Make appropriate referrals.

    6) Provide age-appropriate diversional activities.

N. **Hodgkin's lymphoma:** Cancer of the lymphatic system primarily affecting adolescents and young adults; originates in the lymphoid system. Metastasis may include spleen, liver, bone marrow, and lungs.

  1. Diagnostic Procedure

    a. Computerized axial tomography

    b. Lymph node biopsy, exploratory laparotomy (to stage)

2. Collaborative Care

  a. **Nursing Interventions**

    1) Monitor vital signs, height, and weight.

    2) Monitor I&O and nutritional status.

    3) Monitor for developmental delays related to illness.

  b. Medications

    1) Administer chemotherapeutic agents as prescribed and according to established protocols.

  c. Therapeutic Measures

    1) Radiation and chemotherapy determined by clinical staging

    2) Surgical laparotomy

    3) Splenectomy

  d. Client education

    1) Provide education and support to child and family with a splenectomy regarding increased susceptibility to infection and chronic illness.

    2) Make appropriate referrals.

SECTION 7

CPR Guidelines for Infants and Children

A. **Key BLS Components**

> **NOTE:** Always refer to the American Heart Association for the most current updates and guidelines.

1. Child: Use AED as soon as available; use child pads or a child system for children ages 1 to 8 years, if available; if child pads are not available, use adult AED and pads.

2. Infant: AED is not recommended for infants less than 1 year of age.

B. **Obstructed Airway**

1. With a responsive victim:

  a. Infant: Use a combination of back blows and chest thrusts.

  b. Child and Adolescent: Use abdominal thrusts and Heimlich maneuver.

2. Remove large debris in oral cavity.

3. Do not reach into mouth of an infant unless the object is visible.

4. Place recovered child into recovery position.

5. Use calm approach with victim.

6. Administer oxygen as prescribed.

NURSING CARE OF CHILDREN: WHAT NURSING ACTION IS NEEDED?

Complete the table below for each client.

Client	DOCUMENT IN CHART? (YES/NO)	ADDITIONAL DATA TO COLLECT	REPORT TO RN? (YES/NO)	RATIONALE
1. A 2-day-old newborn exhibits head lag and resists arm extension.				
2. A 12-month-old infant weighs 6.8 kg (15 lb). Birth weight was 3.6 kg (8 lb).				
3. A 2-year-old client has otitis media and attended a birthday party yesterday.				
4. A 4-year-old client burned her left hand by placing it in boiling water.				
5. A 7-year-old child who has diabetes mellitus checks his own blood sugar.				
6. A 12-year-old girl asks how a condom is used.				
7. A 16-year-old who has a parvovirus infection wants to play in a school football game.				

Answers

1. Document in chart? Yes. Additional data to collect: Continue with routine assessment. Report to RN? No. Rationale: These are normal newborn findings in a full-term newborn.

2. Document in chart? Yes. Additional data to collect: Plot weight and height on growth chart. Report to RN? Yes. Rationale: Birth weight should double by 6 months and triple by 12 months. If the baby falls below the 5th percentile for weight/height, the infant might have failure to thrive. The PN should recognize this is a serious condition and report to the RN, who will do further evaluation (such as what the baby is eating at home) and refer as needed.

3. Document in chart? No (birthday party not relevant to condition). Additional data to collect: Eating, sleeping patterns; pain level. Ask if client uses a bottle and if there is smoke in the child's environment. Report to RN? No. Rationale: Otitis media (OM), in the absence of other infection, is not contagious. The child did not risk infecting other children at the birthday party. OM is usually painful and can affect eating and sleeping patterns. Use of a bottle can cause OM and is not recommended after 12 months of age. Cigarette smoke and other allergens can increase the risk of OM..

4. Document in chart? Yes. Additional data to collect: Pain, condition of hand, any other signs of injury. Report to RN? Yes. Rationale: This client might be a victim of abuse. The PN should report this situation to the RN for further assessment.

5. Document in chart? Yes. Additional data to collect: Watch child check blood sugar. Report to RN? No. Rationale: A 7-year-old is often old enough to check blood sugar. The nurse should watch the child to make sure it is done correctly.

6. Document in chart? Yes. Additional data to collect: Ask the girl if she is sexually active. Report to RN? Yes. Rationale: The PN does not do initial teaching, but this client needs more than teaching. The client is 12 and asking about birth control. This raises questions about abuse. Although the client is not unstable, the PN should refer this client to the RN. Additional assessment is required. (For example, has the child been molested?)

7. Document in chart? Yes. Additional data to collect: Ask about contacts while infected, fever, itching, and other discomforts. Report to RN? Yes. Rationale: The RN will need to provide teaching about transmission (droplet and blood). Playing in the game can spread the infection to teammates. In addition, the client needs bedrest. Parvovirus causes erythema infectiosum, or Fifth Disease. A client can exhibit a "slapped" face appearance with a rash. Fever and extreme fatigue may occur.

References

American Diabetes Association. (n.d.). www.diabetes.org.

American Heart Association. (n.d.). www.heart.org.

American Cancer Society. (n.d.). www.cancer.org.

Centers for Disease Control and Prevention. (n.d.). www.cdc.gov.

Hockenberry, M. J., & Winkelstein M. L. (2013). *Wong's essentials of pediatric nursing* (9th ed.). St. Louis, MO: Mosby.

Ignatavicius, D. D., & Workman, M. L. (2013). *Medical-surgical nursing* (7th ed.). St. Louis, MO: Saunders.

Lehne, R. A. (2013). *Pharmacology for nursing care* (8th ed.). St. Louis: Saunders.

Lowdermilk, D. L., Perry, S. E., Cahsion, M. C., & Aldean, K. R. (2012). *Maternity & women's health care* (10th ed.). St. Louis, MO: Mosby.

Marquis, B. L., & Huston, C. J. (2012). *Leadership roles and management functions in nursing: Theory and application* (7th ed.). Philadelphia, PA: Lippincott Williams & Wilkins.

National Institutes of Health. (n.d.). www.nih.gov.

Potter, P. A., Perry, A. G., Stockert, P., & Hall, A. (2013). *Fundamentals of nursing* (8th ed.). St. Louis, MO: Mosby.

Smeltzer, S. C., Bare, B. G., Hinkle, J. L., & Cheever, K. H. (2010). *Brunner and Suddarth's textbook of medical-surgical nursing* (12th ed.). Philadelphia: Lippincott Williams & Wilkins.

Stanhope, M., & Lancaster, J. (2010). *Foundations of nursing in the community* (3rd ed.). St. Louis, MO: Mosby.

Varcarolis, E. M., Carson, V. B., & Shoemaker, N. C. (2010). *Foundations of psychiatric mental health nursing: A clinical approach* (6th ed.). St. Louis, MO: Saunders.

Index

Aplastic anemia, 123

APNs (advanced practice nurses), 14

Appendicitis, 245

Application questions, 4

ARBs (angiotensin II receptor blockers), 32

Arterial blood gases (ABGs), 84, 165

Arthritis, 108–110, 247

Arthroplasties, 113

Aseptic technique, 70

Asian American clients, culturally competent care for, 23–24

Asperger's syndrome, 175

Aspiration, 219, 221

Aspirin (salicylate), 245

Assault, 182

Assessments

of auditory disorders, 154

of burns, 160–161

in community health nursing, 20

in culturally competent care, 22

of disease risk, 73–74

of fall risk, 66, 75–76

of fetal development, 184, 186–187, 195–196

of genitourinary system disorders, 138

of herbal medications, 63

in mental health nursing, 170

of neurosensory disorders, 145–146

of newborns, 205–206

of ocular disorders, 153

of pain, 228

in postpartum care, 201–203

Assignment of duties, 13

Assistive devices for ambulation, 68–69

Assistive personnel (AP), 14

Asthma, 84–85, 246

Atelectasis, 93

ATT (authorization to test) emails, 2

Attention deficit/hyperactivity disorder (ADD/ADHD), 54, 175

Atypical antipsychotics, 174, 177

Audio format questions, 3

Auditory disorders, 154

Augmentation of labor, 199

Auscultatory method for checking feeding tubes, 96

Authorization to test (ATT) emails, 2

Autistic disorder, 175

Automobile safety. *See* Motor vehicle safety

Autonomy, defined, 16

Avoidant personality disorder, 177, 178

B

Bacterial epiglottitis, 241

Bacterial vaginosis (BV), 212

Bandages, 113

Bariatric surgery, 104

Barium series studies, 96

Barlow test, 233

Basilar skull fractures, 147

Battering stage of violence, 181

Behavioral models of development, 168, 169

Behavior disorders, 175–176

Beneficence, defined, 16

Benign prostatic hyperplasia, 143–144

Benzodiazepines, 173

Beta$_2$ adrenergic agonists, 36–37

Beta adrenergic blockers, 33–34

Betamethasone (Celestone), 60

Binge eating-purging, 180

Biophysical profiles (BPPs), 187

Biopsies, 96, 139

Bipolar disorder, 53, 177

Birth. *See* Labor and delivery

Birth control, 58–59, 211

Bisphosphonates, 50–51

Bizarre behaviors, 174

Black tag injuries, 21

Bland diets, 163

Blindness, 153

Blocking agents, 45

Blood and blood products, 42–43

Blood glucose levels, 166

Blood lipid levels, 166

Boards of nursing (BONs), 2, 17

Bodily harm to children, 219, 221, 222, 223

Body fluids and electrolytes, 79–84, 165

Body mass index (BMI), 223

Bone scans, 108

Borderline personality disorder, 177, 178

Bouchard's nodes, 108, 109

BPPs (biophysical profiles), 187

Brachytherapy, 157

"Brain attack," 149–150

Braxton Hicks contractions, 194

Breast cancer, 213

Breastfeeding, 29, 207

Breath tests, 95

Breech presentation, 193

Broad-spectrum antibiotics, 29

Bronchial asthma, 246

Bronchitis, 85–86

Bronchoscopy, 84

B$_{12}$ deficiency anemias, 124

Budget process, 12

Buerger's disease (thromboangiitis obliterans), 132

Bulimia nervosa, 180

Burns

assessment and management of, 160–161

children and, 219–220, 221, 222, 223, 246

Butterfly rash (erythematosus), 159

BV (bacterial vaginosis), 212

C

CAD (coronary artery disease), 127

Calcium channel blockers, 33

Calcium imbalances, 81

Calcium-modified diets, 165

Calculations and conversions, 28

Cancer

breast, 213

cervical, 212

classification of, 156

disease-related consequences of, 155–156

endometrial, 212–213

laryngeal, 87

leukemias, 156, 252

lung, 88

management of, 156–157

manifestations of, 156

ovarian, 213

overview, 155

pancreatic, 107–108

prostate, 144

renal, 252–253

risk factors for, 155

testicular, 144

Canes, 69

CAPD (continuous ambulatory peritoneal dialysis), 142–143

Capital budget, 12

Carbapenem-resistant enterobacteriaceae (CRE), 72

Carbon dioxide toxicity, 86

Carcinomas, 156

Cardiac catheterization, 126–127

Cardiac enzyme testing, 126

Cardiac glycosides, 34

Cardiogenic shock, 132

Cardiopulmonary resuscitation (CPR), 133, 253

Dietary supplements, 61–63

Diets and nutrition, 162–165

Digestive system disorders. *See* Gastrointestinal system disorders

Digoxin toxicity, 34, 232

Dilation of cervix, 193, 194

Disasters and disaster planning, 20–22

Disclosure of information, 16, 17, 18

Disease-modifying antirheumatic drugs (DMARDs), 51

Disease prevention strategies, 73–74. *See also specific types and names of diseases*

Diskectomy, 153

Disorganized schizophrenia, 174

Distributive shock, 132

Diuretics, 47

Diversity. *See* Culturally competent care

Diverticular disease, 102

DMARDs (disease-modifying antirheumatic drugs), 51

Donation of organs and tissue, 16

Door-in-the-face tactics, 11

Dosage calculations, 28

Down syndrome, 233

Drag-and-drop questions, 3

Droplet precautions, 71

Drowning, 220, 221, 222, 223

Drug abuse. *See* Substance abuse and dependence

Drug class suffixes, 31. *See also* Medications; Pharmacology

DSHEA (Dietary Supplement Health and Education Act of 1994), 61

Dual diagnosis, 172

Dual-energy x-ray absorptiometry (DEXA) scans, 108

Due dates, calculation of, 185. *See also* Labor and delivery

Durable power of attorney for health care, 16

DVT (deep-vein thrombosis), 131

Dwarfism, 114–115

Dysentery, 73

Dystocia, 201

E

Ear as route of administration, 229

Ear infections, 240

Eating disorders, 180–181

EBV (Epstein-Barr virus), 241

ECGs (electrocardiograms), 126, 135–137

Echinacea purpurea, 61

Eclampsia, 190

Ecological disasters, 20

Economic abuse, 182

ECT (electroconvulsive therapy), 176, 182

Ectopic pregnancy, 193

Eczema, 246

Effacement, 193, 194

EGD (esophagogastroduodenoscopy), 95

Ego, 168, 169

Elderly populations. *See* Gerontologic considerations

Electrical equipment guidelines, 67

Electrocardiograms (ECGs), 126, 135–137

Electroconvulsive therapy (ECT), 176, 182

Electroencephalograms (EEGs), 147

Electrolytes and fluids, 79–84, 165

Electromyography (EMG), 108

Emergency childbirth, 201

Emergency management systems, 20–22

Emergency Medical Treatment and Active Labor Act of 1986 (EMTALA), 194

Emergent injuries, 21

EMLA (eutectic mixture of local anesthetics), 29, 229

Emotional abuse and neglect, 181, 225

Emphysema, 85

Empirical therapy, 29

Endocrine system functions and disorders, 114–122

  acromegaly, 114

  Addison's disease, 116, 117

  adrenal gland, 116–117

  Cushing's disease and syndrome, 116–117

  diabetes insipidus, 115

  diabetes mellitus, 120–121, 191, 247–248

  diabetic ketoacidosis, 121

  dwarfism, 114–115

  gigantism, 114

  hyperaldosteronism (Conn's syndrome), 117

  hyperglycemic hyperosmolar state, 122

  hyperparathyroidism, 119

  hyperthyroidism, 118–119

  hypoparathyroidism, 119

  hypothyroidism, 118

  medications for, 39–42

  overview, 114

  pancreas, 95, 106–108, 120–122

  parathyroid gland, 119

  pheochromocytoma, 117

  pituitary gland, 114–115

  syndrome of inappropriate secretion of antidiuretic hormone, 115

  thyroid gland, 118–119

End-of-life care, 162, 230–231

Endometrial cancer, 212–213

Endometriosis, 214

Endometritis, 204

Endoscopic retrograde cholangiopancreatography (ERCP), 96

Endoscopy, 95–96

Engorgement, 202

Enteral feeding tubes, 96–97

Enteric precautions, 71

Environmental safety, 67

Epidural blocks, 198

Epidural hematomas, 147

Episiotomy, 199

Epstein-Barr virus (EBV), 241

Equipment guidelines, 67

ERCP (endoscopic retrograde cholangiopancreatography), 96

Ergonomics and client positioning, 67–68

Erikson, Erik, 168, 169, 219, 221, 222, 223, 224

Erythema infectiosum, 241

Erythematosus (butterfly rash), 159

Esophageal disorders, 97–99

Esophagogastroduodenoscopy (EGD), 95

Estrogen, 184

Ethical considerations, 16

Ethnicity. *See* Culturally competent care

Eutectic mixture of local anesthetics (EMLA), 29, 229

Exam day procedures, 7

Exam questions. *See* Test questions

Exam schedule, 2

Exhibit questions, 3

Expectorants, 38

Expert power, 11

Exploration techniques, 171

External disasters, 20

External fixation devices, 111

Extracellular electrolytes, 80

Eye disorders, 57, 153–154

F

FACES pain rating scale, 228

Failure to thrive, 225

Falls, 66, 75–76, 220, 221

Family disaster plans, 21

Farsightedness, 153

FAS (fetal alcohol syndrome), 208

Fat-modified diets, 164

FDA (Food and Drug Administration), 61

Fecal screening tests, 95

Federal disaster areas, 21

Federal Emergency Management Agency (FEMA), 21

Feeding tubes, 96–97

Female reproductive system, 58–60, 184. *See also* Maternal nursing; Women's health

Femoral hernias, 102

Fertilization process, 184

Fetal alcohol syndrome (FAS), 208

Fetal development and assessment, 184, 186–187, 195–196. *See also* Labor and delivery; Pregnancy

Fetal distress, 200

Fetal heart rate (FHR) classification system, 195–196

Fevers, 239

Fiber-modified diets, 163

Fidelity, defined, 16

15/15/15 rule, 121

Figure-8 bandages, 113

Fill-in-the-blank questions, 3

Financial management, 12

Fire response procedures, 67

FLACC postoperative pain tool, 228

Fluids and electrolytes, 79–84, 165

Fluid volume deficit (FVD), 79

Fluid volume excess (FVE), 79–80

Folic acid deficiency anemia, 124

Food and Drug Administration (FDA), 61

Food and nutrition, 162–165

Foot-in-the-door tactics, 11

Forceps, 199

Formal debriefing, 22

Formula-feeding guidelines, 207

Fractures, 110–111, 147, 246

Freud, Sigmund, 168, 169

Full-liquid diets, 163

FVD (fluid volume deficit), 79

FVE (fluid volume excess), 79–80

G

GAD (generalized anxiety disorder), 173

Gallbladder disease, 106

Gastric aspirate, 94

Gastroenteritis, 240

Gastroesophageal reflux disease (GERD), 98

Gastrointestinal system disorders, 94–108
 abdominal hernias, 102–103
 congenital anomalies, 237–238
 Crohn's disease, 100–101
 diagnostic procedures for, 94–96
 diverticular disease, 102
 hepatic disorders, 95, 104–106
 inflammatory bowel disease, 100–102
 intestinal obstructions, 103
 irritable bowel syndrome, 100
 medications for, 45–46
 oral and esophageal disorders, 97–99
 pancreatic disorders, 95, 106–108, 120–122
 peptic ulcer disease, 99–100
 risk factors for, 94
 surgical procedures for, 104
 therapeutic procedures for, 96–97
 ulcerative colitis, 101–102

Generalized anxiety disorder (GAD), 173

Genital herpes, 72, 215

Genitourinary system disorders, 138–145
 assessment of, 138
 benign prostatic hyperplasia, 143–144
 cystitis, 139–140
 diagnostic tests for, 138–139
 dialysis for, 142–143
 glomerulonephritis, 140, 249–250
 incontinence, 144
 kidney disease, 141–142
 medications for, 47–48
 nephrosis, 140, 249–250
 prostate cancer, 144
 renal failure, 141
 surgical procedures for, 143
 testicular cancer, 144
 urinary tract infections, 94
 urine retention, 93, 144
 urolithiasis, 140–141

GERD (gastroesophageal reflux disease), 98

German measles, 243

Gerontologic considerations
 hypertension and, 131
 medications and, 29
 nutrition and, 162

Gestational age, 206, 211

Gestational diabetes mellitus, 191

Gestational hypertension (GH), 190

Gigantism, 114

Ginkgo biloba, 62

Ginseng (panax quinquefolius), 62

Glasgow coma scale, 146

Glaucoma, 154

Glomerulonephritis, 140, 249–250

Glucagon, 120

Glucocorticoids, 37–38, 51

Glucosamine (2-amino-2-deoxyglucose), 62

Glucose levels, 166

Glucose tolerance test, 191

Glycemic agents, 40

Gonadotropin-releasing hormone (GnRH), 213

Gonorrhea, 215

Good Samaritan laws, 17

Gouty arthritis, 110

Graphic options, 3

Graves' disease, 118

Gravidity, 188

Green tag injuries, 21

Group therapy, 172

Growth hormones, 41

Guillain-Barré syndrome, 153

Guilt tactics, 11

H

HAART (highly active antiretroviral therapy) guidelines, 159

HAIs (health care associated infections), 70–73

Half-life, 29

Hallucinations, 174

Hand hygiene, 70

Hazardous material response teams (Hazmat), 21

hCG (human chorionic gonadotropin), 184, 185

hCS (human chorionic somatomammotropin), 184

Head injuries, 147–148

Head lice, 242

Health care associated infections (HAIs), 70–73

Health care facility disaster plans, 22

Health care providers, 14

Health Insurance Portability and Accountability Act of 1996 (HIPAA), 17, 18

Health promotion strategies, 73–74

Hearing disorders, 154

Heart, anatomy of, 133

Heart attack, 128–129

Heart failure (HF), 129, 232

Heberden nodes, 108, 109

HELLP (hemolysis, elevated liver enzymes, and low platelets) syndrome, 190

Hematologic system
  disorders of, 123–125, 248
  medications for, 42–45

Hematomas, 147

Hematophobia, 173

Hematopoietic growth factors, 43

Hemodialysis, 142

Hemolysis, elevated liver enzymes, and low platelets (HELLP) syndrome, 190

Hemolytic anemia, 124

Hemophilia, 248

Hemorrhages, 93, 204

Hemothorax, 89

Hepatic disorders, 72, 95, 104–106

Hepatitis, 72, 105–106

Herbal supplements, 61–63

Hernias, 98–99, 102–103

Herpes, 72, 215

HHS (hyperglycemic hyperosmolar state), 122

Hiatal hernias, 98–99

Hierarchy of Needs (Maslow), 5, 168, 169

High blood pressure, 130–131, 190–191

Highly active antiretroviral therapy (HAART) guidelines, 159

HIPAA (Health Insurance Portability and Accountability Act of 1996), 17, 18

Hirschsprung's disease, 237

Hispanic clients, culturally competent care for, 24

Histamine₂ receptor antagonists, 45

Histrionic personality disorder, 177, 178

HIV/AIDS, 71, 157–159, 215

Hodgkin's lymphoma, 253

Holistic care, 13, 20

Home health settings, 67

Honeymoon stage of violence, 181

Hormone replacement therapy (HRT), 42, 214

Hospice care, 162, 230

Hospitalization
  effects on children, 226, 227
  voluntary vs. involuntary admissions, 182

Hot spot questions, 3

Human chorionic gonadotropin (hCG), 184, 185

Human chorionic somatomammotropin (hCS), 184

Humanistic models of development, 168, 169

Human papillomavirus (HPV), 216

Hydatidiform mole/molar pregnancy, 192

Hydrocarbons, ingestion of, 245

Hydrocephalus, 234–235

Hydrogen breath tests, 95

Hyperaldosteronism (Conn's syndrome), 117

Hyperbilirubinemia, 210–211

Hypercalcemia, 81

Hyperemesis gravidarum, 191

Hyperglycemia, 120–121, 191

Hyperglycemic hyperosmolar state (HHS), 122

Hypericum perforatum (St. John's wort), 61

Hyperkalemia, 80

Hypermagnesemia, 82

Hypernatremia, 81

Hyperopia, 153

Hyperparathyroidism, 119

Hyperphosphatemia, 82

Hypertension, 130–131, 190–191

Hyperthermia, 148

Hyperthyroidism, 118–119

Hypertonic solutions, 79

Hypertrophic pyloric stenosis, 237

Hypnotic medications, 54

Hypocalcemia, 81, 119

Hypoglycemia, 120, 191, 209

Hypoglycemic agents, 39–40

Hypokalemia, 80

Hypomagnesemia, 82

Hypomania, 177

Hyponatremia, 81

Hypoparathyroidism, 119

Hypophosphatemia, 82

Hypostatic pneumonia, 93

Hypothyroidism, 118

Hypotonic solutions, 79

Hypovolemic shock, 132

Hypoxemia, 89

Hypoxia, 89, 93

I

IBS (irritable bowel syndrome), 100

ICP (intracranial pressure), 147

Id, 168, 169

IM injections. See Intramuscular injections

Immunizations, 48–49, 219

Immunologic disorders
  in children, 246
  HIV/AIDS, 71, 157–159, 215
  medications for, 48–50
  systemic lupus erythematosus, 159–160

Impairment of coworkers, 17

Impetigo contagiosa, 241

Incident reports, 12

Incompetent cervix, 192

Incontinence, 144

Indians (American), culturally competent care for, 24–25

Induction of labor, 199

Indwelling urinary catheterization, 139

Infants, 218–220. See also Child and adolescent nursing; Newborn nursing

Infection control, 70–73

Infertility, 211–212

Inflammatory bowel disease, 100–102

Inflammatory medications, 57–58

Influence vs. power, 11

Information systems in nursing profession, 18

Informed consent, 17, 182

Ingestion of toxic substances, 245

Ingratiation, 11

Inhalants, administration to children, 29

Injury levels, 21

Insulin, 40, 120, 121

Intentional torts, 17

Interactions (medication), 29

Internal disasters, 20, 21

Internal uterine pressure catheters (IUPCs), 193

Intestinal obstructions, 103

Intracellular electrolytes, 80

Intracranial pressure (ICP), 147

Intradermal route of administration, 229

Intramuscular (IM) injections, 29, 43, 229

Intraoperative phase, 92

Intravenous (IV) therapy, 28, 30, 79, 97, 229

Intussusception, 238

Involuntary admissions, 182

Iron deficiency anemia, 123

Iron-modified diets, 165

Iron preparations, 43

Irritable bowel syndrome (IBS), 100

Isolation guidelines, 70, 71

Isotonic dehydration, 79

Isotonic solutions, 79

Item types. See Test questions

IUPCs (internal uterine pressure catheters), 193

IV therapy. See Intravenous therapy

J

Jejunostomy feeding tubes, 97

Joint Commission, 20, 92

Joint replacements, 113

Justice, defined, 16

Juvenile rheumatoid arthritis (JRA), 247

Melatonin, 63

Ménière's disease, 154

Meningitis, 242

Meningocele, 235

Meningococcal disease, 72

Menopause, 214

Mental health, defined, 168

Mental health nursing, 167–182

    addictive disorders, 178–179

    anger/violence, abuse, and assault, 181–182

    anxiety and anxiety disorders, 52, 172–173, 219, 226

    assessments in, 170

    for children and adolescents, 175–176

    client-nurse relationship in, 170–171

    cognitive disorders, 56–57, 179–180

    communication techniques in, 171

    crisis intervention and, 22

    defined, 168

    depressive/bipolar disorders, 53, 176–177, 203

    diagnosis in, 170

    eating disorders, 180–181

    group therapy in, 172

    legal considerations in, 182

    personality disorders, 177–178

    PTSD in, 22

    schizophrenia, 174–175

    suicide, 177

    theoretical models of, 168–170

Mental illness, defined, 168

Mental status examinations (MSEs), 170

Meperidine (Demerol), 106, 107

Metabolic acidosis, 83

Metabolic alkalosis, 83

Metabolic syndrome, 120

Metered-space devices, 29

Methicillin-resistant *Staphylococcus aureus* (MRSA), 72, 241

Methylergonovine (Methergine), 60

Methylxanthines, 37

MI (myocardial infarction), 128–129

Microbial disasters, 20

Molar pregnancy, 192

Monoamine oxidase inhibitors (MAOIs), 53, 176

Mood stabilizers, 176

Morbid obesity, bariatric surgery for, 104

Morphine, 102

Morse Fall Scale, 75–76

Motor skill development, 218, 220, 222

Motor vehicle safety, 220, 221, 222, 224, 225

MRI (magnetic resonance imaging), 108, 147

MRSA (methicillin-resistant Staphylococcus aureus), 72, 241

MS (multiple sclerosis), 150–151

MSAFP (maternal serum alpha-fetoprotein screening), 187

MSBP (Munchausen syndrome by proxy), 225

MSEs (mental status examinations), 170

Mucolytics, 38

Mucosal protectants, 46

Mucositis, 156

Multigeneration antibiotics, 49–50

Multiple choice questions, 3

Multiple myeloma, 156

Multiple response questions, 3

Multiple sclerosis (MS), 150–151

Mumps, 242

Munchausen syndrome by proxy (MSBP), 225

Musculoskeletal system disorders, 108–114

    amputations, 113–114

    arthritis, 108–110, 247

    arthroplasties for, 113

    diagnostic tests for, 108

    fractures, 110–111, 147, 246

    gouty arthritis, 110

    medications for, 50–52

    osteoarthritis, 108–109

    osteomyelitis, 112

    osteoporosis, 112

    rheumatoid arthritis, 109–110, 247

Myasthenia gravis, 152

Myelomeningocele (spina bifida), 235

Myocardial infarction (MI), 128–129

Myomas, 213

Myopia, 153

Myxedema coma, 118

N

Nagele's rule of due date calculation, 185

Narcissistic personality disorder, 177, 178

Narcotics Anonymous, 179

Nasogastric feeding tubes, 96

Nasointestinal feeding tubes, 97

National Highway Traffic Safety Administration, 220, 221, 222

Native American clients, culturally competent care for, 24–25

Natural disasters, 20

Nausea, 93

NCLEX-PN®

    day of exam procedures, 7

    format and test plan, 2, 3

    questions. *See* Test questions

    registration process, 2

    study tips, 3–4

    test-taking strategies, 4–6

NDRIs (norepinephrine dopamine reuptake inhibitors), 176

Nearsightedness, 153

Negative symptoms, 174

Neglect, 182, 225

Negligence, defined, 17

Neonatal period, 205–208

Nephroblastoma, 252–253

Nephrosis, 140, 249–250

Nerve conduction studies, 108

Neural tube defects, 235–236

Neurogenic shock, 132

Neurosensory disorders, 145–155

    amyotrophic lateral sclerosis, 151–152

    assessment of, 145–146

    auditory disorders, 154

    cerebrovascular accidents, 149–150

    diagnostic procedures for, 146–147

    Guillain-Barré syndrome, 153

    head injuries, 147–148

    hyperthermia, 148

    medications for, 52–57

    multiple sclerosis, 150–151

    myasthenia gravis, 152

    ocular disorders, 57, 153–154

    Parkinson's disease, 56, 69, 151

    seizure disorders, 56, 66, 148–149, 191

    spinal cord injuries, 150

    status epilepticus, 149

    surgical procedures for, 153

    transient ischemic attacks, 149

New Ballard Score for newborns, 206

Positive symptoms, 174

Posterior pituitary gland, 114, 115

Posterior pituitary hormones, 41

Postmortem care, 162

Postoperative phase, 92–94

Postpartum care, 60, 201–204

Post-term births, 210

Posttraumatic stress disorder (PTSD), 22, 173, 182

Posturing, 146

Potassium imbalances, 80

Potassium-modified diets, 165

Potty training, 221

Power vs. influence, 11

PPE (personal protective equipment), 70, 71

PPN (peripheral parenteral nutrition), 97

Preeclampsia, 190

Pregestational diabetes mellitus, 191

Pregnancy, 184–194. *See also* Labor and delivery

    abortion, 192

    anticipatory care, 188–189

    complications during, 189–193

    delivery dates, calculation of, 185

    fertilization process, 184

    fetal development and assessment during, 184, 186–187

    medications and, 29

    prenatal period and care, 184–187, 188

    psychological and physiological adaptations of, 184–185, 188–189

    signs and symptoms of, 185

    terminology, 188

    verification of, 185

Prenatal period and care, 184–187, 188

Preoperative phase, 92

Presbyopia, 153

Preschoolers, 222. *See also* Child and adolescent nursing

Preterm births, 188, 200, 210

Preventive care, 73–74

Prinzmetal's angina, 127

Prioritization and delegation, 13–15

Priority-setting guidelines, 5

Privacy, 16, 17, 18

Progesterone, 184

Projection, 172

Prostate cancer, 144

Prostatic hyperplasia, 143–144

Protein-modified diets, 164

Proton pump inhibitors, 45

Psychoanalytic models of development, 168, 169

Psychosocial effects of disasters, 22

PTSD. *See* Posttraumatic stress disorder

Puberty, 223

PUBS (percutaneous umbilical blood sampling), 187

PUD (peptic ulcer disease), 99–100

Pudendal blocks, 198

Puerperal infections, 204

Pulmonary embolism (PE), 88–89, 131

Pulmonary emphysema, 85

Pureed diets, 163

Purging, 180

Q

Quality control, 12

QuantiFERON-TB Gold (QFT-G) test, 84

Quasi-intentional torts, 17

Questions. *See* Test questions

R

Rabies, 242

Race. *See* Culturally competent care

Radiation therapy, 67, 157, 213

Radiographic studies, 96

Radiologic tests, 138

Rape and rape trauma syndrome, 182

Raynaud's syndrome, 132

RDS (respiratory distress syndrome), 209–210

Reactions to medications, 29

Reactivity periods of newborns, 206

Red Cross, 21

Red tag injuries, 21

Referent power, 11

Referrals, 13, 20

Reflection techniques, 171

Reflex assessment of newborns, 206

Regional blocks, 198

Registered nurses (RNs), 6, 13, 14, 187, 189

Registration process, 2

Regression, 172

Reimbursement methods, 12

Religious and spiritual considerations, 25–26

Renal angiography, 139

Renal biopsy, 139

Renal cancer, 252–253

Renal disorders in children, 249–250

Renal failure, 141

Renal function tests, 138, 166

Reports, incident, 12

Reproductive system, 58–60, 184. *See also* Maternal nursing; Women's health

Resource management, 12

Respirators, 71

Respiratory acidosis, 83

Respiratory alkalosis, 83

Respiratory distress syndrome (RDS), 209–210

Respiratory syncytial virus (RSV), 72, 242

Respiratory system disorders, 84–91

    airway management for, 89–91

    asthma, 84–85, 246

    bronchitis, 85–86

    carbon dioxide toxicity, 86

    COPD, 85–86

    diagnostic tests for, 84

    hemothorax, 89

    laryngeal cancer, 87

    lung cancer, 88

    medications for, 36–39

    pneumonia, 72, 86–87, 91, 93

    pneumothorax, 89, 91

    pulmonary embolism, 88–89, 131

    pulmonary emphysema, 85

    respiratory distress syndrome, 209–210

    respiratory syncytial virus, 72, 242

    status asthmaticus, 85

    tension pneumothorax, 89

    tuberculosis, 71, 73, 84, 87

Restatement techniques, 171

Restraints, 66, 181, 182

Restricting behaviors, 180

Rett syndrome, 175

Reversal agents, 31

Reward power, 11

Reye syndrome, 242

Rheumatic fever, 242, 247

Rheumatoid arthritis, 109–110, 247

RhoGAM immune globulin, 60, 187, 204

RNs. *See* Registered nurses

Rolling walkers, 69

Room assignments, 70, 71

Root cause analysis, 12

Roseola, 243

Rotavirus, 72

Routes of administration

    intradermal, 229

    intramuscular, 29, 43, 229

    intravenous, 28, 30, 79, 97, 229

    oral, 39–40, 43, 229

    otic, 229

    subcutaneous, 229

RSV (respiratory syncytial virus), 72, 242

Rubella, 73, 243

Rubeola, 243

Rule of Nines, 160